METHODS IN MOLECULAR BIOLOGY

Series Editor
John M. Walker
School of Life and Medical Sciences
University of Hertfordshire
Hatfield, Hertfordshire, UK

For further volumes:
http://www.springer.com/series/7651

For over 35 years, biological scientists have come to rely on the research protocols and methodologies in the critically acclaimed *Methods in Molecular Biology* series. The series was the first to introduce the step-by-step protocols approach that has become the standard in all biomedical protocol publishing. Each protocol is provided in readily-reproducible step-by-step fashion, opening with an introductory overview, a list of the materials and reagents needed to complete the experiment, and followed by a detailed procedure that is supported with a helpful notes section offering tips and tricks of the trade as well as troubleshooting advice. These hallmark features were introduced by series editor Dr. John Walker and constitute the key ingredient in each and every volume of the *Methods in Molecular Biology* series. Tested and trusted, comprehensive and reliable, all protocols from the series are indexed in PubMed.

IMMUNO-model in Cancer

Methods and Protocols

Edited by

Sweta Rani

Department of Science, South East Technological University, Waterford, Cork, Ireland

Lukasz Skalniak

Department of Organic Chemistry, Jagiellonian University, Kraków, Poland

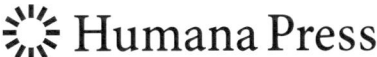 Humana Press

Editors
Sweta Rani
Department of Science
South East Technological University
Waterford, Cork, Ireland

Lukasz Skalniak
Department of Organic Chemistry
Jagiellonian University
Kraków, Poland

European Cooperation in Science and Technology

ISSN 1064-3745   ISSN 1940-6029   (electronic)
Methods in Molecular Biology
ISBN 978-1-0716-4733-2   ISBN 978-1-0716-4734-9   (eBook)
https://doi.org/10.1007/978-1-0716-4734-9

This Humana imprint is published by the registered company Springer Science+Business Media, LLC, part of Springer Nature.
The registered company address is: 1 New York Plaza, New York, NY 10004, U.S.A.

If disposing of this product, please recycle the paper.

Preface

Immuno-model is a model invented to study the immune system. This book describes the computational and experimental models that help researchers understand the responses of the immune system in cancer and test experimental immuno-oncology approaches.

Macrophages can adapt to different phenotypes in response to signals from the microenvironment. This book on immuno-model describes methods to profile polarization in macrophages using ELISA. ELISA is widely used in immunology to detect proteins, antibodies, antigens, or hormones in a sample, including immune checkpoint inhibitors. Immune checkpoints are regulatory molecules that control the activation and intensity of immune responses. Glycosylation is the addition of carbohydrate groups to the proteins. Glycosylation of the immune checkpoint proteins not only promotes immune evasion in tumor cells but also holds therapeutic implications. New immune checkpoint inhibitors are warranted for better cancer treatment. One of the chapters evaluates immune checkpoint inhibitors. One of the most studied immune checkpoints is PD-1/PD-L1. There is one chapter detailing the interaction of PD-1/PD-L1 and T cells. Immune checkpoint inhibitors have significantly improved survival rates in cancers but there are patients who do not respond to these treatments. Induction of immunogenic cell death is another therapeutic option for cancer patients.

A lot of research is underway to study tumor immune microenvironment. There are several well-established in vitro models to study interaction between immune cells and cancer cells and these in vitro models are still evolving. Cells can be co-cultured using cell culture inserts or can be grown as 3D spheroids. 3D co-culture model can be used to study the interaction of immune cells and cancer cells to mimic the in vitro microenvironment. Cells can be grown in 3D using different techniques, and one of the techniques is using scaffolds derived from cancer patients. One of the chapters explores immunocompetent preclinical mouse models to study primary and metastatic brain cancer. CAR T-cell therapy is still evolving, and one of the chapters describes the method to generate CAR T-cells.

Bioinformatics has vast applications and plays a central role in immunology by enabling the analysis of large-scale datasets. Deconvolution analysis can be used to study the epigenetic dysregulation in human tumors and the tumor ecosystem. Computational methods can also be used to study the mutated peptides called neoantigens. Bioinformatics allows us to identify therapeutic targets and develop precision immunotherapies.

Waterford, Cork, Ireland   *Sweta Rani*
Kraków, Poland   *Lukasz Skalniak*

Acknowledgments

This publication is based upon work from COST Action IMMUNO-model, CA21135, supported by COST (European Cooperation in Science and Technology).

COST (European Cooperation in Science and Technology) is a funding agency for research and innovation networks. Our actions help connect research initiatives across Europe and enable scientists to grow their ideas by sharing them with their peers. This boosts their research, career, and innovation.

Please see www.cost.eu for additional information.

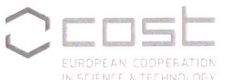 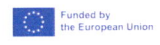

The original version of the book has been revised. A correction to this book can be found at https://doi.org/10.1007/978-1-0716-4734-9_19

Contents

Contributors

PAULA ALAMILLO-MAESO • *Biobizkaia Health Research Institute, Barakaldo, Spain*

ÁNGEL F. ÁLVAREZ-PRADO • *Translational Cancer Immunogenomics Laboratory, Department of Cancer Research, Luxembourg Institute of Health, Luxembourg, Luxembourg*

PILAR BALLESTEROS-CUARTERO • *Departamento de Bioingenieria, Universidad Carlos III de Madrid, Leganés, Spain; Department of Biosystems Science and Engineering, ETH Zürich, Basel, Switzerland*

MARCO BARRECA • *Fondazione Michelangelo, Milan, Italy; Department of Biotechnology and Biosciences, University of Milano-Bicocca, Milan, Italy*

MAGDALENA BOJKO • *Department of Biomedical Chemistry, Faculty of Chemistry, University of Gdańsk, Gdańsk, Poland*

HATIM BOUGHANEM • *Unidad de Gestión Clinica Medicina Interna, Lipids and Atherosclerosis Unit, Maimonides Institute for Biomedical Research in Córdoba, Reina Sofia University Hospital, Córdoba, Spain; Spanish Biomedical Research Center in Physiopathology of Obesity and Nutrition (CIBERObn), Instituto de Salud Carlos III, Madrid, Spain*

IOANA BRIE • *The Oncology Institute "Prof. Dr. I. Chiricuță" Cluj-Napoca, Cluj-Napoca, Romania*

MAURIZIO CALLARI • *Fondazione Michelangelo, Milan, Italy*

TÂNIA B. CRUZ • *i3S-Institute for Research and Innovation in Health, University of Porto, Porto, Portugal*

MARIUS EIDSAA • *Department of Biotechnology and Nanomedicine, SINTEF Industry, Trondheim, Norway*

MAITE EMALDI • *Biobizkaia Health Research Institute, Barakaldo, Spain; CIBERER, ISCIII, Madrid, Spain*

AGUSTINA ERCOLE • *Departamento de Biología Molecular, Facultad de Ciencias Exactas, Físico-Químicas y Naturales, Universidad Nacional de Río Cuarto, Río Cuarto, Córdoba, Argentina*

DIOGO ESTÊVÃO • *i3S-Institute for Research and Innovation in Health, University of Porto, Porto, Portugal; ICBAS—Institute of Biomedical Sciences Abel Salazar, University of Porto, Porto, Portugal*

ROBERTO FORNELINO-GONZÁLEZ • *Cancer Heterogeneity and Immunomics (CHI) Group, University Hospital Lozano Blesa, Aragon Health Research Institute (IISA), Zaragoza, Spain*

PAOLO GANDELLINI • *Department of Biosciences, University of Milan, Milan, Italy*

SANDRA GARCÍA-MULERO • *Department of Pathology and Experimental Therapy, ONCOBELL Program, Institut d'Investigacio Biomedica de Bellvitge (IDIBELL), University of Barcelona, L'Hospitalet de Llobregat, Spain*

DANIEL GÓMEZ-GARRIDO • *Centro Nacional de Biotecnología, Consejo Superior de Investigaciones Científicas, Madrid, Spain*

HANNE HASLENE-HOX • *Department of Biotechnology and Nanomedicine, SINTEF Industry, Trondheim, Norway*

MUHAMMET KARAMAN • *Department of Biology, Faculty of Science, Dokuz Eylul University, Izmir, Turkey; Department of Basic Science, Faculty of Engineering, Architecture and Design, Bartin University, Bartin, Turkey*

THEODORA KATSILA • *Institute of Chemical Biology, National Hellenic Research Foundation, Athens, Greece*

GEIR KLINKENBERG • *Department of Biotechnology and Nanomedicine, SINTEF Industry, Trondheim, Norway*

JUSTYNA KOCIK-KROL • *Department of Organic Chemistry, Faculty of Chemistry, Jagiellonian University, Krakow, Poland; Real Research S.A., Krakow, Poland*

MARCIN KRZYKAWSKI • *Real Research S.A., Krakow, Poland*

KATARZYNA KUNCEWICZ • *Department of Biomedical Chemistry, Faculty of Chemistry, University of Gdańsk, Gdańsk, Poland*

MARÍA JULIA LAMBERTI • *INBIAS-UNRC-CONICET, Río Cuarto, Córdoba, Argentina; Departamento de Biología Molecular, Facultad de Ciencias Exactas, Físico-Químicas y Naturales, Universidad Nacional de Río Cuarto, Río Cuarto, Córdoba, Argentina*

NGUYEN QUOC KHANH LE • *AIBioMed Research Group, Taipei Medical University, Taipei, Taiwan; In-Service Master Program in Artificial Intelligence in Medicine, College of Medicine, Taipei Medical University, Taipei, Taiwan*

JUDITH LEITNER • *Division of Immune Receptors and T Cell Activation, Institute of Immunology, Medical University of Vienna, Vienna, Austria*

SIMON LOEVENICH • *Department of Biotechnology and Nanomedicine, SINTEF Industry, Trondheim, Norway*

MANUEL MACIAS-GONZALEZ • *Spanish Biomedical Research Center in Physiopathology of Obesity and Nutrition (CIBERObn), Instituto de Salud Carlos III, Madrid, Spain; Department of Endocrinology and Nutrition, Virgen de la Victoria University Hospital, Institute of Biomedical Research in Malaga (IBIMA)-Bionand Platform, University of Malaga, Malaga, Spain*

MAIDER MADARIAGA • *Biobizkaia Health Research Institute, Barakaldo, Spain*

SUNIL MARTIN • *Laboratory of Synthetic Immunology, Cancer Research Division, Rajiv Gandhi Centre for Biotechnology, Biotechnology Research Innovation Council, Thiruvananthapuram, Kerala, India*

EDEL A. MCNEELA • *Department of Science, School of Science and Computing, South East Technological University, Waterford, Ireland; Pharmaceutical and Molecular Biotechnology Research Center, South East Technological University, Waterford, Ireland*

JAI PRAKASH MEHTA • *Department of Applied Science, South East Technological University, Carlow, Ireland*

AMIE MENTON • *Department of Science, School of Science and Computing, South East Technological University, Waterford, Ireland*

FÁTIMA MARÍA MENTUCCI • *INBIAS-UNRC-CONICET, Río Cuarto, Córdoba, Argentina*

ANDREA MORENO-MANUEL • *Cancer Heterogeneity and Immunomics (CHI) Group, University Hospital Lozano Blesa, Aragon Health Research Institute (IISA), Zaragoza, Spain*

ARRATE MUÑOZ-BARRUTIA • *Departamento de Bioingenieria, Universidad Carlos III de Madrid, Leganés, Spain; Área de Ingeniería Biomédica, Instituto de Investigación Sanitaria Gregrorio Marañón, Madrid, Spain*

MUTHUGANESH MUTHUVEL • *Laboratory of Synthetic Immunology, Cancer Research Division, Rajiv Gandhi Centre for Biotechnology, Biotechnology Research Innovation Council, Thiruvananthapuram, Kerala, India; Manipal Academy of Higher Education (MAHE), Manipal, Karnataka, India*

GURO KRUGE NÆRDAL • *Department of Biotechnology and Nanomedicine, SINTEF Industry, Trondheim, Norway*

VU TO NAKSTAD • *Department of Biotechnology and Nanomedicine, SINTEF Industry, Trondheim, Norway*

MAI HANH NGUYEN • *International Ph.D. Program in Cell Therapy and Regenerative Medicine, College of Medicine, Taipei Medical University, Taipei, Taiwan; Pathology and Forensic Medicine Department, 103 Military Hospital, Hanoi, Vietnam; AIBioMed Research Group, Taipei Medical University, Taipei, Taiwan*

CAROLINE E. NUNES-XAVIER • *Biobizkaia Health Research Institute, Barakaldo, Spain; CIBERER, ISCIII, Madrid, Spain; Institute for Cancer Research, Oslo University Hospital, Oslo, Norway*

ORLA O'DONOVAN • *Department of Science, School of Science and Computing, South East Technological University, Waterford, Ireland; Pharmaceutical and Molecular Biotechnology Research Center, South East Technological University, Waterford, Ireland*

MARIA J. OLIVEIRA • *i3S-Institute for Research and Innovation in Health, University of Porto, Porto, Portugal; ICBAS—Institute of Biomedical Sciences Abel Salazar, University of Porto, Porto, Portugal*

SOTIRIS OUZOUNIS • *Institute of Chemical Biology, National Hellenic Research Foundation, Athens, Greece*

MARIA PERDE-SCHREPLER • *The Oncology Institute "Prof. Dr. I. Chiricuță" Cluj-Napoca, Cluj-Napoca, Romania*

RAFAEL PULIDO • *Biobizkaia Health Research Institute, Barakaldo, Spain; CIBERER, ISCIII, Madrid, Spain; Ikerbasque, Basque Foundation for Science, Bilbao, Spain*

SWETA RANI • *Pharmaceutical and Molecular Biotechnology Research Center, South East Technological University, Waterford, Ireland; Department of Science, School of Science and Computing, South East Technological University, Waterford, Ireland*

ESTHER REY-IBORRA • *Biobizkaia Health Research Institute, Barakaldo, Spain; CIBERER, ISCIII, Madrid, Spain*

NATALIA BELÉN RUMIE VITTAR • *INBIAS-UNRC-CONICET, Río Cuarto, Córdoba, Argentina; Departamento de Biología Molecular, Facultad de Ciencias Exactas, Físico-Químicas y Naturales, Universidad Nacional de Río Cuarto, Río Cuarto, Córdoba, Argentina*

REBECA SANZ-PAMPLONA • *Cancer Heterogeneity and Immunomics (CHI) Group, University Hospital Lozano Blesa, Aragon Health Research Institute (IISA), Zaragoza, Spain; Centro de Investigación Biomédica en Red en Epidemiología y Salud Pública (CIBERESP), Instituto de Salud Carlos III, Madrid, Spain; Aragonese Foundation for Research and Development (ARAID), Zaragoza, Spain*

MACIEJ SIEDLAR • *Department of Clinical Immunology, Jagiellonian University Medical College, Institute of Pediatrics, Krakow, Poland*

MARGRÉT SYLVÍA SIGFÚSDÓTTIR • *Department of Biotechnology and Nanomedicine, SINTEF Industry, Trondheim, Norway*

LUKASZ SKALNIAK • *Department of Organic Chemistry, Faculty of Chemistry, Jagiellonian University, Krakow, Poland*

HÅVARD SLETTA • *Department of Biotechnology and Nanomedicine, SINTEF Industry, Trondheim, Norway*

KRISTINE SLETTA • *Department of Biotechnology and Nanomedicine, SINTEF Industry, Trondheim, Norway; Department of Clinical Science, University of Bergen, Bergen, Norway*

MARTA SPODZIEJA • *Department of Biomedical Chemistry, Faculty of Chemistry, University of Gdańsk, Gdańsk, Poland*

MALGORZATA STEC • *Department of Clinical Immunology, Jagiellonian University Medical College, Institute of Pediatrics, Krakow, Poland*

PETER STEINBERGER • *Division of Immune Receptors and T Cell Activation, Institute of Immunology, Medical University of Vienna, Vienna, Austria*

HANNE HEIN TRØEN • *Department of Biotechnology and Nanomedicine, SINTEF Industry, Trondheim, Norway*

ESTEBAN VEIGA-CHACÓN • *Centro Nacional de Biotecnología, Consejo Superior de Investigaciones Científicas, Madrid, Spain*

PIROSKA VIRÁG • *The Oncology Institute "Prof. Dr. I. Chiricuță" Cluj-Napoca, Cluj-Napoca, Romania*

TORKILD VISNES • *Department of Biotechnology and Nanomedicine, SINTEF Industry, Trondheim, Norway*

THANH HOA VO • *Pharmaceutical and Molecular Biotechnology Research Center, South East Technological University, Waterford, Ireland; Department of Science, School of Science and Computing, South East Technological University, Waterford, Ireland*

DONYA ZOJAJI • *Fondazione Michelangelo, Milan, Italy*

Chapter 1

Profiling of Macrophage Polarization Using Automated Enzyme-Linked Immunosorbent Assay

Simon Loevenich, Vu To Nakstad, Hanne Hein Trøen, Margrét Sylvía Sigfúsdóttir, Kristine Sletta, Guro Kruge Nærdal, Håvard Sletta, Geir Klinkenberg, Hanne Haslene-Hox, and Torkild Visnes

Abstract

Macrophage activation has emerged as a key area in immunology, in which they are polarized to adopt different functional phenotypes in response to various environmental signals. Here, we describe the procedure of isolating human primary CD14+ monocytes and polarization toward M1 (pro-inflammatory) and M2 (anti-inflammatory) phenotypes. Relevant cytokine levels can be detected by manual and automated enzyme-linked immunosorbent assays (ELISA).

Key words Macrophage, ELISA, Monocyte, Differentiation, Polarization, Human, Blood, Cytokine, Antibody

1 Introduction

Macrophages are innate immune cells with critical roles in immunity, tissue development, homeostasis, and tissue repair, and account for 10% of all immune cells in the human body [1, 2].

Macrophage subpopulations/phenotypes are conventionally described based on their function, using a spectrum ranging from M1 (pro-inflammatory) to M2 (anti-inflammatory) [3, 4]. Immunological research commonly uses monocyte-derived macrophages (MDMs) as an in vitro model for biological assays. These cells are isolated as monocytes from human blood and differentiated to macrophages in vitro. Additionally, these macrophages can be further polarized to specific subtypes to resemble a specific in vivo macrophage population (Fig. 1).

Supplementary Information The online version contains supplementary material available at https://doi.org/10.1007/978-1-0716-4734-9_1.

Sweta Rani and Lukasz Skalniak (eds.), *IMMUNO-model in Cancer: Methods and Protocols*, Methods in Molecular Biology, vol. 2959, https://doi.org/10.1007/978-1-0716-4734-9_1, © The Author(s) 2026

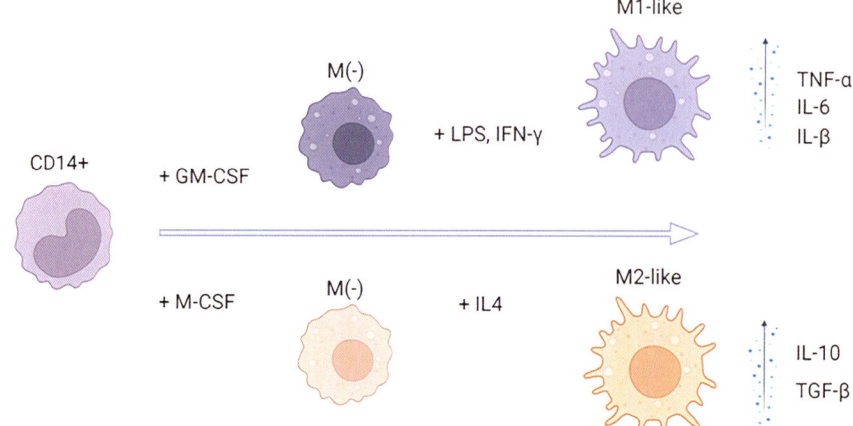

Fig. 1 Schematic overview of macrophage differentiation and polarization from human CD14+ blood monocytes. The resulting M1-like and M2-like phenotype produce different cytokine production profiles that can be verified with ELISA (Figure made with Biorender)

Here, we describe a workflow spanning from isolation of monocytes from human blood to functional analysis by ELISA (enzyme-linked immunosorbent assays). This procedure consists of four parts: (1) the isolation of peripheral blood mononuclear cells (PBMCs) from human blood, (2) the enrichment of CD14+ monocytes, (3II) macrophage differentiation and polarization toward desired phenotypes, and (4) analysis of cytokine expression by ELISA.

In brief, PBMCs are isolated from human blood anticoagulated with Li-heparin using standard density centrifugation with Ficoll-Paque [5]. CD14+ cells are then enriched via positive selection by magnetic labeling with CD14MicroBeads [6]. CD14 belongs to the lipopolysaccharides (LPS) receptor complex and is mainly expressed on monocytes and macrophages [7]. As CD14 itself lacks a cytoplasmatic domain, antibody (CD14MicroBead) binding to CD14 does not trigger signal transduction [8]. Enriched populations of human CD14+ monocytes can be differentiated to MDMs using either granulocyte-macrophage colony-stimulating factor (GM-CSF) or macrophage colony-stimulating factor (M-CSF). Depending on the desired phenotype, these MDMs can be further polarized using Interferon-γ (IFN-γ), LPS, or Interleukin-4 (IL-4). As there is a plethora of possible differentiation and polarization regimes, one must consider which monocyte/macrophage model is biologically most relevant for the intended assay. This protocol states selected regimes to obtain certain general MDM phenotypes, for example, "M1", or to obtain MDM phenotypes suitable for particular assays (e.g., phagocytosis). However, it should always be considered beforehand if a generated MDM-phenotype is a suitable biological model for a specific biological context. In addition, it is important to keep in mind not to overstimulate MDMs during differentiation/polarization (by too high doses of the respective agents) as this may lead, for example, to "saturated" cytokine responses, which will make it difficult to assay any additional effects in functional assays afterward.

Last, we describe a method for cytokine measurement (e.g., TNF-α, IL-1β, IL-6) in the MDM cell culture supernatants via ELISA. It includes detailed procedures both for manual and automated ELISA analysis. ELISAs are a type of immunoassay that are commonly used to quantify levels of a specific target within a sample. Samples routinely used in ELISAs include serum, plasma, cell culture supernatants, cell lysates, saliva, tissue lysates, and urine [9]. Sandwich ELISAs are the most common type of ELISA. Two specific antibodies are used to sandwich the antigen, commonly referred to as matched antibody pairs. The capture antibody is coated on a microplate, sample is added, and the protein of interest binds and is immobilized on the plate. An enzyme-conjugated detection antibody is then added and binds to an additional epitope on the target protein. Substrate is added and produces a signal that is proportional to the amount of analyte present in the sample. Sandwich ELISAs are highly specific, since two antibodies are required to bind to the protein of interest [10]. Our protocol uses DuoSet sandwich ELISA kits from R&D (Biotechne), which use horseradish peroxidase to catalyze the conversion of the chromogenic substrate into a coloured product. However, the protocol can be adjusted for use of other ELISA or multiplex kits.

2   Materials

2.1   Monocyte Isolation

1. Centrifuge for 15 mL and 50 mL tubes.
2. Refrigerator, 2–8 °C.
3. Cell culture incubator 37 °C, 5% CO_2, and 95% humidity.
4. Water bath.
5. Biohazard safety cabinet approved for biosafety level 2.
6. Cell counter.
7. Inverted microscope.
8. Pipet boy.
9. Pipettes covering a range of 0.05 to 1 mL.
10. Sterile serological pipettes, 1 mL to 50 mL.
11. Sterile microcentrifuge tubes, 1.5 or 2 mL.
12. Sterile polypropylene tubes, 15 and 50 mL.
13. Scissors or surgical knife.

14. Spray bottles with 80% ethanol.

15. Ficoll-Paque Plus medium.

16. Hanks′ balanced salt solution (HBSS).

2.2 Enrichment of CD14+ Monocytes

1. Centrifuge for 15 mL and 50 mL tubes.

2. Refrigerator, 2–8 °C.

3. Cell culture incubator 37 °C, 5% CO_2, and 95% humidity.

4. Water bath.

5. Biohazard safety cabinet approved for biosafety level 2.

6. Cell counter.

7. Inverted microscope.

8. Vortex.

9. Pipet boy.

10. Pipettes covering a range of 0.05 to 1 mL.

11. Sterile serological pipettes, covering a range of 1 mL to 50 mL.

12. Sterile microcentrifuge tubes, 1.5 or 2 mL.

13. Sterile polypropylene tubes, 15 and 50 mL.

14. Cell culture-coated tissue culture plates and/or flasks.

15. MACS® MultiStand.

16. QuadroMACS® Separator.

17. LS Columns.

18. MACS® 15 mL Tube Rack.

19. CD14 MicroBeads, human.

20. MACS BSA Stock Solution, 20×.

21. autoMACS Rinsing Solution.

22. Rinsing solution: 5% (v/v) BSA stock solution in 1× auto-MACS Rinsing Solution. Keep buffer cold (2–8 °C). The solution contains PBS, pH 7.2, 0.5% BSA, and 2 mM EDTA (*see* **Note 1**).

2.3 Macrophage Differentiation and Polarization

1. Centrifuge for 15 mL and 50 mL tubes.

2. Refrigerator, 2–8 °C.

3. Freezer, −20 °C.

4. Cell culture incubator 37 °C, 5% CO_2, and 95% humidity.

5. Water bath.

6. Biohazard safety cabinet approved for biosafety level 2.

7. Cell counter.

8. Inverted microscope.

9. Pipet boy.

10. Sterile pipettes covering a range of 0.05 to 1 mL.

11. Sterile serological pipettes covering a range of 1 mL to 50 mL.

12. Sterile microcentrifuge tubes, 1.5 or 2 mL.

13. Polypropylene tubes, 15 and 50 mL.

14. Cell culture-coated tissue culture plates and/or flasks (e.g., 96-well plates).

15. RPMI 1640 medium.

16. Fetal bovine serum (FBS).

17. Penicillin/Streptomycin antibiotics mix.

18. L-glutamine (200 mM).

19. Basal monocyte medium: 10% (v/v) FBS, 100 U/mL penicillin/streptomycin, 2 mM L-glutamine in RPMI 1640 medium.

20. Macrophage colony-stimulating factor.

21. Granulocyte-macrophage colony-stimulating factor.

22. Interleukin-4.

23. Interferon-γ.

24. Lipopolysaccharides (LPS) from *Escherichia coli* O111:B4.

25. Macrophage differentiation medium: 10 ng/mL M-CSF or 10 ng/mL GM-CSF in basal monocyte medium.

26. Macrophage polarization medium: dilute cytokines according to Table 2 in macrophage differentiation medium to achieve the intended macrophage polarization (*see* **Note 2**).

2.4 ELISA

1. Centrifuge.

2. Refrigerator, 2–8 °C.

3. Freezer, −20 °C.

4. Plate reader for wavelength 450 nm and 540/570 nm.

5. Plate washer, or, for example, MultiFlo Fx dispenser with washing module.

6. Vortex.

7. Pipet boy.

8. Pipettes covering a range of 0.05 to 1 mL.

9. Serological pipettes covering a range of 1 mL to 50 mL.

10. Microcentrifuge tubes, 1.5 or 2 mL.

11. Polypropylene tubes, 15 and 50 mL.

12. Sterile plastic reservoirs.

13. High-adsorption 96-well half-area plate for plate reader.

14. ELISA kits for IL-1β, TNF-α, IL-6.

15. Dulbecco's phosphate buffered saline (PBS).

16. Tween-20.

17. Bovine serum albumin (BSA), heat shock fraction, protease free.

18. Stop solution: H_2SO_4, 2 N. Aliquot required volume on day of analysis.

19. Wash buffer: 0.05% (v/v) Tween-20 in PBS.

20. Reagent diluent: 1% w/v BSA in PBS, sterile filter with 0.2 μm filter.

21. HRP-substrate.

2.5 Automated ELISA

1. Biomek i7 (Beckman Coulter) liquid handling system integrated with hotel, MultiFloX, and plate reader.

2. Assay plate (high-adsorption 96-well half-area).

3. Plate lid.

4. Reservoir 300 mL.

5. Tips 180–250 μL (e.g., BioMek AP250).

6. 96-well deep well (DW) plate 2 mL.

7. 96-well polypropylene V-shaped.

8. Sterile container with low excess volume for STR_HRP and substrate (e.g., T75 cell culture plates, placed in a tilted position in a container with iced water).

3 Methods

Blood or buffy coat is ordered from the blood bank at the local hospital. Please be aware that use of human biological material requires informed donor consent and approval from relevant ethical committees (*see* **Note 3**). The following protocol consists of four parts: lymphocyte isolation (1), enrichment of CD14+ monocytes (2), macrophage differentiation and polarization (3), and ELISA (4). The workflow of the method and connection to relevant assays is depicted in Fig. 2. For use in monocyte activation assays, CD14+ monocytes can be used immediately after seeding. Subheading 3.4 describes the workflow for manual ELISA. For automated ELISA, refer to Subheading 3.5. It is imperative to pay heed to health and safety aspects related to the use of potentially harmful substances (*see* **Note 4**) and biosafety level 2 materials (*see* **Note 5**).

3.1 Lymphocyte Isolation from Human Blood

Until mononuclear cells are isolated, all work should be performed according to biosafety level (BSL) 2 regulations. Isolated cells can be handled as BSL-1 material. Fresh blood or buffy coats should be kept at room temperature (RT) until processing.

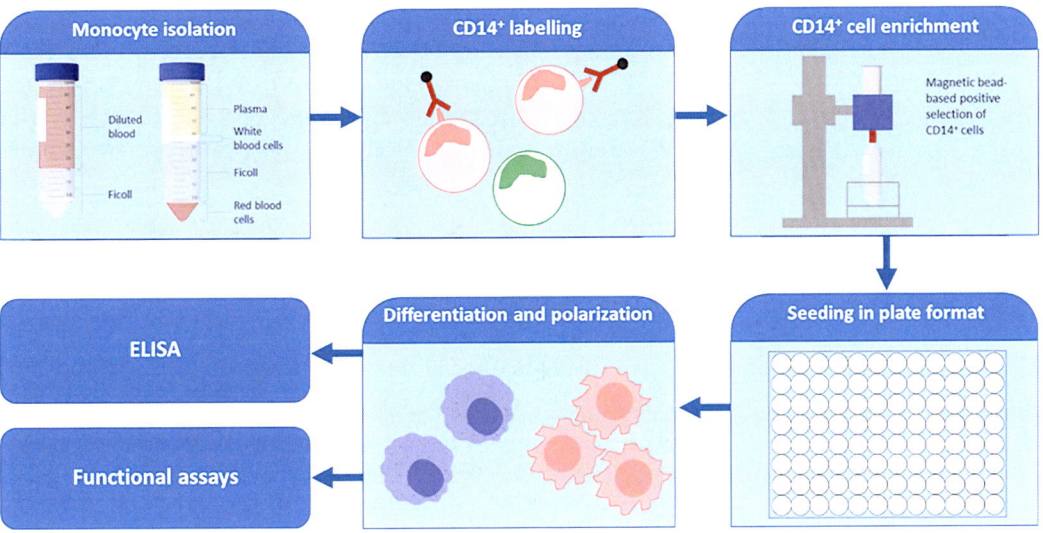

Fig. 2 Schematic workflow of monocyte isolation from buffy coats and macrophage differentiation and polarization

1. Sterilize biosafety cabinet and equipment using 80% ethanol. It is recommended to use bench paper in biosafety cabinet (can be easily discarded in case of spillage).

2. Sterilize buffy coat bag with ethanol, and place it into the cabinet.

3. Use scissors to cut tubes. Collect buffy coat (usually about ~40 mL) in 50 mL tube.

4. Assess blood volume and dilute 1:1 with RT HBSS.

5. Transfer 15 mL Ficoll-Pacque from glass bottle to 50 mL tubes (prepare 4 tubes per buffy coat). Tilt the tube at 45°, then carefully layer 20 mL blood-HBSS on top of Ficoll, using a 25 mL pipette and pipet boy set at lowest speed.

6. Centrifuge at $400 \times g$ for 30 min at RT with centrifuge brakes turned off. Too fast breaking after centrifugation may disturb the white blood cell layer. Reset rotor brakes.

7. Observe the tube. Three to four separate layers will have formed; red blood cells at the bottom, then a clear layer of Ficoll, followed by a layer of white blood cells precisely at the interphase between Ficoll and water, and finally a beige opaque layer of plasma on the top (Fig. 2).

8. Remove the top plasma layer using a serological pipette. This contains platelets and serum proteins.

9. Pipette the white blood cells into two 50 mL tubes.

10. Spin at $100 \times g$ for 10 min at RT and remove supernatant.

11. Resuspend each cell pellet in 1 mL warm HBSS (37 °C). Merge the different white blood cell fractions into one tube. Add warm HBSS to a total volume of 25 mL and repeat centrifugation. Remove supernatant and resuspend in 25 mL warm HBSS. Repeat centrifugation and resuspension two more times.

12. Resuspend in 25 mL of warm HBSS and count cells.

13. If viability is >90%, proceed with cells for experimental use (*see* **Notes 6**, **7**, and **8**).

3.2 Enrichment of CD14+ Monocytes

Several different types of columns are offered for cell sorting. For example, Milenyi biotech "LS" columns are used for positive <u>S</u>election and are size "**L**" in terms of loading capacity (number of cells), which is sufficient for this application. Columns with 10× lower ("MS") and 10× higher (XS) capacity are also available. The LS columns are single-use, flow-stop-controlled, and do not run dry. They have a void volume of 400 µL and a reservoir volume of 8 mL. A typical flow rate for PBS containing 0.5% BSA, in our hands, is in the range of 1.2–2.1 mL/min. During this part it is recommended to work fast, keep cells cold, and use precooled solutions. This will prevent capping of antibodies on the cell surface and nonspecific cell labelling. The volumes for magnetic labelling given below are for up to 10^7 cells. When working with fewer than 10^7 cells, use the same volumes as indicated. When working with higher cell numbers, scale up all reagent volumes and total volumes accordingly (e.g., for 2×10^7 total cells, use twice the volume of all indicated reagent volumes and total volumes; *see* **Notes 9** and **10**).

1. Attach QuadroMACS Separator to the MACS MultiStand and place LS Column in the separator. Place a collection tube under the LS Column (Fig. **3**).

2. Check that the ejection blocks in the gap of the magnet are attached before placing the MACS Column into the magnetic field of the QuadroMACS Separator.

3. Be careful when attaching the QuadroMACS Separator to the MultiStand to avoid trapping your fingers (for details see QuadroMACS Starting Kit data sheet).

4. Determine cell number (from **Step 12** in Subheading 3.1).

5. Centrifuge cell suspension at $300 \times g$ for 10 min at RT. Aspirate supernatant completely.

6. Resuspend cell pellet in 80 µL of buffer per 10^7 total cells.

7. Add 20 µL of CD14 MicroBeads per 10^7 total cells.

8. Mix well by pipetting and incubate for 15 min in the refrigerator (2–8 °C).

9. Wash cells by adding 1–2 mL buffer per 10^7 cells and centrifuge at $300 \times g$ for 10 min at RT. Aspirate supernatant completely.

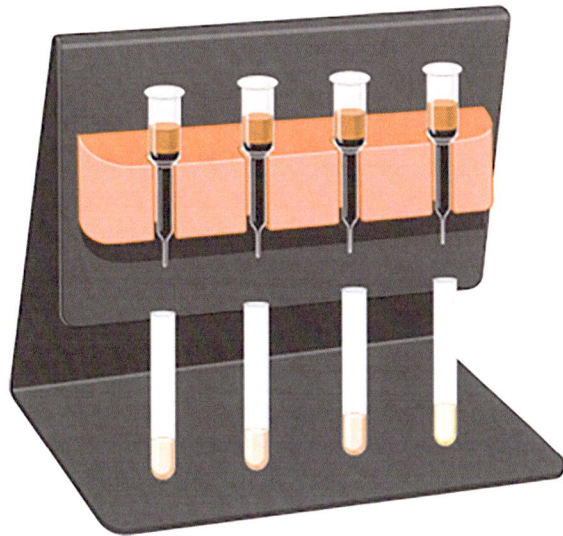

Fig. 3 Setup of magnetic cell separator, stand and column (Figure made with Biorender)

Resuspend up to 10^8 cells in 500 μL buffer. For higher cells numbers, scale up buffer volume accordingly.

10. Proceed to magnetic separation. Choose an appropriate MACS column and MACS Separator according to the number of total cells and the number of CD14+ cells.

11. Place column in the magnetic field of a suitable MACS Separator (*see* **Note 11**).

12. Rinse column with the appropriate amount of buffer (3 mL for an LS column).

13. Apply cell suspension onto column.

14. Collect unlabeled cells that pass through and wash column with the appropriate amount of buffer (LS: 3 mL). Collect total effluent; this is the unlabeled cell fraction. Perform washing steps by adding buffer three times. Only add new buffer when the column reservoir is empty.

15. Remove column from the separator and place it on a suitable collection tube.

16. Pipette the appropriate amount of buffer onto the column (LS: 5 mL). Immediately flush out the magnetically labeled cells by firmly pushing the plunger (supplied with the column) into the column (*see* **Note 12**).

3.3 Macrophage Differentiation and Polarization

Macrophage differentiation is performed with freshly isolated CD14+ monocytes (**Step 16** from Subheading 3.2). Macrophage polarization is performed on day 5 of differentiation. For many applications, M-SCF- or GM-CSF-*differentiated* cells are sufficient, but this depends on the exact experimental strategy.

Table 1
Parameters for seeding cells

Size	Culture volume	Monocytes/well
6-well plate	4 mL/well	4×10^6 cells
24-well plate	1 mL/well	1×10^6 cells
96-well plate	200 μL/well	2×10^5 cells

Table 2
Overview of differentiation and polarization agents

Cytokine	Stock concentration	Final concentration	Resulting phenotype
M-CSF	10 μg/mL (50 μL)	10–25 ng/mL	M(−)
GM-CSF	10 μg/mL (50 μL)	10–25 ng/mL	M(−)
IL-4	10 μg/mL (50 μL)	10–20 ng/mL	M2
IFN-γ	10 μg/mL (50 μL)	20 ng/mL	M1
LPS	1 mg/mL	0.1–1 ng/mL	M1

1. Count cell numbers from **step 16** of Subheading 3.2.

2. Centrifuge monocytes at $300 \times g$ for 10 min at RT.

3. Dilute CD14+ monocytes to 10^6 cells/mL in warm basal monocyte medium (37 °C) and seed cells in multiwell-plates according to Table 1.

4. Incubate for 1.5 h at 37 °C, 5% CO_2 in a humidified incubator to allow monocytes to adhere.

5. Wash away nonbinding cells with warm HBSS (37 °C), using equivalent volumes as specified in Table 1. Wash wells a total of three times.

6. Add the desired macrophage differentiation medium.

7. Incubate cells for 3 days at 37 °C, 5% CO_2 in a humidified incubator. Monitor cell viability and morphology daily under microscope.

8. Replace medium with fresh macrophage differentiation medium (37 °C).

9. Prepare stocks of the needed differentiation and polarization agents in PBS (according to Table 2) and store at −20 °C until use.

10. Prepare working solutions of the chosen polarization agent in warm (37 °C) basal monocyte medium (="polarization medium"). Table 2 provides an overview over suitable concentrations.

11. Remove medium from wells and replace with polarization medium. Incubate for 24 h.

12. After 24 h, cells can be used for experiments, assays, etc.

3.4 ELISA

For easier downstream handling, it is strongly recommended to match layouts from cell culture/experiment plate(s) with the ELISA plate(s). One approach is to (1) set up samples in plate columns and (2) using sample plates instead of single tubes for collecting samples (Fig. 4). This allows the use of multichannel pipettes (or robotic systems) both for sample collection and transfer to the assay plate. If using parallels/replicates in the original experiment, for example, in cell culture, decide whether pooled replicates or single replicates should be analyzed by ELISA. For the latter case, identical sample plates could be created for each set of replicates. Please be aware that in case of the automated ELISA, two columns on the sample plate need to be kept empty for the standard curve. Standards and capture/detection antibodies are provided as powder in vials (amount specified in data sheet), take 1 vial of each and reconstitute and aliquot in 1.5 mL microcentrifuge tubes or smaller. Use the resuspension volumes and buffers as specified by the manufacturer. A suggestion for aliquoted volumes is given in Table 3. For a whole assay plate, several aliquots will be required. Calculate the required volumes prior to starting the assay. The whole assay is performed at RT.

1. Dilute the capture antibody to the working concentration in PBS without carrier protein (in a tube). See Table 4 for details. Immediately coat a 96-well microplate with 50 µL per well of the diluted capture antibody. Seal the plate (either parafilm or adhesive strip) and incubate overnight at RT.

2. Aspirate each well and wash with Wash Buffer, repeating the process two times for a total of three washes. Wash by filling each well with Wash Buffer (100 µL) using a squirt bottle, manifold dispenser, or autowasher. Complete removal of liquid at each step is essential for good performance. After the last wash, remove any remaining Wash Buffer by aspirating or by inverting the plate and blotting it against clean paper towels.

3. Block plates by adding 100 µL Reagent Diluent (RD) to each well. Incubate at RT for 1–2 h (*see* **Note 13**).

4. Repeat the aspiration/wash as in **step 2**. The plates are now ready for sample addition.

5. Add 50 µL of sample or standards in Reagent Diluent, or an appropriate diluent, per well (samples/standards prepared in microcentrifuge tubes). Cover with a plate lid (alternatively adhesive strip).

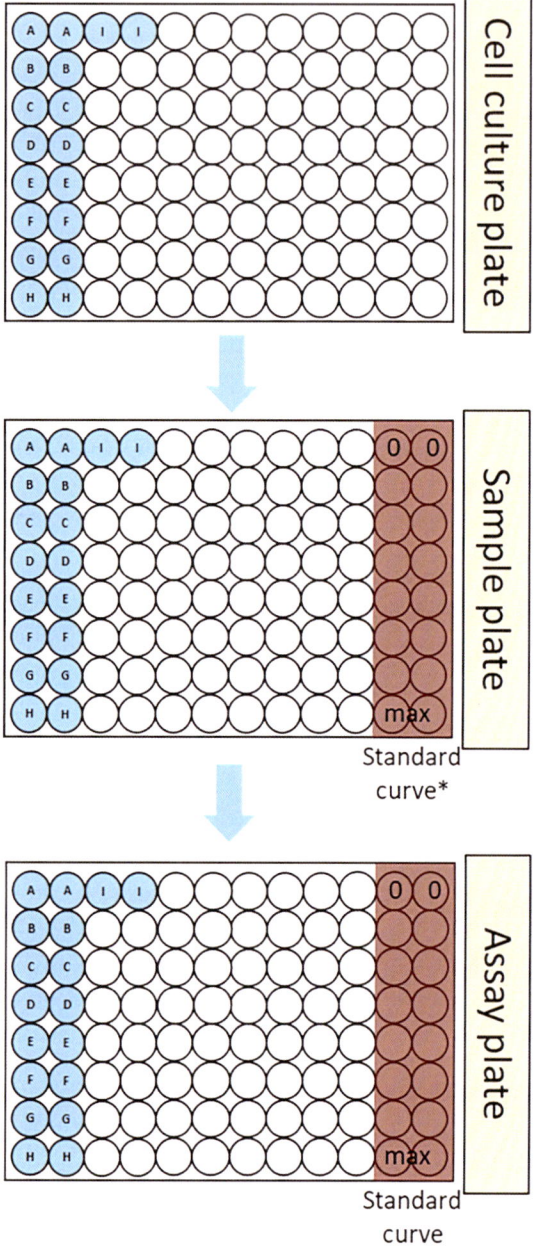

Fig. 4 Example of optimized experimental design for ELISA. The experiment is performed in cell culture plates, with nine different treatments/samples (A-I) run in duplicate. In this example workflow, cell culture replicates are pooled in the cell culture plate before transfer in duplicate to the sample plate (for storage or immediate use). Defined sample volumes are then transferred to the ELISA assay plate on the day of analysis. (*) The standard curve is prepared fresh on the day of ELISA analysis and directly added to the assay plate (for manual ELISA) or added to the sample plate (automated ELISA)

Table 3
Suggestions for reagent stock preparations

		Resuspend in	Stock concentration	µL per aliquot	# aliquots
IL-1β	Capture	500 µL PBS	480 µg/mL	22	22
	Detection	1 mL reagent diluent	12 µg/mL	45	22
	Standard	500 µL ddH$_2$O	95 ng/mL	15	33
TNF-α	Capture	500 µL PBS	480 µg/mL	22	22
	Detection	1 mL reagent diluent	3 µg/mL	45	22
	Standard	500 µL ddH$_2$O	130 ng/mL	15	33
IL-6	Capture	500 µL PBS	240 µg/mL	22	22
	Detection	1 mL reagent diluent	3 µg/mL	45	22
	Standard	500 µL ddH$_2$O	180 ng/mL	15	33

Table 4
Instructions for dilution from aliquoted stock to working concentration

		Stock concentration	µL per aliquot	Working concentration	Dilution factor for working conc.	Add [µL]
IL-1β	Capture	480 µg/mL	22	4 µg/mL	120	2618 (PBS)
	Detection	12 µg/mL	40	200 ng/mL	60	2360 (RD)
	Standard	95 ng/mL	15	250 pg/mL	380	see Table below
TNF-α	Capture	480 µg/mL	22	4 µg/mL	120	2618 (PBS)
	Detection	3 µg/mL	40	200 ng/mL	60	2360 (RD)
	Standard	130 ng/mL	15	1000 pg/mL	130	see Table below
IL-6	Capture	240 µg/mL	22	2 µg/mL	120	2618 (PBS)
	Detection	3 µg/mL	40	200 ng/mL	60	2360 (RD)
	Standard	180 ng/mL	15	600 pg/mL	300	see Table below

6. Sample preparation: Keep tubes/plates with sample and standard solutions on ice. Spin down samples before use. Add 50 µL sample directly to well.

7. Standard preparation. Follow instructions on data sheet to prepare highest standard concentration (summary in Table 5), thereafter make 1:2 dilution series in microcentrifuge tubes (total of 7 concentrations). 8th "dilution" is 0 pg/mL, that is, pure reagent diluent equal to zero standard value.

8. Repeat the aspiration/wash as in **step 2**.

9. Add 50 µL of the Detection Antibody diluted in Reagent Diluent (from microcentrifuge tube) to each well. Cover with a new adhesive strip and incubate 2 h at RT.

Table 5
Instructions for initial dilution of recombinant standard

	Stock concentration	µL per aliquot	Working concentration	1st dilution	2nd dilution
IL-1β	95 ng/mL	15	250 pg/mL 1:380	1:76 1.25 ng/mL Add 1125 µL RD to aliquot	1:5 250 pg/mL Mix 200 µL first, add 800 µL RD
TNF-α	130 ng/mL	15	1000 pg/mL 1:130	1:65 2 ng/mL Add 960 µL RD to aliquot	1:2 1000 pg/mL Add 500 µL first, add 500 µl RD
IL-6	180 ng/mL	15	600 pg/mL 1:300	1:60 3 ng/mL Add 885 µL RD to aliquot	1:5 600 pg/mL Mix 200 µL first, add 800 µL RD

10. Repeat the aspiration/wash as in **step 2**.

11. Add 50 µL of the working dilution of Streptavidin-HRP (from microcentrifuge tube) to each well. Cover the plate and incubate for 20 min at RT. Avoid placing the plate in direct light.

12. Repeat the aspiration/wash as in **step 2**.

13. Add 50 µL of Substrate Solution (from tube) to each well. Incubate for 20 min at RT. Avoid placing the plate in direct light. Substrate converted by HRP should turn blue.

14. Add 25 µL of Stop Solution (2 N H_2SO_4) to each well. This should turn the blue HRP product yellow. Gently tap the plate to ensure thorough mixing.

15. Determine the optical density of each well immediately, using a microplate reader set to 450 nm. If wavelength correction is available, set to 540 nm or 570 nm. If wavelength correction is not available, subtract readings at 540 nm or 570 nm from the readings at 450 nm. This subtraction will correct for optical imperfections in the plate. Readings made directly at 450 nm without correction may be higher and less accurate.

16. Calculation of results (*see* **Notes 14–21**).

17. For each standard, control, and sample, subtract the average zero standard value.

18. Create a standard curve.

19. Option 1: Reduce the data using computer software capable of generating a four-parameter logistic (4-PL) curve-fit.

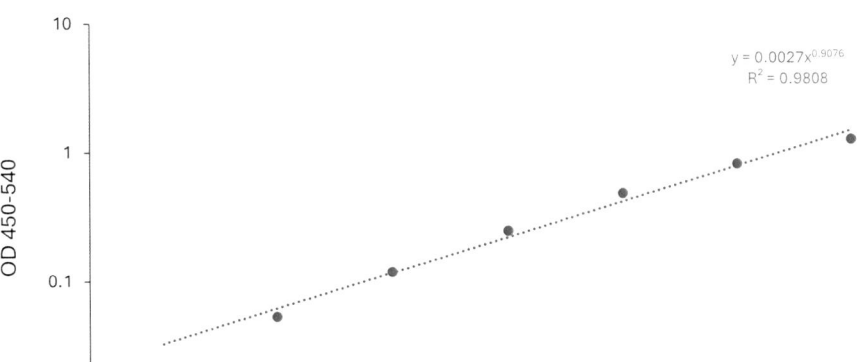

TNF-α calibration curve

$y = 0.0027x^{0.9076}$
$R^2 = 0.9808$

OD 450–540 (y-axis)

Concentration [pg/mL] (x-axis)

Fig. 5 Example standard curve for TNF-α (same donor as in Fig. 7A and 7B). Generated with option 2: plotting the mean absorbance for each standard on the *y*-axis against the concentration on the *x*-axis and draw a best-fit curve through the points on the graph

20. Option 2: Construct a standard curve by plotting the mean absorbance for each standard on the *y*-axis against the concentration on the *x*-axis, and draw a best fit curve through the points on the graph. The data may be linearized by plotting the log of the human TNF-α concentrations versus the log of the absorption and the best fit line can be determined by regression analysis (Fig. 5).

21. If samples have been diluted, the concentration read from the standard curve must be multiplied by the dilution factor.

3.5 Automated ELISA Refer to Subheading 3.4 for overview of the manual assay procedure. This section describes the automated handling of assay plates after the second step in Subheading 3.4. After overnight incubation with Capture Antibody, the assay plate is transferred to a Beckman i7 robotic system, the rest of the steps are automated with a series of automated processes recapitulating the steps in Subheading 3.4. The automated method is run from the SAMI software, using, for example, the configuration file in Supplementary File 1. A table of labware and solutions used in the automated method is found in Table 6 (*see* **Note 22**). All well plates are prepared and placed before the method is started, except well plates containing detection antibody and samples.

1. Open SAMI EX Editor Software and open the relevant protocol (Table 7).

2. Schedule the number of assay plates to be run, press OK.

Table 6
Labware and solutions required for processing of 1 assay plate

Solution	Position	Container/ vessel	Minimum excess volume	Estimated consumption for each assay plate (wo excess)	Temp	Shared/ unique
Wash buffer	P8 (Biomek)	Reservoir (300 mL)	100 mL	144 mL (100 µL/well × 15 rep)	RT	S
Blocking solution	P6 (Biomek)	Greiner 96 DW without lid	200 µL/ well	9.6 mL (100 µL/well)	RT	S
Stop solution	P14 (Biomek)	Greiner 96 DW with lid	200 µL/ well	2.4 mL (25 µL/well)	RT	S
Detection AB[a]	P9 (Biomek)	Greiner 96 DW	200 µL/ well	5.8 mL (50 µL/well)	4 °C	S
Samples[a]	Deck hotel, rack 1	96 PPV With lid	50 µL/ well	4.8 mL (50 µL/well)	4 °C	U
Assay plate (precoated)	Carousel Holder1	96 half area With lid		Manually processed	RT	U
STR_HRP[a]	MultiFloX, peri1	T75	~100 mL (incl priming)	4.8 mL (50 µL/well)	4 °C	S
Substrate[a]	MultiFloX, peri2	T75	Ca 100 mL	4.8 mL (50 µL/well)	4 ° C/ RT	S

[a]Cooled solutions are placed on Beckman i7 directly before use. Solutions dispensed by MultiFloX can be placed in container with iced water; however, priming of the tubes must be executed directly before addition of these

Table 7
Overview of Biomek nodes in the SAMI method

Node	Biomek Method	
1	Washplate_lid_block_Halv_area_V2	Supplementary material 1
2	Washplate_lid_block_Halv_area_add_samples_V2	Supplementary material 2
3	Washplate_lid_block_Halv_area_add_detection_AB_V4	Supplementary material 3
4	Washplate_lid_block_Halv_area_add_STR_HRP_V2	Supplementary material 4
5	Washplate_lid_block_Halv_area_add_substrate_V2	Supplementary material 5
6	Add_25ul_STOP_halv_Area	Supplementary material 6

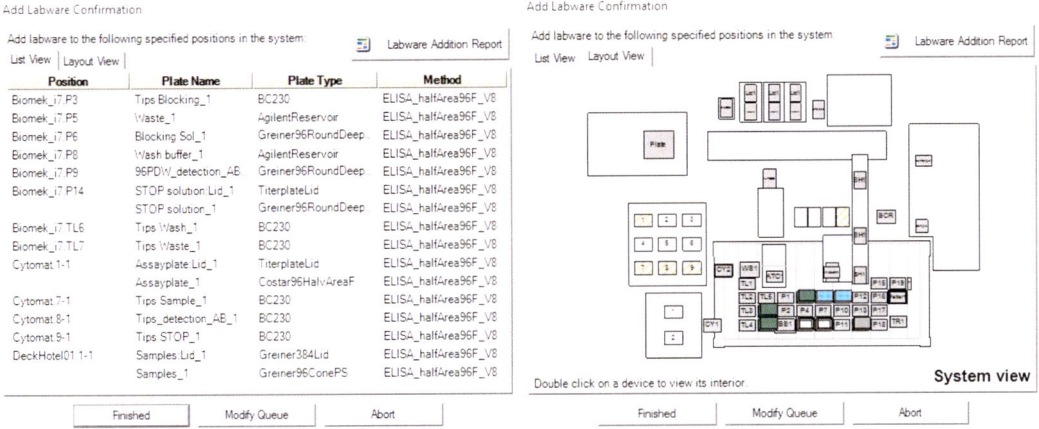

Fig. 6 Pipetting robot setup. Labware pipetting tips, plates, and solutions are added in defined and specified positions (right). Refer to Supplementary materials for the relevant robot scripts

3. Press Run (Green symbol), before the method starts a list of required consumables will appear (can be viewed in list form or System view), refer to Fig. 6.

4. Install cassettes on the MultiFloX (5 μL, 8 channels) on pump 1 and 2.

5. Wash cassettes by priming a 5% solution of Deconex, if some of the tips are clogged let the system incubate with Deconex for 30 min.

6. Rinse the system by priming with PBS or water to make sure that no Deconex remains in the system.

7. Test both cassettes by dispensing 200 μL in a 96-well test plate, and check that all wells contain the same volume by ocular inspection.

8. Transfer the inlet tubings to their respective solutions (STR_HRP in pump1, and substrate in pump2), prime both solutions, the priming must be repeated just before addition of both solutions to ensure that dispensed solutions are cooled (the volumes that are in the tubings while the first part of the method is run will no longer be cooled).

9. Make sure to place the inlets at the bottom corner and tilt the containers so that excess volume is reduced.

The outcome of the experimental procedures described in this report can be evaluated in two ways: (1) cell morphology and (2) functional assays. Cell morphology will be more commonly used to monitor the process. Monocytes will appear round when examined under a microscope. Macrophage differentiation and polarization will lead (depending on the regime) to larger (a) more spread-out roundish cells ("fried egg"), (b) spindle-like cells, or (c) a mix of the aforementioned.

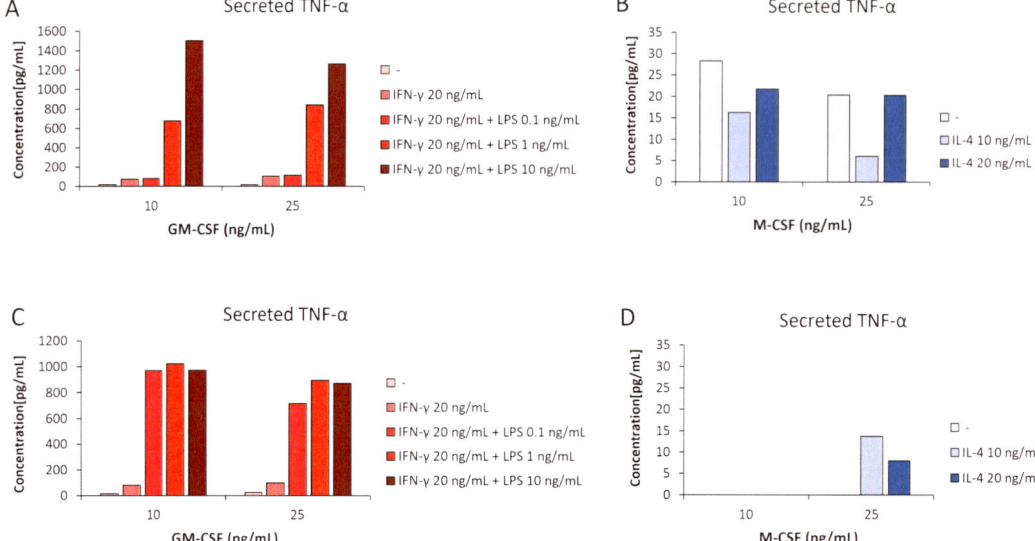

Fig. 7 TNF-α levels in differentiated and polarized macrophages. Monocytes from two separate donors (A and B, and C and D, respectively) were differentiated with the indicated concentration of M-CSF or GM-CSF for 5 days, followed by 24 h of the indicated regime ("-": plain). The bars show average values from $n = 2$ technical replicates

Functional assays are not usually used for controlling or monitoring the generated cell population but are mainly used to answer research question (utilizing the generated cells). A usual functional readout in monocytes and macrophages is analysis of cytokine production using ELISA.

In macrophages, cytokine responses can, for example, be used to assay effects of compounds on polarisation, i.e., anti-inflammatory vs. inflammatory phenotypes. An example of baseline expression of TNF-α (marker cytokine for inflammatory phenotypes) after different polarization regimes is presented in Fig. 7. Note the pronounced difference in TNF-α levels between macrophages polarized toward M2 (via M-CSF and IL-4, Fig. 7B) and M1 macrophages (via IFN-γ and LPS, Fig. 7A).

4   Notes

1. Degas rinsing solution before use, since air bubbles could block the column.

2. If further macrophage polarization is intended (as specified in Subheading 3.3), use M-CSF for cells which will be treated with IL-4.

3. In most jurisdictions, work with and access to human blood may require prior approval by the relevant ethical committee and informed consent from the donors to use donated materials for research.

4. The stop solution ($2 N H_2SO_4$) is a concentrated acid. Aliquot the required volume with adequate safety measures (fume hood, heavy duty acid proof gloves, protective goggles). Small amounts can then be used on the lab bench (or fume hood) using gloves, which are "short-term" acid-resistant. Neutralize leftovers of aliquoted acid by adding them to water or to the reagent/buffer leftovers before disposing them.

5. Biological samples need to be handled according to their biosafety level at least until addition of the detection antibody (at that point, all unbound sample material should have been washed away). Donated human blood from healthy donors is classified as biosafety level 2.

6. Poor lymphocyte viability ($<90\%$) can be caused by errors in cell counting, such as out-of-focus samples, the presence of large numbers of platelets, or dead cells due to improper treatment. Observe cells under the microscope to distinguish between these possibilities. Healthy cells will appear as round and shiny ~10 μm diameter spheres. Dead cells will appear as irregular grains of the same size, while platelets can be seen as irregular, small cells that will be stained by trypan blue.

7. ELISA can be run on monocytes, if desired. If so, stop the procedure before CD14+ enrichment and add basal monocyte medium instead of differentiation agents after **step 4** in Subheading 3.2.

8. Potential causes for failed isolation of monocytes:

   (a) Gradient centrifugation (Ficoll-Paque): No/insufficient separation due to layer mixing. May be due to improper preparation of layers or using a centrifuge with active braking.

   (b) No/few attached cells after incubation on cell culture surface (plate/flask): Too short or too long incubation.

   (c) CD14 selection not properly performed due improper/incomplete magnetic labelling (possible causes: wrong temperature, incomplete mixing of beads and cells, wrong ratio reagents/cells).

9. For optimal performance, it is important to obtain a single-cell suspension before magnetic separation. Pass cells through 30 μm nylon mesh (e.g., Pre-Separation Filters) to remove cell clumps which may clog the column.

10. Working on ice may require increased incubation times. Higher temperatures and/or longer incubation times may lead to nonspecific cell labeling.

11. Refer to the instructions, manuals, or data sheets from MACS Column manufacturer for details regarding column and magnet assembly.

12. To increase the purity of CD14+ cells, the eluted fraction can be enriched over a second LS Column. Repeat the magnetic separation procedure as described in **step 10** to **16** by using a new column.

13. 2 h is recommended unless increased background is not a concern for the intended ELISA analysis.

14. If you observe a poor standard curve (low absorbance signal, loss of signal for lower concentrations, pronounced variations), check the following:

    (a) Impure BSA used for Reagent Diluent preparation?

    (b) Improper reconstitution and/or storage of standard?

    (c) Improper dilution of highest standard and standard curve?

    (d) Incomplete washing and/or aspiration of wells?

    (e) Unequal volumes added to wells/pipetting error?

    (f) Incorrect incubation times or temperatures?

15. If the assay precision is poor, check the following:

    (a) Unequal volumes added to wells/pipetting error?

    (b) Incomplete washing and/or aspiration of wells?

    (c) Unequal mixing of reagents?

16. If no or only weak color is developed:

    (a) Inadequate volume of substrate added to wells?

    (b) Incorrect incubation times or temperatures?

    (c) Impure BSA used for Reagent Diluent preparation?

17. There are the following check points for quality control:

    (a) Cell count of isolated lymphocytes should be $>10^7$ (best $>10^8$ cells), with $>90\%$ viability.

    (b) Cell count after CD14 selection is expected to be ca. 10% of original cell count. Significant deviation from this may be reason for aborting the isolation.

    (c) Cell survival after 3–5 days of macrophage differentiation should be closely observed. If a marked loss of cells (relative to seeding count) is observed, the batch of cells should be discarded and not used in experiment.

18. A first checkpoint for quality control is color development for the diluted standard series (and potentially reference samples with expected high levels of target peptide). In particular, the color intensity should correspond with the concentration gradient.

19. A second checkpoint for quality control is the R^2 value of the standard curve. The R^2 value should be at least 0.98, even better 0.99. Check whether the standard curve contains obvious outliers that may be removed.

20. When analyzing the sample data, discard all datapoints with absorbance values below or above the range covered by the standard curve.

21. For best assay results, it is strongly recommended to use high-adsorption assay plates and heat shock fraction, protease-free BSA.

22. The maximum capacity of the reservoirs used for wash and waste solutions are 300 mL, if more than 1 assay plate is scheduled for run it will be necessary to refill the wash reservoir and empty the waste during the run.

Acknowledgments

This chapter is based upon work from COST Action IMMUNO-model, CA21135, supported by COST (European Cooperation in Science and Technology) and a SINTEF (strategic institute project on immunotherapy 102020958). T.V. and H.H-H. acknowledges funding from the Research Council of Norway (projects 303369 and 353112).

References

1. Sender R, Weiss Y, Navon Y et al (2023) The total mass, number, and distribution of immune cells in the human body. Proc Natl Acad Sci 120:e2308511120. https://doi.org/10.1073/pnas.2308511120

2. Watanabe S, Alexander M, Misharin AV, Budinger GRS (2019) The role of macrophages in the resolution of inflammation. J Clin Invest 129:2619–2628. https://doi.org/10.1172/JCI124615

3. Murray PJ, Allen JE, Biswas SK et al (2014) Macrophage activation and polarization: nomenclature and experimental guidelines. Immunity 41:14. https://doi.org/10.1016/j.immuni.2014.06.008

4. Xue J, Schmidt SV, Sander J et al (2014) Transcriptome-based network analysis reveals a Spectrum model of human macrophage activation. Immunity 40:274–288. https://doi.org/10.1016/j.immuni.2014.01.006

5. Bøyum A (1964) Separation of white blood cells. Nature 204:793–794. https://doi.org/10.1038/204793a0

6. Bhattacharjee J, Das B, Mishra A et al (2018) Monocytes isolated by positive and negative magnetic sorting techniques show different molecular characteristics and immunophenotypic behaviour. F1000Res 6:2045. https://doi.org/10.12688/f1000research.12802.3

7. Ziegler-Heitbrock L, Ancuta P, Crowe S et al (2010) Nomenclature of monocytes and dendritic cells in blood. Blood 116:e74–e80. https://doi.org/10.1182/blood-2010-02-258558

8. Wu Z, Zhang Z, Lei Z, Lei P (2019) CD14: biology and role in the pathogenesis of disease. Cytokine Growth Factor Rev 48:24–31. https://doi.org/10.1016/j.cytogfr.2019.06.003

9. Lequin RM (2005) Enzyme immunoassay (EIA)/enzyme-linked immunosorbent assay (ELISA). Clin Chem 51:2415–2418. https://doi.org/10.1373/clinchem.2005.051532

10. Enzyme-linked immunosorbent assay (ELISA) | British Society for Immunology. https://www.immunology.org/public-information/bitesized-immunology/experimental-techniques/enzyme-linked-immunosorbent-assay. Accessed 30 May 2024

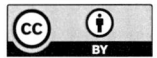

Determination of the Inhibitory Properties of Compounds Toward Immune Checkpoint Complex Formation Using ELISA

Katarzyna Kuncewicz and Marta Spodzieja

Abstract

ELISA is one of the most widely used methods in immunology, molecular biology, and medical diagnostics. It enables the detection and quantification of specific proteins, antibodies, antigens, or hormones in biological samples such as blood serum, urine, or cerebrospinal fluid. ELISA is highly sensitive and specific, which makes it extremely useful in various fields of scientific research and clinical diagnosis. In recent years, this method has gained importance in the context of research on immune checkpoint inhibitors. Immune checkpoint inhibitors, such as antibodies, peptides, or small-molecule compounds that block receptor/ligand complex formation, have become modern therapeutic tools in immuno-oncology. Therefore, more and more research is being conducted in this field. ELISA is a relatively cheap and rapid method that can be effectively used to verify the initial inhibitory potential of compounds before more expensive and much more sophisticated cell-based assays are performed. In this protocol, we described how the inhibitory properties of compounds toward immune checkpoint complex formation can be investigated using ELISA and provided a detailed procedure that was used to evaluate the inhibitory properties of peptides toward the BTLA/HVEM complex formation.

Key words Peptide inhibitors, Competitive ELISA, Immune checkpoints, Protein-protein interactions, Protein-peptide interactions

1 Introduction

The enzyme-linked immunosorbent assay (ELISA) method is based on a specific antigen-antibody interaction, where enzyme-bound antibodies are used to detect antigens in the test sample. As a result of this process, in the presence of a suitable substrate, the enzyme catalyzes a chemical reaction, the product of which can be easily measured, usually using a spectrophotometer. There are four major types of ELISA—direct, indirect, sandwich, and competitive (Fig. 1) [1–3].

Sweta Rani and Lukasz Skalniak (eds.), *IMMUNO-model in Cancer: Methods and Protocols*, Methods in Molecular Biology, vol. 2959, https://doi.org/10.1007/978-1-0716-4734-9_2, © The Author(s) 2026

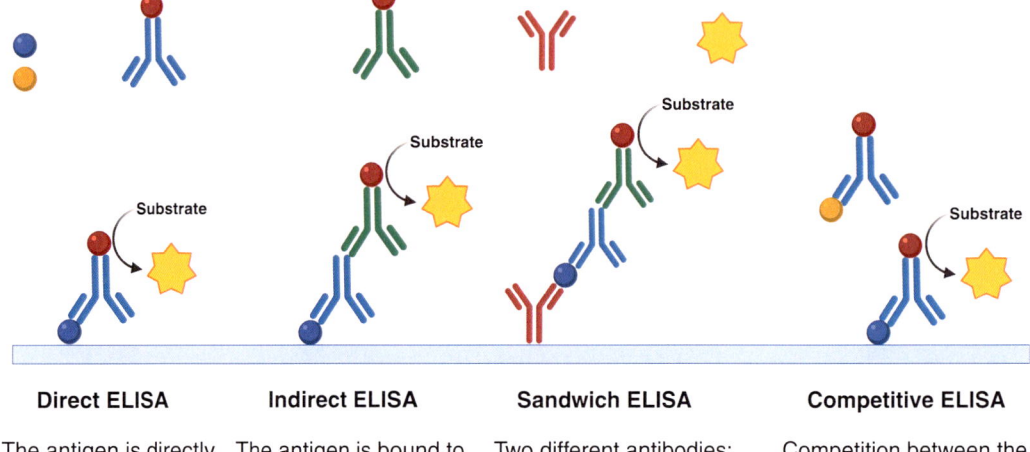

Direct ELISA	Indirect ELISA	Sandwich ELISA	Competitive ELISA
The antigen is directly bound to the solid phase and detection is performed with an enzyme-labelled antibody	The antigen is bound to the solid phase and then detected by a primary antibody, which is later recognised by an enzyme-labelled secondary antibody	Two different antibodies: one for antigen capture (bound to the solid phase) and the other for antigen detection, which increases the specificity and sensitivity of the method	Competition between the antigen present in the sample and the reference antigen for binding sites on the antibody, allowing low antigen concentrations to be measured

Fig. 1 ELISA types

In research on immune checkpoint inhibitors, a modified competitive ELISA can be used to test the potential of the compounds. In our research group, we are concerned with testing the inhibitory properties of the peptides on B- and T-lymphocyte attenuator (BTLA)/Herpesvirus entry mediator (HVEM) complex formation, but this test could also be used for other proteins [4–7]. If the molecular target of inhibitors is HVEM performing this assay involves the following steps: (a) coating the plate with the HVEM, (b) blocking the sites on the plate unoccupied by HVEM, (c) incubation of HVEM protein with the peptides—potential inhibitors, (d) adding the BTLA with Fc tag, and (e) detection of BTLA using antibodies conjugated with enzyme (Fig. 2).

The individual steps of this assay will be discussed below, not only in the context of our research but more generally. This description is intended to help researchers plan their experiments appropriately, depending on the availability of plates, proteins, buffers, and detection equipment.

1.1 Coating the Plate with Protein

In ELISA, one of the molecules is immobilized on a solid phase, which is usually a 96-well polystyrene or polypropylene plate. The plate type is chosen depending on the type of molecule to be immobilized on it. Four main methods of immobilizing compounds on a plate could be distinguished: physical adsorption, binding by His-tag, binding by biotin, and covalent immobilization [8].

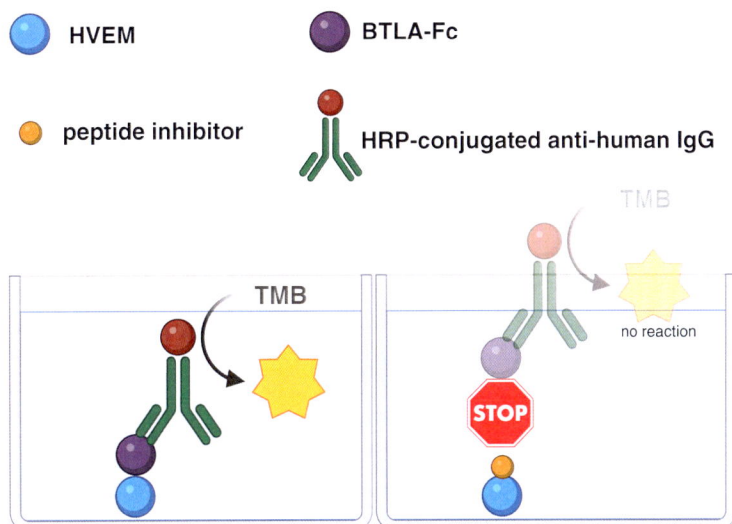

Fig. 2 Schematic of the competitive ELISA used to study the blocking properties of peptides—potential immune checkpoints inhibitors. (**a**) If HVEM interacts with BTLA protein, HRP-conjugated antibody recognizes the BTLA protein, and the enzyme converts the substrate to the colored product; (**b**) If a peptide inhibitor blocks the binding of BTLA to HVEM, the reaction does not occur

Physical adsorption is the most commonly used method for protein immobilization, and it is based on hydrophobic and electrostatic interactions between the protein and the surface of the plate. Depending on the chemical nature of the molecules, different plates are used for their immobilization. Hydrophilic plates are useful when working with polar molecules, such as some proteins, while hydrophobic plates are adapted to bind hydrophobic compounds, such as lipids. Moreover, the plates can also be divided into high-binding and low-binding plates. The surface of high-binding plates is modified to increase the binding capacity of proteins and other molecules. Low-binding plates have a reduced ability to bind proteins, which is useful when the compound under investigation must remain free or when nonspecific interactions need to be minimized. In physical adsorption, the protein is dissolved in a suitable buffer (usually of low ionic strength), applied to the surface of the plate, and incubated for 2 h at room temperature or at 4 °C overnight [3, 8, 9].

His-tag binding plates contain immobilized nickel ions (Ni^{2+}) on the surface, which are capable of binding proteins with a histidine tag (His-tag). Proteins with such a tag, due to the high affinity of histidine for metal ions, can be easily and selectively bound to the plate surface. Biotin-binding plates coated with streptavidin or avidin are also commonly used. These plates allow the binding of biotinylated proteins, antibodies, or other molecules that have a strong affinity for streptavidin or avidin. This method of immobilization is often used in analyses requiring high sensitivity due to the stability of the biotin-streptavidin complex [3, 8, 9].

In the case of covalent binding plates, biomolecules are covalently bound to the surface, providing extremely stable immobilization of biomolecules. Molecules can bind to a range of functional groups, such as amine (-NH$_2$), sulfhydryl (-SH), and carboxyl (-COOH). Such plates are ideal when long-term and stable retention of molecules on the plate surface is required, without the risk of them washing out during the following steps of ELISA [3, 8, 9].

In ELISA, not only the type of plate is important, but also the buffer in which the protein is dissolved and immobilized. The choice of the right buffer is crucial for the successful immobilization of a protein on a plate. Buffers must stabilize the protein, preserve its activity, and provide suitable conditions for adsorption or chemical reactions. The commonly used buffers used to dissolve and immobilize the protein are:

- Carbonate-bicarbonate buffer (pH 9.5)—this is the most commonly used buffer for protein adsorption. The higher pH of sodium carbonate favors the binding of the protein to the polystyrene surface.

- Phosphate buffered saline (PBS, pH 7.2–7.4)—this is used as a milder buffer to stabilize proteins during adsorption, especially when there is a need to minimize changes in protein structure.

- Tris-buffered saline (pH 7.5–8.5)—used where a more alkaline pH is required, which can increase the affinity of the protein to the surface [3, 8, 9].

It should be noted that optimal coating conditions and plate binding capacity can vary with proteins and must be determined experimentally. The plates are usually coated with more capture protein than can be bound to the plate to ensure the largest possible working range of detection.

1.2   Plate Blocking   In ELISA, once a protein has been immobilized on a plate, it is necessary to block the remaining sites on the plate surface that are unoccupied by protein. This prevents the non-specific binding of other molecules used in the next steps of the test, which could lead to false positives. The choice of blocker is important to minimize background and ensure high specificity of the ELISA, which affects the accuracy and reliability of the results. The most commonly used compounds for blocking are proteins, such as bovine serum albumin (BSA) and casein. BSA is available in a variety of purity grades and is relatively inexpensive. In addition to blocking unoccupied sites on a plate, it also stabilizes immobilized proteins, improving the reproducibility of results. Another agent is skimmed milk powder containing casein. It is a cheap and widely available blocker, particularly useful in tests where BSA interacts with the other molecules used in the next ELISA steps. In experiments where skimmed milk may not be effective enough or where blocking conditions need to be precisely controlled, pure casein is used. For blocking also gelatin is used, particularly in cases where other blockers may not be suitable due to their interaction with test components, but it requires higher temperatures for dissolution, which may limit its use [3, 8]. Detergents (such as Tween-20 and Triton X-100) might also be components of blocking solutions in combination with proteins or polymers to further reduce nonspecific interactions and eliminate background. Tween-20 (polysorbate 20) is a nonionic detergent that helps to minimize nonspecific binding by reducing surface forces and background in ELISA readings. Triton X-100 is another nonionic detergent similar to Tween-20, although it is less commonly used in blocking and more frequently in washing processes [3, 8, 10].

In the case of His-tag and biotin-binding plates, plate blocking is not required due to the specific interaction between protein and the surface of the plate.

1.3 Incubation with Inhibitors

Potential inhibitors are dissolved as standard in PBS or other buffer in which the plate-coated protein is stable. If there is a problem with the solubility of compounds, they are dissolved in DMSO, and a concentration of up to 5% DMSO is used for the test. It is also necessary to choose the appropriate time for incubating the compounds; usually, it is 1.5–2 h. Moreover, the potential inhibitor should not be used at only one concentration, but in serial dilutions (at least 3 concentrations) to check whether the observed effect is nonspecific and whether a dose-dependent response will be observed [1, 3].

1.4 Incubation with Protein

It is important that the protein contains a suitable tag that will be recognized by the antibody used in the next ELISA step (detection). Commonly used tags include His tag, Fc-tag, and biotin. The standard buffers in which the protein is dissolved are Tris and PBS. The proteins are incubated for 1–2 h as standard [1, 3].

1.5 Protein Detection

In ELISA, detection of the protein is based on the use of antibody-conjugated enzymes that first recognize the specific tag conjugated with the protein and, secondly, catalyze chemical reactions, leading to a signal such as color change, luminescence, or fluorescence. The detection modalities in ELISA can be divided into several main categories. The choice of the appropriate detection method depends on a number of factors, such as the sensitivity requirements of the assay, the available measuring equipment, the type of sample to be tested, as well as the cost and convenience of performing the assay. Depending on the type of detection, it is also necessary to select the appropriate color of the plate on which the protein is immobilized. For ELISA, transparent (colorimetric detection), black (fluorescence and less commonly luminescence detection), and white plates (luminescence detection) are used. In practice, colorimetric detection is most commonly used due to its simplicity, availability, and low cost, while fluorescent and luminescent detection is chosen when higher sensitivity is required. The most important detection methods are described below.

- Colorimetric detection—involving the generation of a colored product by an enzymatic reaction. The change in color is proportional to the amount of the target protein bound to the molecule immobilized on the plate. The typical enzyme used in this method is horseradish peroxidase (HRP), used with substrates such as 3,3′,5,5′-tetramethylbenzidine (TMB). In this enzymatic reaction, TMB is turned from a colorless substrate to a blue product, which turns yellow upon the addition of sulfuric acid. The second commonly used enzyme is an alkaline phosphatase (AP) converting substrate such as p-nitrophenyl phosphate (pNPP) from colorless to yellow product.

- Fluorescence detection—this method uses enzymes and fluorophores to produce a fluorescence signal. It is a more sensitive method than colorimetric detection, allowing the detection of lower concentrations of protein. A typical enzyme used in this method is AP and 4-methylumbelliferyl phosphate (4-MUP) substrate. After conversion by AP, MUP generates 4-methylumbelliferone, which emits fluorescence at around 450 nm when excited at 360 nm. Fluorescence is measured using a plate reader with fluorescence detection at a specific excitation and emission wavelength.

- Luminescence detection—is characterized by high sensitivity and specificity. Signal detection is based on the emission of light, which is generated during the reaction of substrate with an enzyme conjugated with antibody. The use of luminescence allows highly sensitive detection, which is particularly important for assays requiring the detection of low concentrations of analytes. A typical enzyme used in this detection method is HRP with substrates such as luminol and hydrogen peroxide. In this reaction, intense light is produced, which is read by a plate reader with luminescence detection [8, 11–13].

2   Materials

Equipment: Immunograde plates (Brand, Wertheim, Germany), multichannel pipette, plate thermo-shaker, vacuum aspirator bottle, microplate reader (such as Infinite M200 Pro Tecan Life Sciences, Männedorf, Switzerland).

Reagents: In ELISA, always use freshly prepared buffers and individual test components. This allows for correct, reproducible results and further reduces nonspecific interactions.

1. Coating buffer—PBS: 5 mM Na_2HPO_4, 150 mM NaCl (*see* **Note 1**).

2. HVEM-His protein (ACROBiosystems, USA)—prepare 5 µg/mL in PBS (*see* **Note 2**).

3. Washing buffer—PBS-T: 5 mM Na_2HPO_4, 150 mM NaCl, with the addition of 0.3 M NaCl and 0.05% Tween-20, pH 7.4 (*see* **Note 3**).

4. Blocking buffer—PBS-T with 5% BSA (v/w) (*see* **Note 4**).

5. Peptide inhibitor—prepare each peptide in PBS in stock at the highest concentration to be used in the assay (*see* **Note 5**).

6. Positive control—anti-HVEM antibody (Abnova, Taiwan)—prepare 1 µg/mL in PBS.

7. BTLA-Fc protein (Novoprotein, USA)—prepare 5 µg/mL in PBS.

8. HRP-conjugated goat antihuman IgG (Bio-Rad, Hercules, CA, USA)—concentrations 1:3000 in PBS-T.

9. TMB—ready to use.

3   Methods

It is very important to perform control tests before starting the final experiment. To begin with, it is necessary to check cross-reactivity between all components used in the experiment, for example, that the antibody used for detection does not interact with the immobilized protein, inhibitor, or blocking agent that the inhibitor or second protein does not bind to the blocking agent, resulting in a false result. Moreover, duplicate wells should be used to improve assay reproducibility.

Protocol (Fig. 3):

1. Coat 96-well immunograde plate with HVEM-His protein dissolved in PBS at a concentration of 5 µg/mL, 100 µL/well, and incubate overnight at 4 °C (*see* **Notes 6** and **7**).

2. Wash each well 5 times with 200 µL of PBS-T (0.05% Tween-20 in PBS buffer supplemented with 0.3 M NaCl, pH 7.4) (*see* **Note 8**).

3. Apply 200 µL per well of 5% BSA in PBS-T and incubate for 2 h at 37 °C using continuous shaking (*see* **Note 9**).

4. Wash wells 5 times with 200 µL of PBS-T.

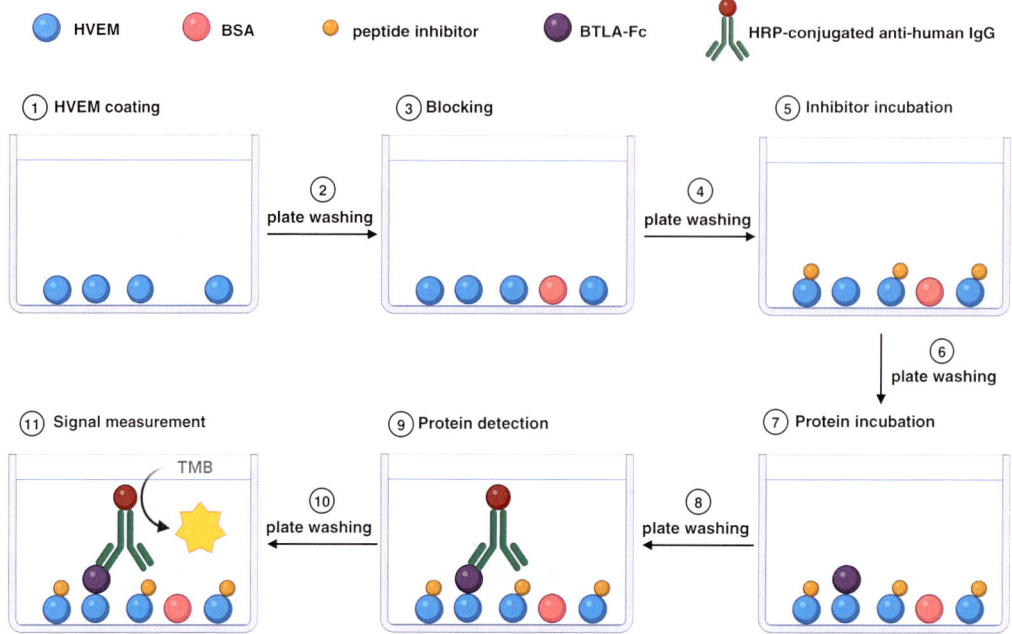

Fig. 3 ELISA step by step

5. Add antihuman HVEM antibody as a positive control (*see* **Note 10**), peptide inhibitors at 3 concentrations (1.5 mg/mL, 750 µg/mL, 375 µg/mL) (*see* **Note 11**), and PBS as a negative control (*see* **Note 12**), 100 µL of each solution per well and incubate the plate for 2 h at 37 °C using continuous shaking.

6. Wash wells 5 times with 200 µL PBS-T.

7. Add 100 µL each of BTLA-Fc protein at 5 µg/mL to the wells and incubate for 2 h at 37 °C with continuous shaking.

8. Wash wells 5 times with 200 µL PBS-T.

9. Add 100 µL of HRP-conjugated goat antihuman IgG at 1:3000 (v:v) to each well and incubate for 1 h at 37 °C using continuous shaking.

10. Wash wells 5 times with 200 µL PBS-T.

11. Apply 100 µL of commercial TMB substrate to each well; after 15 min of light-free incubation, measure absorbance at 650 nm using a plate reader [6].

The result of the experiment is measured at wavelengths 650 nm with a plate reader and is presented as an absorbance measurement reflecting the intensity of the enzymatic reaction. In the case described, when the substrate TMB is added to the samples, a colored (blue) product is produced by reaction with the enzyme HRP-conjugated antibodies. The intensity of the color is proportional to the amount of antibody bound to the BTLA

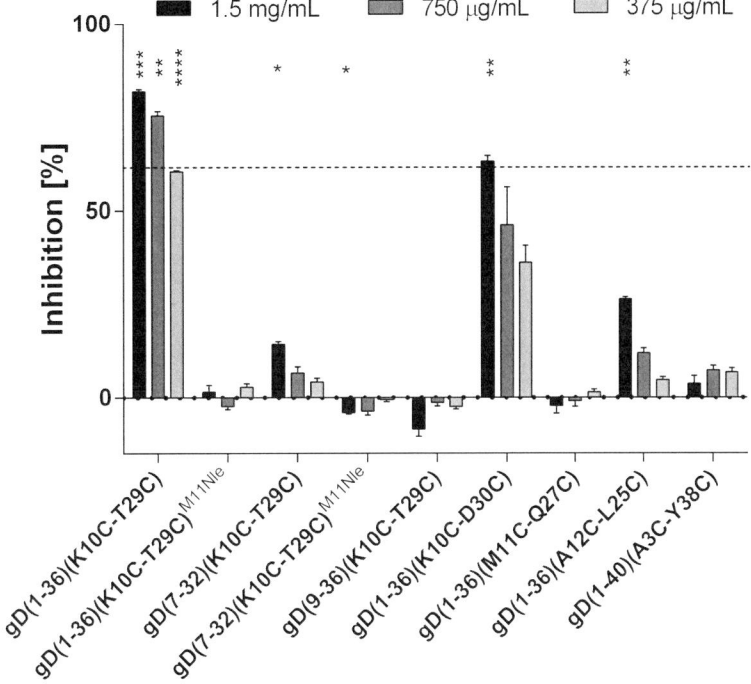

Fig. 4 The inhibitory properties of the peptides—fragments of gD protein toward BTLA/HVEM complex formation determined by ELISA [6]

protein interacting with HVEM. A higher absorbance value indicates a greater amount of BTLA protein bound to the HVEM protein, indicating that the inhibitor did not block the formation of the HVEM/BTLA complex. In contrast, a lower absorbance value indicates a lack of interaction between BTLA and HVEM, showing that the inhibitor blocks the binding of these proteins. In Fig. 4, the results are presented as a percentage of inhibition and were calculated assuming that PBS-T (negative control) does not inhibit BTLA/HVEM complex formation. The corresponding background was subtracted from the absorbance value in each well (*see* **Note 6**) [6].

4 Notes

1. When the protein is immobilized on the hydrophobic plate, it is essential to pay attention to its isoelectric point (pI)—an immobilization buffer with a pH close to the protein's pI can reduce its surface charge, which promotes stronger binding to the plate surface.

2. When planning an ELISA, it is important to consider which tags the proteins should possess. In the case of the immunograde plate, there is no need for the protein with a His-tag;

there can be the protein without any tag. The second protein should not have the same tag, because it may lead to false results, as the second protein could not only bind to the first protein but also to the plate surface.

3. 0.3 M NaCl is often added to the wash buffer to enhance the effective removal of nonspecifically bound proteins and other components that can lead to false positive results.

4. Before the final experiments, a series of tests should be performed to check which blocking agent will be most effective. The suitable concentration of it should also be selected.

5. The inhibitor is usually prepared in PBS, but can also be prepared in water or washing buffer. Difficult-to-solubilize compounds can be dissolved with up to a maximum of 5% DMSO. The concentration of the inhibitor is always adjusted experimentally and will be different for each test. It is important to test a wide enough range of concentrations in order to select those that are appropriate. The final test result should indicate a correlation between % of inhibition and inhibitor concentration.

6. Prepare the same number of wells containing only coating buffer (without HVEM). These wells should be used to monitor the ELISA background. Perform all other steps of the test in the same way as for the wells in which the HVEM protein is present.

7. Before applying the protein to the plate, ensure that it is well dissolved and does not form aggregates. If not removed, these aggregates will bind to surfaces in a manner different from single protein molecules and adversely affect precision. Typical biomolecule concentrations destined for immobilization to a plastic surface are in the μg/mL range. The best incubation conditions for the initial surface coating step is 4 °C overnight (16 h).

8. In ELISA, washing is a very important step in which unbound molecules must be thoroughly washed away after each step. This has a very important impact on the results obtained and determines their correctness. Typically, a volume of 200–300 μL of washing buffer per well is used (it must be at least twice the volume of the reagents used during the experiment), which is sufficient to cover the entire well surface and effectively remove unbound molecules.

9. For blocking, use a volume of blocking solution larger than that used for protein immobilization, with a minimum of 200 μL/well. During the development of a blocking procedure, the blockers should be evaluated for cross-reactivity with all other assay reactants.

10. This control only indicates if the test is working properly. This value is not taken into account by us in the calculation of the inhibitory properties of the compounds.

11. Serial dilutions of peptides are best performed directly on the plate. This allows serial dilutions to be carried out easily in each well, resulting in a consistent concentration gradient. To prepare twofold dilutions of peptides, add 200 μL of a 1.5 mg/mL peptide solution in the first well, then transfer 100 μL to the next well and add 100 μL of PBS. The same procedure should be followed for the remaining wells. Remove 100 μL from the well with the lowest concentration of peptide. Each further dilution in the same plate reduces the risk of errors due to sample transfer between different tubes, which affects the accuracy of concentrations.

12. A negative control in which there is only buffer used to dissolve the inhibitor. This control shows that the HVEM protein interacts with the BTLA protein.

5 Additional Remarks

Various problems can be experienced when performing ELISA that can affect the accuracy, precision, and reliability of the results. We outline the most common problems and potential causes and solutions:

5.1 Low Reproducibility of the Results

– Variations in test technique, such as irregular pipetting, inhomogeneous washes, or variable incubation times. It is very important to use pipettes that are regularly calibrated and to strictly follow the established protocol including careful control of incubation times and number of plate washes between each step of the experiment. A very important factor for the reproducibility of the results is also a constant temperature. Always perform the tests at the same temperature, using preferably plate thermo-shakers [1, 3, 14–16].

5.2 High Signal Background

– Insufficient blocking of the plate surface, leading to nonspecific binding of the other compounds added in the next steps of the tests. Try other blocking compounds or a higher concentration of the currently used blocking agent.

– Too high a concentration of antibodies or too long an incubation time, which can cause excessive nonspecific binding. Reduce the concentration of antibodies or shorten the incubation time.

– Insufficient washes, leading to unbound antibodies conjugated with enzymes remaining. Increase the number of washes [1, 3, 8, 15, 16].

5.3 Low or No Signal
- the protein did not coat on the plate. Change the buffer used for coating, the pH of this buffer, the temperature, or increase the protein concentration.
- Too low a concentration of antibodies or proteins that may not be sufficient for detection. Increase the concentration of antibodies or proteins.
- Incubation times are too short, limiting the ability of the experimental components to bind. Optimize incubation conditions, such as increasing incubation time or changing temperature [1, 3, 14, 15].

Acknowledgments

The study is supported by the National Science Centre in Poland, OPUS 22 grant (no. UMO 2021/43/B/NZ7/01022) "New immunomodulators of BTLA-HVEM complex as potential therapeutics in systemic lupus erythematosus." This publication is based upon work from COST Action IMMUNO-model, CA21135, supported by COST (European Cooperation in Science and Technology).

References

1. Crowther JR (2000) The ELISA guidebook. In: Methods in Molecular Biology, p 149
2. Gan SD, Patel KR (2013) Enzyme immunoassay and enzyme-linked immunosorbent assay. J Invest Dermatol 133:1–3
3. Hosseini S, Vázquez-Villegas P, Rito-Palomares M et al (2018) Enzyme-linked immunosorbent assay (ELISA): from A to Z. Springer Singapore, Singapore
4. Kuncewicz K, Battin C, Sieradzan A et al (2020) Fragments of gD protein as inhibitors of BTLA/HVEM complex formation—design, synthesis, and cellular studies. Int J Mol Sci 21: 1–19
5. Kuncewicz K, Bojko M, Battin C et al (2023) BTLA-derived peptides as inhibitors of BTLA/HVEM complex formation—design, synthesis and biological evaluation. Biomed Pharmacother 165:115161
6. Kuncewicz K, Battin C, Węgrzyn K et al (2022) Targeting the HVEM protein using a fragment of glycoprotein D to inhibit formation of the BTLA/HVEM complex. Bioorg Chem 122: 105748
7. Spodzieja M, Kuncewicz K, Sieradzan A et al (2020) Disulfide-linked peptides for blocking BTLA/HVEM binding. Int J Mol Sci 21:636

8. Wild D (2013) The immunoassay handbook: theory and applications of ligand binding, ELISA and related techniques, pp 1–1013
9. Gibbs J, Vessels M, Rothenberg M. Immobilization principles—selecting the surface for ELISA assays. Corning Incorporated, Life Sciences, Application Note
10. Gibbs J (2001) Effective blocking procedures. Application Note. pp 1–6
11. Hayrapetyan H, Tran T, Tellez-Corrales E et al (2023) Enzyme-linked immunosorbent assay: types and applications. Methods Mol Biol 2612:1–17
12. Matson RS (2023) ELISA essentials: surfaces, antibodies, enzymes, and substrates. Methods Mol Biol 2612:19–31
13. Gibbs J, Vessels M, Rothenberg M. Selecting the detection system—colorimetric, fluorescent, luminescent methods for ELISA assays. Application Note
14. RnDSystems (2012) ELISA Development Guide, pp 1–41
15. Daven S (2009) Technical guide for ELISA—protocols—troubleshooting, pp 1–40
16. Thermo Scientific (2010) ELISA technical guide and protocols, vol 65, pp 1–14

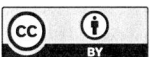

## Chapter 3

The Nucleic Acids' Immunoprecipitation Method for DNA Repair Research

Muhammet Karaman

Abstract

Typically, the goal of molecular research is to obtain a highly pure target for study. The affinity principle may generally be used to achieve biomolecules that have high purity. Significant benefits come from an antibody's affinity for its antigen, including the ability to obtain a very pure target antigen and time savings from a single application. Based on the idea of affinity, immunoprecipitation (IP) is a precipitation technique used to purify biomolecules, including proteins, nucleic acids, lipids, and carbohydrates. Nucleic acids are biomolecules responsible for preserving, transferring, and expressing an organism's genetic information. Therefore, obtaining nucleic acids in high purity is of great importance to scientists. This section covers critical topics such as the basic principles of IP, application types of IP, and the selection of the solid phase and antibodies. In addition, the purification process of repair products resulting from the nucleotide excision repair mechanism of UVC-induced DNA damage is described step by step, serving as an example of nucleic acid purification.

Key words Immunological methods, Immunoprecipitation, Nucleic acid purification, DNA damage, DNA repair

1 Introduction

Organisms have evolved to have immune systems capable of identifying pathogens and destroying them. Bacteria and Archaea generally possess immune systems including restriction-modification (R-M), CRISPR, and prokaryotic Argonaute (pAgo) systems that target pathogen DNA or RNA [1]. There exists an evolutionary connection between prokaryotic and eukaryotic immune systems [2]. When a eukaryotic organism is infected by a pathogen, two successive phases of the immune response are activated. Initially, it is determined whether the entity is part of the organism or a foreign entity. Upon determining that the entity is foreign, the protective immune response is initiated to eliminate the threat. This process not only addresses the immediate infection but also establishes

Sweta Rani and Lukasz Skalniak (eds.), *IMMUNO-model in Cancer: Methods and Protocols*, Methods in Molecular Biology, vol. 2959, https://doi.org/10.1007/978-1-0716-4734-9_3, © The Author(s) 2026

long-term immunity. In eukaryotes, the immune system mediates protective responses through two distinct processes: cell-mediated immunity and antibody-mediated immunity. In the antibody-mediated response, a specific antibody is produced that targets a foreign material associated with the pathogen, known as an antigen and the antibody ensures the elimination of the pathogen [3]. The specific interaction between antibodies and antigens is used to conduct a wide range of biochemical and molecular analyses.

All organisms transmit the information necessary for the survival of subsequent generations through nucleic acids, which are deoxyribonucleic acid (DNA) and ribonucleic acid (RNA). This transferred information enables the organisms to regulate all metabolic activities. All processes, including an organism's growth and development, are considered metabolic activities. Numerous disorders will arise as a result of abnormalities in metabolic activity. For this reason, any processes that may occur in the genome, such as mutations, gene expression changes, and DNA damage, are monitored carefully and with great interest by scientists.

In research with nucleic acids, there is a need to obtain either the nucleic acid in its pure form or its complex form with another biomolecule, like a protein. The immunoprecipitation (IP) method is one of the most effective techniques that can be applied in this situation.

1.1 The Immunoprecipitation (IP)

IP is based on small-scale affinity purification using the specific interaction between antigen and antibody. An antigen, such as proteins, DNA, and RNA, precipitates out of solution using a specific antibody that binds to that particular antigen. This unique interaction permits the target antigen to be isolated and separated from all other macromolecules in pure form. For effective purification and separation, the antibody must be immobilized on a solid surface that does not interfere with biomolecules or the antigen-antibody interaction. IP is a preferred technique across a wide range of research fields, including posttranslational modifications, protein–DNA/RNA binding, intracellular signaling, autophagic responses, cell surface molecules, as well as disease diagnostics. The majority of IP applications are utilized to purify the specific antigen recognized by the antibody, a process referred to as direct immunoprecipitation (DIP). In addition to individual antigen IP, this technique is also employed for purifying desired targets and elucidating molecular interactions, including protein-protein, protein-DNA, and protein-RNA interactions. Depending on the type of target antigen, advanced IP methods such as complex immunoprecipitation (Co-IP), chromatin immunoprecipitation (ChIP), and RNA immunoprecipitation (RIP) can be used. Principles of all IP application types are shown in Fig. 1.

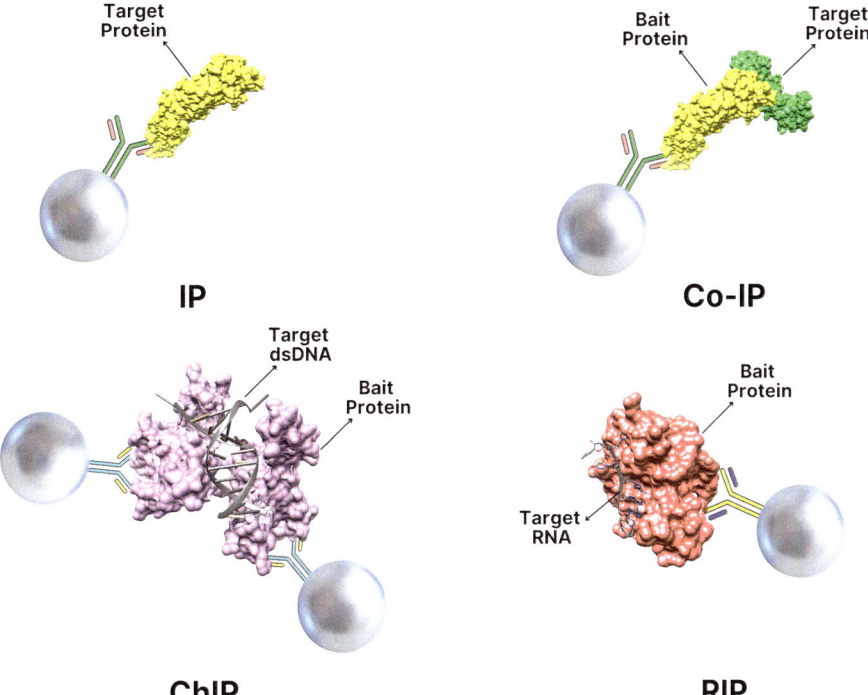

Fig. 1 IP application types. 3D structures of protein, DNA, and RNA are produced using UCFC Chimera [4]. PDB structure (4HXI [5], 6LAE [6], 5DNO [7]) are obtained from RCSB Protein Data Bank [8]

1.2 Application of IP for DNA Damage Detection Research

The purification of a biomolecule using IP, irrespective of the specific biomolecule type to be obtained in pure form, is conducted in five distinct stages. These stages include cell/tissue lysis, preparation of beads conjugated with the antigen-specific antibody, sample application, washing, and elution. In this section, we will discuss each stage in detail. Additionally, we will highlight the critical points that must be considered to ensure the method's effectiveness, ensuring that no important details are overlooked. DIP method will be discussed step by step, using a scenario to illustrate its application in detecting repair product of the nucleotide excision repair mechanism (NER), which is activated by UV radiation or platinum-based chemotherapy drug. This method can also be adapted with minor modifications for the precipitation of different DNA repair products or other biomolecules, such as proteins.

When cells are exposed to UVC/UVB radiation or cisplatin, the resulting CPD, 6–4PP, or Pt-DNA lesions in the genome (Fig. 2) are repaired by NER within a specific time frame, thereby maintaining genomic stability. For analysis processes such as the repair time of damage, repair efficiency, and particularly the mechanism by which the damage is repaired, the repair products must be obtained in a pure form. The complete methodology for obtaining pure repair products is comprehensively detailed in a step-by-step manner.

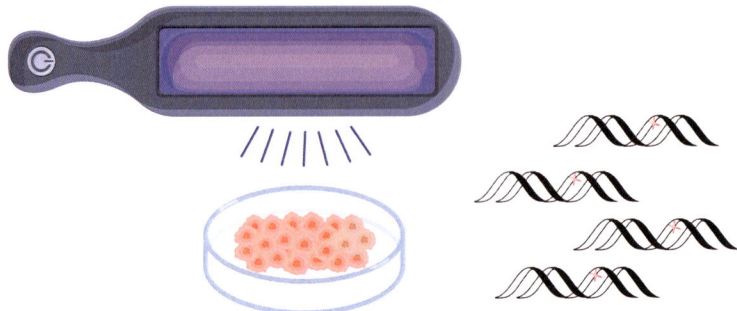

Fig. 2 UV-induced damage on DNA

A sufficient quantity of repair product can be obtained from 500,000 to 1,000,000 HeLa cells. DNA damage is induced by irradiating cells with UVA/UVB radiation at appropriate doses and for an adequate duration. In order to produce UV lesions on DNA, an average UV fluence of 10–25 j/m^2 is used using a lamp generating light at 254 nm. Immediately after irradiation, DNA repair commences, and repair products begin to form. However, a sufficient quantity of repair products is typically obtained after an incubation period of 60 min [9].

2   Materials

Mouse anti-CPD (Kamiya Biomedical, # MC-062), mouse anti-(6-4)PP (Cosmo Bio, #CAC-NM-DND-002), rabbit anti-mouse IgG (Invitrogen, #31450), Dynabeads M-280 sheep anti-rabbit IgG (Invitrogen, #11203D) ethanol, ethylenediaminetetraacetic acid (EDTA), glycogen (20 μg/mL, molecular biology grade), lithium chloride (LiCl), Nonidet P-40 (NP-40, Thermo Scientific, #85124), phosphate-buffered solution (PBS), phenol:chloroform: isoamyl alcohol (25:24:1), proteinase K (20 mg/mL), RNase A/T1 (2 mg/mL of RNase A and 5000 U/mL of RNase T1), sodium acetate (CH_3COONa), sodium bicarbonate ($NaHCO_3$), sodium dodecyl sulfate (SDS), sodium deoxycholate, Tris base, sodium chloride (NaCl), and Triton X-100. UVC lamp (254 nm), refrigerated centrifuge, ice maker, cortex, magnetic rack, tube rotator, heating block.

2.1   Receipt of Solutions

Lysis buffer: 10 mm Tris-Cl (pH:8.0), 1 mm EDTA should be sterilized by filtration or autoclaving.

Salt solution: 5 M NaCl should be sterilized by filtration or autoclaving.

SDS solution: 10% SDS solution should be sterilized by filtration.

Sodium acetate buffer: 3 M CH₃COONa (pH:5.2) should be sterilized by filtration or autoclaving.

TE buffer: 10 mm Tris-Cl (pH:8.0), 1 mm EDTA should be sterilized by filtration or autoclaving.

Reaction buffer: 20 mM Tris-HCl, 2 mM EDTA, 1% Triton X-100, 150 mM NaCl, 0.5% sodium deoxycholate should be sterilized by filtering.

Wash Buffer I: 20 mM Tris-Cl (pH: 8.0), 2 mM EDTA, **150 mM NaCl**, 1% Triton X-100, and 0.1% SDS should be sterilized by filtration.

Wash Buffer II: 20 mM Tris-Cl (pH: 8.0), 2 mM EDTA, **500 mM NaCl**, 1% Triton X-100, and 0.1% SDS should be sterilized by filtration.

Wash Buffer III: 10 mM Tris-Cl (pH 8.0), 1 mM EDTA, **150 mM LiCl**, 1% Nonidet P-40, and 1% sodium deoxycholate should be sterilized by filtration.

Wash Buffer IV: 100 mM Tris-Cl (pH: 8.0), 1 mM EDTA, **500 mM LiCl**, 1% Nonidet P-40, and 1% sodium deoxycholate should be sterilized by filtration.

Elution buffer: 50 mM NaHCO₃, 1% SDS, 20 μg/mL glycogen.

3   Methods

3.1   Stage 1: Cell/ Tissue Lysis and DNA Extraction

Prior to separation from genomic DNA, RNA, and other biomolecules, repair products must be extracted from the cell nucleus and the cell itself. In order to isolate the repair products, the standard cell lysis and low-molecular-weight DNA extraction method [9] is employed.

1. After post-UV incubation, pour cold phosphate-buffered solution (PBS) on the cells and detach the cells from the petri dish surface using a cell scraper.

   Prior to the cell scraping process, the petri dish should be placed on ice to halt the DNA repair process.

2. Transfer the scraped cells to clean Eppendorf tubes kept on ice.

3. Centrifuge the tubes at 2800 × *g* for 5 min at +4 °C and pour supernatant.

4. Add cell lysis buffer at 4 × volume of precipitated cell pellet, and the tubes are incubated on ice for 15 min.

5. During this period, vortex the tubes to ensure thorough access of the lysis buffer to the cells, thereby enhancing the efficiency of the lysis process.

   Cell pellets can be stored at −80 °C until genomic DNA extraction is performed.

6. Following the lysis process, centrifuge the tubes including the lysed cells at 22,000 × *g* for 30 min at +4 °C.

7. Carefully transfer the supernatant to clean Eppendorf tubes kept on ice.

8. Add 1:500 (v:v) RNase A/T1on the cell lysate and mix it with pipette.

9. Incubate the tubes for 10 min at room temperature.

10. Add the 10% SDS stock solution to the mixture to achieve a final concentration of 1%.

11. Incubate the tubes for 15 min at room temperature.

12. Add 5 M salt solution to achieve a final concentration of 1 M and invert the tube 5–10 times.

13. Incubate the tubes at 4 °C for 8 h.

14. Centrifuge the tube at 22,000 × *g* and 4 °C for 1 h, resulting in the precipitation of genomic DNA.

    In this step, genomic DNA is removed from cell lysate.

15. Transfer the supernatant to clean Eppendorf tubes and add proteinase K to the mixture at a 1:100 (v:v) ratio.

16. Incubate the tubes at 55 °C for 30 min.

    In this step, protein denaturation and hydrolysis are carried out, providing the release of DNA from its histone packaging and the denaturation and protection of DNase from hydrolysis. Proteinase K (20 mg/mL).

17. Add an equal volume of phenol:chloroform:isoamyl alcohol (25:24:1) to the mixture and briefly vortex.

18. Centrifuge the mixture at 22,000 × *g* for 2 min.

19. Transfer the upper aqueous phase to clean Eppendorf tubes kept on ice.

    Subsequent to denaturation and hydrolysis of proteins, nucleic acids are decontaminated from proteins and cell debris using phenol-chloroform-isoamyl alcohol extraction. This procedure should be repeated two to three times to ensure minimal protein contamination in the aqueous phase.

20. For each 1 μL sample of the aqueous phase containing DNA, add 0.4 μL of glycogen, 1:10 (v/v) sodium acetate buffer, and 3:1 (v/v) ice-cold 95% ethanol to each tube.

21. Incubate the mixture at −20 °C for a minimum of 30 min.

    In this step, glycogen helps to precipitate DNA and also provide visible pellet. Very low amounts of DNA precipitation require more visibility. Consequently, glycogen conjugated with a covalently bound dye is recommended as an alternative to standard glycogen in order to enhance the visibility of precipitated DNA. Concentrated sodium acetate buffer supplies abundant sodium and acetate ions. The acetate ions interact with water, enhancing DNA solubility, while the Na+ions interact with the phosphate groups in DNA. Ammonium acetate, sodium chloride, lithium chloride, and potassium acetate can be preferred as alternative salts. The addition of alcohol to the aqueous phase neutralizes water and enhances the interaction between Na+ions and DNA, thereby increasing the precipitation efficiency.

22. At the end of the incubation, centrifuge the mixture at 22,000 × *g* at 4 °C for 15 min, and carefully remove the supernatant to obtain the DNA pellet.

23. Add 1 mL of 70% ethanol solution to the DNA pellet and centrifuge the mixture at 22,000 × *g* at 4 °C for 5 min.

    At this stage, the sodium acetate salt used for precipitation is removed. Given the low solubility of sodium acetate in absolute ethanol, an ethanol-water mixture is prepared to effectively remove the salt from the pellet.

24. Carefully remove the supernatant to obtain the DNA pellet.

25. Air-dry the resulting pellet and suspend in an appropriate volume of TE buffer or nuclease-free water.

    DNA solution can be stored at −20°C until performing the next step.

3.2 Stage 2: Preparation of Beads Conjugated with Specific Antibody

In this step, antibody-conjugated beads are prepared to isolate repair products from the DNA solution, effectively separating them from other DNA and oligonucleotides, thereby ensuring their purification. This stage is the most critical in the IP process, as it requires the selection of an appropriate and effective solid phase (*see* **Note 1**) and the correct antibody (*see* **Note 2**), which must be compatible with both the solid phase and the target antigen for purification. You can determine the most appropriate solid phase for your research by referring to the information in the "Critical Details for IP Application" section. In this instance, magnetic beads, which facilitate effective and straightforward purification, were chosen as the solid phase.

1. Mix 10 μL of sheep anti-rabbit IgG-conjugated Dynabeads in an Eppendorf tube.

   The primary antibodies for 6,4 photo product ([6-4] PP) and cyclobutene pyrimidine dimer (CPD), which are repair products of UV-induced DNA damage, are produced in mice. Therefore, a magnetic sphere containing anti-rabbit IgG that specifically binds to the rabbit anti-mouse IgG.

2. In order to remove the original buffers from the beads, place the tubes in a magnetic rack, allowing the magnetic beads to collect on the side walls of the tube.

3. Carefully remove the liquid with an automatic pipette.

4. Remove the tubes from the magnet, add 50 μL of wash buffer I, and mix it by pipetting.

5. Place the tubes back on the magnet and remove Wash Buffer I.

6. Repeat **steps** 4 and **5** two more times, and the washing process with Wash Buffer I is done three times in total.

7. Remove the tubes from the magnet, add 200 μL of reaction buffer on washed mixture, and mix it by pipetting.

8. Place the tubes back on the magnet and remove the reaction buffer.

9. At the end of the wash, the beads are suspended with a reaction buffer in twice their initial volume (**Step 1**).

10. Add 1 μL of rabbit anti-mouse IgG (secondary antibody) and 1 μL of the primary antibody (mouse anti-CPD or mouse anti-[6-4] PP) to the bead suspension.

11. Mix the tubes on a rotator at 4 °C for 2 h.

    During this time, rabbit anti-mouse IgG binds to the magnetic beads and forms a beads IgG-IgG complex. The primary antibody then binds to this beads IgG-IgG complex through its specific interaction with the anti-mouse IgG.

12. Following incubation, place the tubes in a magnetic rack, allowing the magnetic beads to collect on the side walls of the tube.

13. Carefully remove the liquid with an automatic pipette.

    In this step, magnetic beads capable of binding repair products are prepared.

The preparation process of beads is illustrated in Fig. 3.

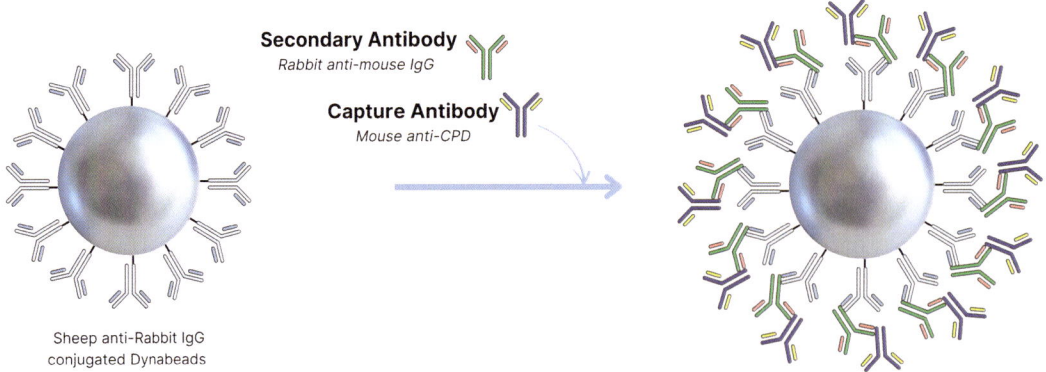

Fig. 3 Preparation of beads conjugated with capture antibody

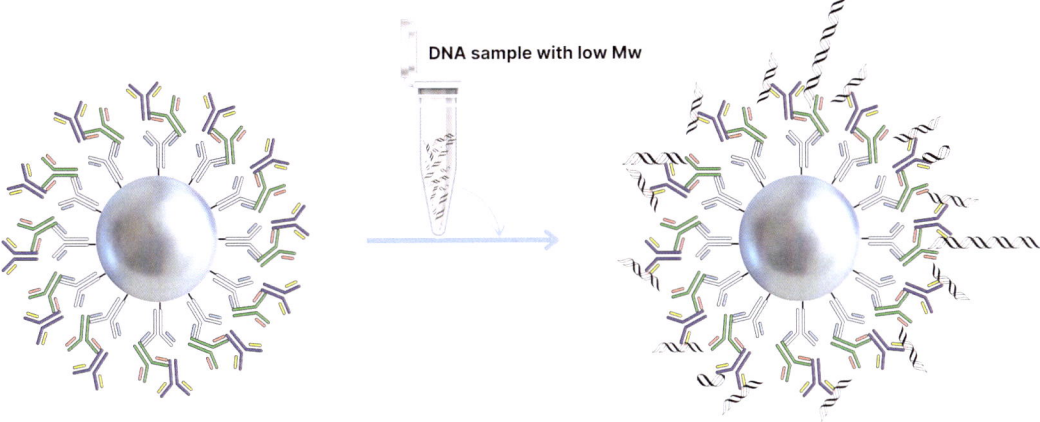

Fig. 4 Application of DNA sample with low Mw onto beads-capture antibody conjugate

3.3 Stage 3: Sample Application

1. Resuspend the prepared beads in 90 μL of reaction buffer, add 10 μL of the DNA solution to the prepared beads.

2. Incubate the DNA-beads mixture overnight at 4 °C while being continuously mixed on a tube rotator.

   In this step, the repair products bind to the magnetic beads due to the affinity between the primary antibody and the DNA solution containing the repair products.

3. Following incubation, place the tubes in a magnetic rack, allowing the magnetic beads to collect on the side walls of the tube.

4. Carefully remove the liquid with an automatic pipette.

   The sample application process is illustrated in Fig. 4.

3.4 Stage 4: Washing of Nonspecific Bound DNA or Oligonucleotides

1. Resuspend the beads that interacted with DNA with 200 μL each of Wash Buffer I.

2. Incubate the tubes on a rotator for 2 min.

3. Centrifuge the mixture at $22,000 \times g$ for 2 min.

4. Place the tubes in a magnetic rack, allowing the magnetic beads to collect on the side walls of the tube.

5. Carefully remove the liquid with an automatic pipette.

6. Resuspend the beads that interacted with DNA with 200 μL each of Wash Buffer II.

7. Incubate the tubes on a rotator for 2 min.

8. Centrifuge the mixture at $22,000 \times g$ for 2 min.

9. Place the tubes in a magnetic rack, allowing the magnetic beads to collect on the side walls of the tube.

10. Carefully remove the liquid with an automatic pipette.

11. Resuspend the beads that intraced with DNA with 200 μL each of Wash Buffer III.

12. Incubate the tubes on a rotator for 2 min.

13. Centrifuge the mixture at $22,000 \times g$ for 2 min.

14. Place the tubes in a magnetic rack, allowing the magnetic beads to collect on the side walls of the tube.

15. Carefully remove the liquid with an automatic pipette.

16. Resuspend the beads that intraced with DNA with 200 μL each of Wash Buffer IV.

17. Incubate the tubes on a rotator for 2 min.

18. Centrifuge the mixture at $22,000 \times g$ for 2 min.

19. Place the tubes in a magnetic rack, allowing the magnetic beads to collect on the side walls of the tube.

20. Carefully remove the liquid with an automatic pipette.

21. Resuspend the beads that intraced with DNA with 200 μL each of Wash Buffer IV.

22. Incubate the tubes on a rotator for 2 min.

23. Centrifuge the mixture at $22,000 \times g$ for 2 min.

24. Place the tubes in a magnetic rack, allowing the magnetic beads to collect on the side walls of the tube.

25. Carefully remove the liquid with an automatic pipette.

    All wash buffers remove other DNA or oligonucleotides that interact with the beads complex due to nonspecific interactions without damaging the interaction between the repair products and the primary antibody. This step is crucial. If appropriate wash buffers are not used in sufficient quantities, other DNA or oligonucleotides interacting with the bead complex through nonspecific interactions will remain with the repair products, albeit in small amounts. This contamination will prevent the repair products from being obtained in pure form in the subsequent step.

The washing process is illustrated in Fig. 5.

3.5 Stage 5: Elution of Repair Product and DNA Precipitation

1. Resuspend beads bound to repair products with 100 μL of elution buffer.

2. Incubate tubes at 65 °C for 15 min.

3. During this period, vortex the tubes to ensure that the specific interaction between antibody and antigen is disrupted.

   The elution process performed in this step is known as denaturing elution. The buffer solution and temperature applied to the repair products in complex with the beads disrupt both the binding between the repair products and the capture

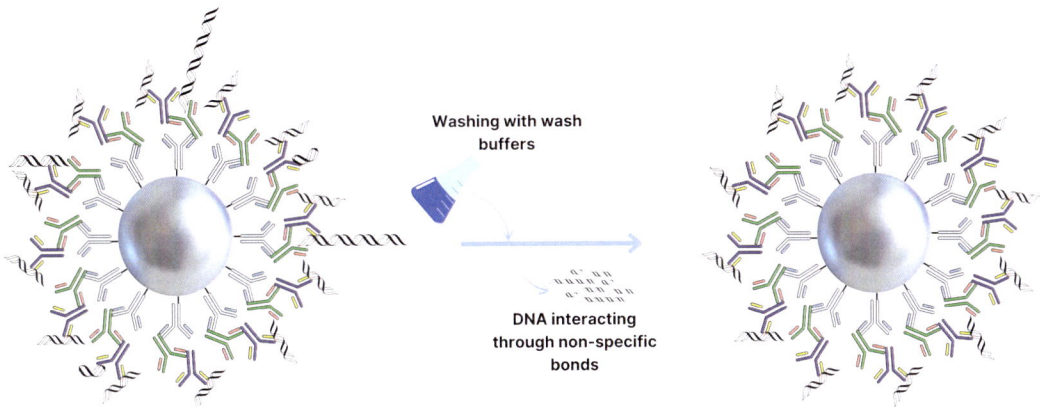

Fig. 5 Washing of DNA interacting through nonspecific bonds

antibody, as well as the binding between the secondary anti-body and the beads and capture antibody. Consequently, in the subsequent step, a DNA isolation method is applied again to separate the repair products from the antibodies in the eluates, achieving the final purity of the repair products.

4. Place the tubes in a magnetic rack, allowing the magnetic beads to collect on the side walls of the tube.

5. Carefully transfer the solution which contain repair products to clean Eppendorf tubes kept on ice.

6. Complete the elution process by repeating all **steps** from **1** to **6** twice. The elution process of repair products is illustrated in Fig. 6.

7. In order to enrich the repair products in an elution solution, perform again the standard DNA precipitation method for genomic DNA extraction without any modifications. For this purpose, the DNA precipitation process is repeated exactly as from **step** 5 of the Stage 1.

Only the solution containing oligonucleotides with [6-4] photoproduct (PP) or cyclobutene pyrimidine dimer (CPD) damage, which are DNA repair products, can be directly analyzed. For instance, an ELISA assay can be applied to solutions containing repair products [10] obtained from various treatments to assess the effects of UV irradiation or to determine the impact of any treatment that modulates NER activity in cells post-UV irradiation. Additionally, repair products can be labeled with tags such as biotin [11] or ^{32}P [9] and visualized on a sequencing gel to assess in vitro/ex vivo NER activity.

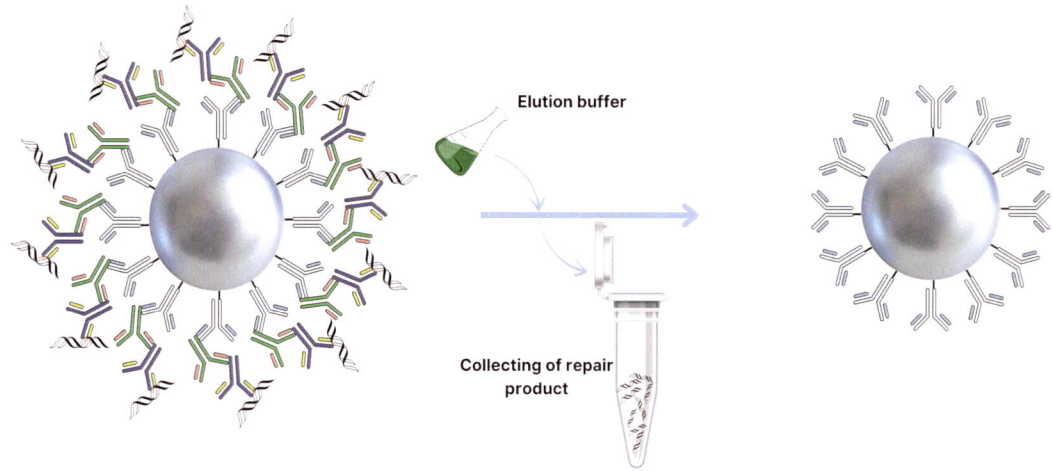

Fig. 6 Elution of repair product

4   Notes

Note 1. Solid-phase selection and functionalization.

IP is a purification technique that employs antibodies bound to a solid phase, which may exhibit varying specificities. Solid phases, referred to as beads, are produced from polysaccharide materials such as agarose and sepharose that are resistant to nonspecific interactions with biomolecules and can be reused after repeated cleaning. Polysaccharides are materials that facilitate the formation of porous spheres with a large surface area. This provides a significant advantage as it facilitates the purification of large quantities of the target antigen. The high surface area of polysaccharide-based beads, while beneficial for binding capacity, can also pose a disadvantage by promoting nonspecific binding. If the secondary or primary antibody specific to the target antigen does not fully occupy the bead surface, biomolecules in the lysate may bind nonspecifically, resulting in the target antigen being obtained with insufficient purity. This issue can be addressed in two different ways. The first approach is to fully occupy the bead surface by using high amounts of primary and secondary antibodies. The second approach involves subjecting the lysate to a preclearing process to prevent nonspecific binding. However, these methods increase the cost of the procedure and compromise its ease of application.

On the other hand, solid phases are also produced from polystyrene materials with magnetic properties. Polystyrene material, unlike polysaccharide material, possesses a smaller surface area due to its nonporous nature. Despite this limited surface area, a higher number of polystyrene magnetic beads can be accommodated within a given volume. This is attributed to their significantly smaller size (1–4 μm), which is 10–40 times smaller than that of polysaccharide beads. Consequently, the separation capacity of polystyrene magnetic beads is comparable to that of polysaccharide beads. Furthermore, the magnetic properties of the beads significantly reduce the experimental time and enhance the applicability of the experimental process. Instead of the material composition of the beads, the type of ligand used for binding to the beads significantly contributes to the effectiveness of the immunoprecipitation (IP) technique.

Beads that are not functionalized with structures such as proteins, antibodies, or compounds can bind biomolecules nonspecifically through weak interactions, thereby limiting their utility for purification purposes. The specific binding properties of beads are achieved through the immobilization of various structures such as ligand, protein, capture (primary) antibody, or secondary antibody. The antibody intended to capture the antigen is immobilized on the solid phase either directly or via the structures. Three different proteins are preferred for those in protein form among these structures. The most commonly used proteins are Protein A and Protein G, both of which are cell surface proteins derived from *Staphylococcus* sp. [12]. These proteins possess the capacity to bind various types of different type of immunoglobulins. Although they can bind different types of immunoglobulins, their affinities vary. Specifically, they exhibit no affinity for human immunoglobulin M (IgM) and immunoglobulin D (IgD) [13]. Protein L obtained from *Peptostreptococcus* sp. is utilized for the binding of IgM and IgD [14]. The protein binds to the kappa light chain of the antibody unlike Protein A and Protein G [15]. This protein also lacks binding affinity for antibodies from goat, sheep, or cow sources. This characteristic provides an advantage in cell culture studies, as it minimizes unwanted binding to antibodies present in serum supplemented in the medium. Understanding the organism and IgG specificity of the proteins immobilized on the beads is crucial for selecting the appropriate secondary antibody and/or capture antibody for subsequent binding. The literature provides extensive information on the organism and IgG specificities of these proteins. A critical step involves reviewing some articles [16–18] to identify antibodies that are suitable both for the target antigen and for the protein immobilized on the beads. The other protein immobilized on the beads is streptavidin from *Streptomyces* sp. However, instead of utilizing streptavidin's affinity for immunoglobulins, its high affinity for biotin is exploited in IP [19]. The capture antibody specific to the biomolecule must be conjugated with biotin for binding via streptavidin. The strong and specific interaction between biotin and streptavidin ensures robust binding of the capture antibody to the beads, thereby facilitating efficient elution of the antigen in subsequent steps. Another method for tightly binding the capture antibody to the beads is covalent

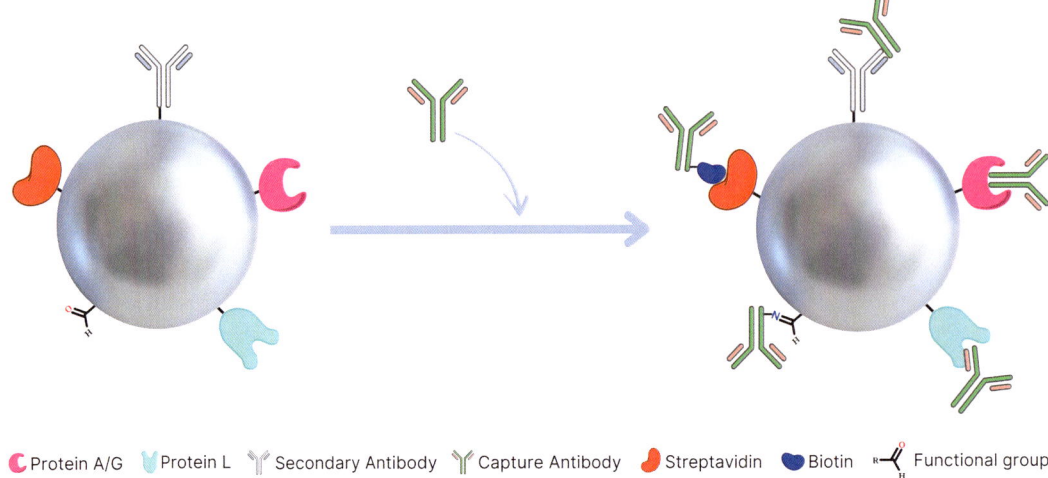

Protein A/G   Protein L   Secondary Antibody   Capture Antibody   Streptavidin   Biotin   Functional group

Fig. 7 Immobilization of some structures on beads

immobilization, where the capture antibody is directly bound to the beads via a covalent bond. The bioconjugation is achieved through a chemical bonding process between the functional groups on the beads and the functional groups on heavy chain of the capture antibody [20–22]. The covalent immobilization method is not typically preferred for the solid phase, as it requires separate preparation for each capture antibody. However, in cases where there is incompatibility with secondary or capture antibodies suitable for Protein A/G and Protein L, this solid phase is used as an alternative. In addition to the capture antibody, a secondary antibody specific to the capture antibody can also be covalently immobilized on the beads. The immobilized secondary antibody in the solid phase allows the host to specifically bind to the capture antibody. Therefore, if the capture antibody is a rabbit antibody, the secondary antibody must have anti-rabbit specificity. Solid-phase functionalization type is illustrated in Fig. 7.

Note 2. Antibody selection.

Antibody selection is another critical consideration in IP. The primary antibody, known as the capture antibody, must be specific to the target antigen. Antibody selection should be guided not only by the antigen but also by the characteristics of the solid phase. The higher the specificity of the primary antibody to the antigen, the greater the purity of the target. Additionally, this high specificity minimizes nonspecific binding with other biomolecules, thereby preventing background formation in subsequent analyses. Antibodies can be produced in many different species including rabbit, goat, mouse, rat, chicken, and donkey. Any of these host species can be used in IP. However, it is important to note that both rabbits and mice produce primary antibodies specific to a wide range of antigens.

The first and most important criterion in selecting the primary antibody is that it should be produced in a different species from the one in which the target antigen is obtained. This ensures that if the primary antibody is to be bound to the beads via a secondary antibody, the secondary antibody conjugated to the beads will not bind to the immunoglobulins in the sample containing the antigen. We can clarify this with the following example. Mouse samples are frequently used in biochemical studies, second only to human samples. If you are analyzing a biomolecule from a mouse immunologically, the primary antibody should be produced in a species other than a mouse. For instance, an antibody specific to a mouse biomolecule but produced in a rabbit would be an appropriate choice. At this point, it is useful to clarify the concepts of target species and host species for antibodies. As demonstrated in the example above, the host species is the organism in which the secondary antibody is produced. If the target antigen-specific primary antibody is a mouse antibody, then a secondary antibody that is immune to the primary antibody can be produced in a rabbit as the host. In this case, the antibody is referred to as a rabbit anti-mouse secondary antibody. However, this is not necessary for IP without the use of secondary antibodies; in such cases, the target antigen and antibody can be of the same species. Unlike secondary antibodies, the organism in which the primary antibody is produced does not influence its specificity for the antigen. For example, a primary antibody produced in a mouse can recognize the same antigen in other model organisms, such as humans and rats, as well as in mice. The specific antigen reactivity of the antibody is typically indicated in the commercial product catalog or on the company's website. If the antibody is to be used in a species other than the one specified by the company, it is essential to confirm that the antibody is reactive to that species. The most practical way to do this is by determining the similarity in protein sequence between the target proteins (antigens) in the species where the antibody is known to be reactive and the target protein (antigen) in the desired species. The Basic Local Alignment Search Tool (BLAST) is used to assess the homology between the target protein in the species in which the antibody is reactive and the target protein in the desired species. When the sequence homology between the proteins of these two species is 75% or higher, it suggests that the primary antibody may be reactive against target protein in the desired species. However, this reactivity must be experimentally confirmed.

Either monoclonal or polyclonal antibodies can be used at IP application. However, unlike western blotting, IP requires the antigen to be in its native (non-denatured) conformation. Therefore, irrespective of the clonality, the primary antibody should be validated for IP compatibility. If efficient purification is the goal, polyclonal antibodies are preferred over monoclonal antibodies, as polyclonal antibodies recognize multiple epitopes on the antigen, thereby exhibiting greater antigen-binding capacity. Denaturation and mild elution are two distinct elution methods that can be used to acquire the pure form of an antigen coupled to the solid phase.

Note 3. Elution type of target antigen.

Denaturing and mild elution are two distinct elution methods that can be used to obtain the pure form of an antigen coupled to the solid phase. The choice between the two elution methods depends on the desired form of the target antigen post-immunoprecipitation. If the objective is to retain the target antigen in its native form, a mild elution process is preferred. Consequently, mild elution is generally the favored method for elution. Mild elution can be achieved by initially using a solution with either a high salt concentration (2 M NaCl) or a high pH (pH 6), followed by stepwise elution to progressively decrease the salt concentration or the pH value of the solutions. The denaturing elution method can be employed when preserving the native form of the target antigen is unnecessary. In these cases, the antigen-antibody interaction is disrupted by subjecting the complex to circumstances like high concentrations of salt, low pH, or higher temperatures, which affect the three-dimensional conformation of both the antigen and the antibody.

Acknowledgments

I wish to express my profound gratitude to Prof. Aziz Sancar for providing me the opportunity to investigate the NER mechanism in plants in his laboratory at the University of North Carolina at Chapel Hill. I also extend my sincere thanks to Dr. Michael G. Kemp, Dr. Christopher P. Selby, Dr. Laura A. Lindsey-Boltz, Dr. Jinchuan Hu, and the entire research team for generously sharing their expertise and experience with me regarding the IP method during this research. This publication is based upon work from COST Action IMMUNO-model, CA21135, supported by COST (European Cooperation in Science and Technology).

References

1. Gao L, Altae-Tran H, Bohning F et al (2020) Diverse enzymatic activities mediate antiviral immunity in prokaryotes. Science 369:1077–1084

2. Cohen D, Melamed S, Millman A et al (2019) Cyclic GMP-AMP signalling protects bacteria against viral infection. Nature 574:691–695

3. Yu H-W, Halonen MJ, Pepper IL (2015) Immunological methods. In: Pepper IL, Gerba CP, Gentry TJ (eds) Environmental microbiology, 3rd edn. Elsevier, London

4. Pettersen EF, Goddard TD, Huang CC et al (2004) UCSF Chimera—a visualization system for exploratory research and analysis. J Comput Chem 25:1605–1612

5. Ji AX, Prive GG (2013) Crystal structure of KLHL3 in complex with Cullin3. PLoS One 8:e60445

6. Lian FM, Yang X, Jiang YL et al (2020) New structural insights into the recognition of undamaged splayed-arm DNA with a single pair of non-complementary nucleotides by human nucleotide excision repair protein XPA. Int J Biol Macromol 148:466–474

7. Wang C, Zhu Y, Bao H et al (2016) A novel RNA-binding mode of the YTH domain reveals the mechanism for recognition of determinant of selective removal by Mmi1. Nucleic Acids Res 44:969–982

8. RCSB Protein data bank (2025) Available from: https://www.rcsb.org/.

9. Hu J, Choi JH, Gaddameedhi S et al (2013) Nucleotide excision repair in human cells: fate of the excised oligonucleotide carrying DNA damage in vivo. J Biol Chem 288:20918–20926

10. Fang C, Chen W, Li C et al (2016) Methyl-CpG binding domain protein acts to regulate the repair of cyclobutane pyrimidine dimers on rice DNA. Sci Rep 6:34569

11. Choi JH, Gaddameedhi S, Kim SY et al (2014) Highly specific and sensitive method for measuring nucleotide excision repair kinetics of ultraviolet photoproducts in human cells. Nucleic Acids Res 42:e29

12. Bilitewski U (2006) Protein-sensing assay formats and devices. Anal Chim Acta 568:232–247

13. Guss B, Eliasson M, Olsson A et al (1986) Structure of the IgG-binding regions of streptococcal protein G. EMBO J 5:1567–1575

14. Björck L (1988) Protein L. a novel bacterial cell wall protein with affinity for Ig L chains. J Immunol 140:1194–1197

15. Kastern W, Sjöbring U, Björck L (1992) Structure of peptostreptococcal protein L and identification of a repeated immunoglobulin light chain-binding domain. J Biol Chem 267:12820–12825

16. Murphy C, Devine T, O'Kennedy R (2016) Technology advancements in antibody purification. Antibody Technol J 2016:17–32

17. Sviatenko OV, Gorbatiuk OB, Vasylchenko OA (2014) Application of immunoglobulin-binding proteins a, G, L in the affinity chromatography. Biotechnol Acta 7:34–45

18. Reese H, Bordelon T, Odeh F et al (2020) Purification of animal immunoglobulin G (IgG) using peptoid affinity ligands. Biotechnol Prog 36:e2994

19. Taylor CR, Shi S-R, Barr NJ (2011) Techniques of immunohistochemistry: principles, pitfalls, and standardization. In: Dabbs DJ (ed) Diagnostic immunohistochemistry, 3rd edn. Elsevier, Amsterdam

20. Foubert A, Beloglazova NV, Rajkovic A et al (2016) Bioconjugation of quantum dots: review & impact on future application. TrAC Trends Anal Chem 83:31–48

21. Hermanson GT (2013) Introduction to bioconjugation, bioconjugate techniques, 3rd edn. Academic Press, New York

22. Hermanson GT (2013) Immobilization of ligands on chromatography supports, bioconjugate techniques, 3rd edn. Academic Press, New York

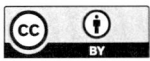

Chapter 4

Analysis of the Functional Impact of Glycosylation on Immune Checkpoint Proteins

Maite Emaldi, Esther Rey-Iborra, Paula Alamillo-Maeso, Rafael Pulido, and Caroline E. Nunes-Xavier

Abstract

B7 immune checkpoint proteins play an important role in modulating antitumor immune response. These proteins interact with co-inhibitory or co-stimulatory receptors on immune and tumor cells, and their expression associates with cancer progression and poor prognosis. B7 proteins are highly glycosylated, as part of their posttranslational modification process. This process consists of the covalent addition of glycans to proteins, which directly affects protein expression, stability, localization, and interaction with partners. Protein glycosylation of immune checkpoint proteins has also been linked to therapy response and immune evasion. Here, we describe experimental methodologies to study the molecular and clinical impact of glycosylation on the B7 family of glycoproteins. We summarize experimental protocols and technical notes to assess the N-glycosylation of B7 proteins, and to study the functional effect of glycosylation on the expression and localization of B7 proteins.

Key words N-glycosylation, Glycanase, Deglycosylation, Protein expression and stability, Protein localization, B7 immune checkpoint proteins

1 Introduction

Cancer occurs due to the accumulation of a variable number of genetic alterations. During cancer progression, tumor cells acquire pro-oncogenic properties that enable them to evade the immune elimination. Different factors in the tumor microenvironment can modulate the antitumor immune activity. Proteins belonging to the B7 immune checkpoint family are modulators of the immune response, including antitumor immunity [1, 2].

The B7 family includes B7-1 (*CD80*), B7-2 (*CD86*), PD-L1/B7-H1 (*CD274*), PD-L2/B7-DC (*PDCD1LG2*), B7-H2 (*ICOSLG*), B7-H3 (*CD276*), B7-H4 (*VTCN1*), B7-H5/VISTA (*VSIR*), B7-H6 (*NCR3LG1*), and B7-H7 (*HHLA2*) [2, 3] (Fig. 1). All members are type I transmembrane proteins containing immunoglobulin (Ig)-like domains in their extracellular region.

Sweta Rani and Lukasz Skalniak (eds.), *IMMUNO-model in Cancer: Methods and Protocols*, Methods in Molecular Biology, vol. 2959, https://doi.org/10.1007/978-1-0716-4734-9_4, © The Author(s) 2026

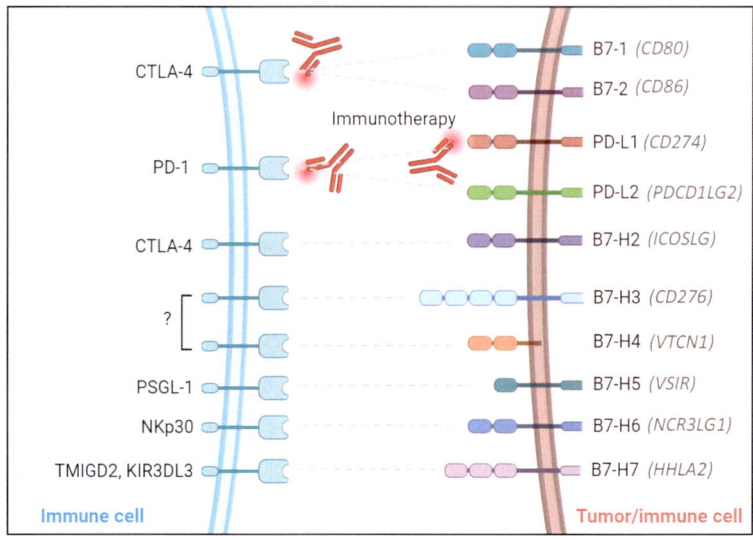

Fig. 1 Diagram illustrating immune checkpoint interactions between immune cells and tumor/immune cells. On the left, immune cell receptors such as CTLA-4, PD-1, PSGL-1, NKp30, and TMIGD2/KIR3DL3 are shown. On the right, corresponding ligands on tumor/immune cells include B7-1 (CD80), B7-2 (CD86), PD-L1 (CD274), PD-L2 (PDCD1LG2), and others. Immunotherapy antibodies are depicted targeting CTLA-4 and PD-1 pathways. Unknown receptors are indicated with a question mark. The diagram highlights the role of these interactions in immune response modulation. (Created with BioRender.com)

However, B7-H4 is predicted to have only two amino acids in the cytosolic portion, and it has been proposed to be anchored to the membrane by glycophosphatidylinositol linkage [4, 5]. B7 immune checkpoint proteins play an important role in immune regulation, as they can act as co-inhibitory regulators, by creating negative signals and suppressing T/NK-cell activity, or as co-stimulatory regulators, providing positive signals to support T/NK-cell activation, depending on the receptor they bind to [2, 6]. B7 proteins are expressed both on tumor and immune cells [7–15]. Besides their immunoregulatory role, some B7 proteins also induce pro-oncogenic traits such as cancer cell proliferation, resistance to drugs and metastasis [16]. High expression of B7 proteins has been associated with poor prognosis in several cancers, making these proteins suitable targets for immunotherapy [17]. Blockage of the binding between B7 proteins and their receptors by monoclonal antibodies is used in cancer immunotherapy, with a positive effect on the survival of cancer patients [18]. However, the complex interactions among the immune checkpoint molecules of the B7 family are still not fully understood.

Like most transmembrane proteins, B7 proteins undergo glycosylation as part of their posttranslational modification process. Protein glycosylation consists of sequential attachment of glycans by around 200 glycosyltransferase enzymes that determine the position and structure of the glycans on the immature proteins, leading to the most abundant posttranslational modification in eukaryotic cells. This process is carried out as proteins go through the endoplasmic reticulum and Golgi apparatus during and after translation [19, 20]. Depending on the amino acid residue that glycans attach to, two types of protein glycosylation are described. N-glycosylation occurs by glycan attachment to Asn (N) residues at the consensus motif N-X-S(Ser)/T(Thr) (where X is any amino acid). O-glycosylation occurs when the glycan is attached to the hydroxyl group side chain of Ser (S) or Thr (T) residues. In mammals, the primary glycans are composed of 10 monosaccharide building blocks: D-glucose (Glc), D-galactose (Gal), N-acetyl-D-glucosamine (GlcNAc), D-mannose (Man), L-fucose (Fuc), N-acetylneuraminic sialic acid (Neu5Ac), D-glucuronic acid (GlcA), L-iduronic acid (IdoA), and D-xylose (Xyl) [20, 21].

Once on the cell surface, glycans modulate developmental biological processes by regulating protein folding, cell adhesion, inflammation, metabolism, and protein-protein and cell-cell interactions [22]. Glycosylation plays a pivotal role in protein quality control and it is essential for the functionality of mature membrane proteins. Thus, glycosylation malfunction has been related to different genetic diseases, including cancer [23]. When compared to healthy tissue cells, tumor cells display a broad range of glycosylation alterations. Aberrant protein glycosylation increases molecular and functional heterogeneity among cell populations, as these modifications are protein-, site-, and cell-specific [24]. Two major mechanisms for the generation of tumor-associated carbohydrate have been proposed, incomplete synthesis and neosynthesis. The incomplete synthesis usually occurs in the early stages of the tumor, and disrupts the process of the sequential glycan attachment, leading to the appearance of truncated forms of glycans. On the other hand, neosynthesis takes place in the advanced stages of cancer and involves an increase in the expression of genes associated with carbohydrate synthesis, leading to the de novo formation of antigens [25]. The most common cancer-associated changes in glycosylation are N- and O-glycosylation branching, fucosylation, and sialyation [26, 27].

Immune cells play a protective role against carcinogenesis by attacking the transformed cancer cells. Tumor-specific glycans have been described to interact with the immune effector cells and modulate the tumor microenvironment, gaining resistance against the tumor suppression response [27]. All B7 proteins are highly glycosylated proteins, and they present multiple potential N-glycosylation Asn residues, as summarized in Table 1. N-glycosylation of B7 proteins in several of the predicted residues has been experimentally verified [28–32]. In this regard, PD-L1, an important B7 family immunosuppressor, is a highly N-glycosylated protein, and

Table 1
Potential N-glycosylation sites in the extracellular region of the B7 proteins

Protein Gene	NCBI entry	Amino acid/potential glycosylation							
B7-1 CD80	NP_005182.1	N53 ++	N89 +	N98 ++	N186 +	N207 +	N211 −	N226 +	N232 ++
B7-2 CD86	NP_787058.5	N33 +	N47 +	N135 +	N146 +	N154 ++	N177 +	N192 +	N213 +
PD-L1/B7-H1 CD274	NP_054862.1	N35 ++	N192 +++	N200 +	N219 −				
PD-L2/B7-DC PDCD1LG2	NP_079515.2	N37 +++	N64 ++	N157 +	N163 −	N189 +			
B7-H2 ICOSLG	NP_056074.1	N70 ++	N102 −	N137 ++	N173 −	N186 +	N225 +		
B7-H3 CD276	NP_001019907.1	N91 +	N104 ++	N189 +++	N215 ++	N309 +	N322 +	N407 ++	N433 +
B7-H4 VTCN1	NP_078902.2	N112 +	N160 +	N190 −	N196 −	N205 +	N216 ++	N220 −	
B7-H5/VISTA VSIR	NP_071436.1	N49 +++	N91 ++	N108 +	N128 ++	N135 +	N190 +		
B7-H6 NCR3LG1	NP_001189368.1	N43 +++	N57 +++	N174 +	N208 ++	N216 ++	N242 +++	N260 ++	
B7-H7 HHLA2	NP_009003.1	N90 ++	N103 ++	N200 +	N205 −	N284 +	N296 −	N308 +	N318 ++

Amino acids are indicated with the one-letter code. Numbering is according to the indicated NCBI entries. Potential glycosylation is indicated according to Net-N-Glyc web server https://services.healthtech.dtu.dk/services/NetNGlyc-1.0/. Note that experimental verification is necessary to identify the N-glycosylated Asn residues

its glycosylation at various Asn residues has been shown to be important for antagonizing its proteasomal degradation [33]. PD-L2 N-glycosylation has also been described to promote immune evasion in tumors [34]. Antibodies targeting PD-L1 are currently used as an immunotherapy treatment for a variety of cancers, but it has been demonstrated that heavy PD-L1 N-glycosylation hinders recognition by anti-PD-L1 antibodies, leading to reduced therapeutic efficacy [35]. Moreover, N-glycosylation of B7-H3 protein has been described to correlate with tumor development and progression in a variety of cancers, and B7-H4 glycosylation has been proposed as a potential therapeutic intervention in PD-L1 negative tumors [32]. It has also been described that N-glycosylation of B7-H5 has an impact on protein expression levels and localization, suggesting a potential effect on its immunosuppressive role [36].

N-glycosylation is known to alter protein conformation and structure, modulating the protein functional activity and protein-protein interaction. Deciphering the biological impact of glycan-based intra- and intermolecular interactions will contribute to unraveling the complex functional interactions of the B7 immune checkpoint proteins, their pro-oncogenic roles in cancer, and their precise recognition by monoclonal antibodies for precision immunotherapy.

In this chapter, we describe experimental methodologies to study the molecular and clinical impact of N-glycosylation on B7 family glycoproteins.

2 Materials

All plasticware used for laboratory protocols is previously auto-claved. Cell culture and transfection procedures are performed under sterile conditions, and all solutions are prepared in deionized, double-distilled MilliQ filtered water.

2.1 Assessing the Enzymatic Removal of N-Linked Oligosaccharides by PNGase F

1. Tissue culture plates.

2. HEK293 human embryonic kidney cells for transient ectopic expression of proteins of interest (*see* **Note 1**).

3. *DMEM* medium (Dulbecco's Modified Eagle Medium) supplemented with 5% heat-inactivated FBS (Fetal Bovine Serum), 1% L-glutamine, and 1% penicillin/streptomycin.

4. Trypsin-EDTA (0.05%) solution.

5. cDNAs of protein of interest, cloned into a suitable mammalian expression vector (*see* **Note 2**).

6. Transfection reagent (*see* **Note 3**).

7. Lysis buffer: *M-PER* (Mammalian Protein Extraction Reagent, Thermo Scientific) supplemented with *PhosSTOP* phosphatase inhibitor cocktail tablets (Roche) and *cOmplete* EDTA-free protease inhibitor cocktail tablets (Roche).

8. PNGase F glycan cleavage kit (*see* **Note 4**).

9. Loading buffer (4×): *NuPAGE™* sample buffer (Life Technologies) with 5% 2-mercaptoethanol.

10. Prestained molecular weight marker (Sigma-Aldrich).

11. Polyvinylidene fluoride (PVDF) protein transfer membrane: *Immobilon-FL Transfer Membrane* (Merck Millipore), suitable with the detection system used (*see* **Note 5**).

12. Immunoblot transfer buffer: 48 mM Tris base, 39 mM glycine, 0.037% SDS, 20% methanol.

13. Immunoblot blocking buffer: 1:1 *Odyssey Blocking Buffer* (OBB, LI-COR®) diluted in phosphate buffer saline (PBS).

14. Primary antibodies recognizing the proteins of interest or recognizing a suitable artificial tag, and primary antibodies against an endogenous protein for reference (*see* **Note 6**).

15. Fluorochrome-conjugated secondary antibodies, suitable with the detection system used (*see* **Note 5**).

16. Immunoblot washing buffer: 50 mM Tris-HCl, pH 7.5, 150 mM NaCl, 5 mM EDTA, 0.05% Triton X-100, and 0.25% gelatine.

2.2 Site-Directed Mutagenesis and Study of the Effect of N-Glycosylation on B7 Protein Expression

1. Plasmid template containing the cDNA of interest (*see* **Note 7**).

2. Synthetic mutagenic oligonucleotide primers (*see* **Note 8**).

3. dNTP mix.

4. High-fidelity Pwo DNA polymerase (Roche) (*see* **Note 9**).

5. DpnI restriction enzyme.

6. *E. coli* competent cells (*see* **Note 10**).

7. LB-ampicillin medium and LB-ampicillin plates.

8. Plasmid DNA purification kit: *NucleoSpin® Plasmid EasyPure* (Macherey-Nagel).

9. Agarose gel electrophoresis and DNA visualization reagents.

10. Materials for transient transfection and immunoblot protocol listed above (*see* Subheading 2.1).

11. Software for protein band quantification (*see* **Note 5**).

2.3 Study of the Effect of N-Glycosylation on Protein Localization by Immunofluorescence Staining

1. Materials for transient transfection protocol listed above (*see* Subheading 2.1).

2. Methanol 100%.

3. Blocking solution: PBS with 3% BSA (bovine serum albumin).

4. Primary antibodies recognizing the proteins of interest or recognizing a suitable artificial tag (*see* **Note 6**).

5. Fluorophore-conjugated secondary antibodies compatible with the microscopy system employed. Here, we used Alexa Fluor 546 (Thermo Scientific)-conjugated antibody for red staining (*see* **Notes 6** and **11**).

6. Mounting fluid containing DAPI (4′6–diamidino-2-phenylindole) (Abcam) (*see* **Note 12**).

7. Microscopy system for fluorescence detection (*see* **Note 11**).

3   Methods

Glycans are essential in fundamental molecular and cellular processes both in physiology and in pathology. The importance of glycans in cancer is highlighted by the fact that changes in glycosylation influence cancer development and progression, making them relevant biomarkers and potential targets for precision therapy, including immunotherapy [24]. Thus, functional characterization of glycans present in B7 immune checkpoint proteins is clinically relevant.

The *first method* explained in this chapter (*see* Subheading 3.1) illustrates the methodology used to enzymatically remove the N-linked oligosaccharides from B7 glycoproteins and to monitor the glycan removal by immunoblot with specific antibodies. We used PNGase F, a commercially available glycanase, to digest highly glycosylated B7 immune checkpoint proteins. PNGase F enzymes are secreted by gram-negative bacteria and are widely used to remove N-linked glycans from proteins [37]. For this purpose, we transiently transfected mammalian cells with cDNAs encoding the B7 proteins of interest, to ectopically express the proteins for subsequent PNGase F digestion. After digesting protein lysates with PNGase F, we assessed the extent of deglycosylation by mobility shifts on SDS-PAGE (Fig. 2).

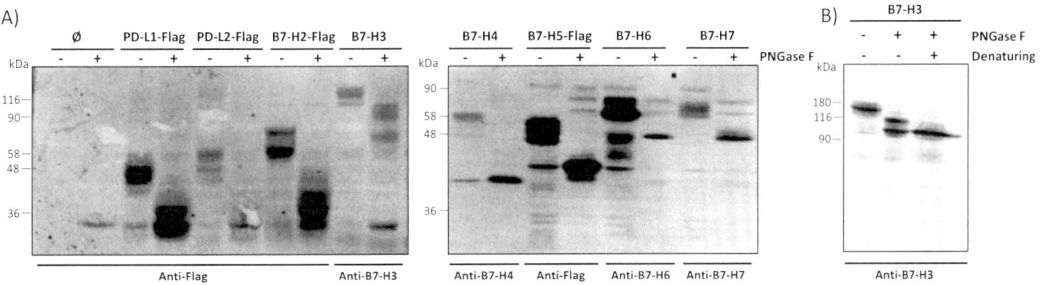

Fig. 2 Protein deglycosylation by PNGase F digestion. Panel A displays representative immunoblots of total HEK293 cell lysates containing PD-L1-Flag, PD-L2-Flag, B7-H2-Flag, B7-H3, B7-H4, B7-H5-Flag, B7-H6, and B7-H7, untreated or treated with PNGase F. Cells were transfected with pcDNA3.1 empty vector or the plasmid containing the indicated B7 proteins. Lysates were processed for PNGase F protocol in the absence (−) or presence (+) of PNGase F enzyme. Proteins containing the Flag-tag were visualized using anti-Flag antibody, and proteins lacking the epitope were visualized by antibodies recognizing the corresponding B7 proteins. Panel B displays a representative immunoblot of total HEK293 cell lysates ectopically expressing B7-H3, processed for PNGase F protocol in the absence (−) or presence (+) of PNGase F enzyme under denaturing (+) or non-denaturing (−) conditions. Proteins were detected by immunoblot using anti-B7-H3 antibody. Molecular weights are marked in kilodaltons (kDa) on the left

3.1 Assessing the Enzymatic Removal of N-Linked Oligosaccharides by PNGase F

1. Plate cells in 6-well culture plates (2×10^5 cells/well) (*see* **Notes 1** and **13**).

2. 24 h after plating the cells, transfect each well with 1 μg of plasmid containing the cDNA of interest (*see* **Notes 2** and **3**). One well should always be transfected in parallel with an empty vector as a negative control.

3. 48 h after transfection, put the plates on ice, wash twice with PBS, and lyse the cells by directly adding 150 μL of cold lysis buffer to each well. Keep the plate on ice for 10 min under rocking and recover lysate from each well in an Eppendorf tube by carefully scratching the wells with a pipette.

4. Centrifuge the lysates at $10,000 \times g$ for 10 min at 4 °C. Transfer the cellular protein extract containing supernatant to a new Eppendorf tube. Cell lysates can be frozen at this step.

5. Digest total cell lysates with PNGase F (*see* **Notes 4**, **14**, **15**, and **16**).

6. Mix 45 μL of cell lysate (including PNGase F and PNGase F buffers) with 10 μL sample buffer (*see* **Note 17**).

7. Boil for 5 min, spin, and load the mix in a 10% SDS-PAGE (*see* **Note 18**).

8. Run the gel (*see* **Note 19**) and transfer to a PVDF membrane. Cut a piece of the membrane in the range of migration of the glycosylated and deglycosylated form of the protein. Be aware that highly glycosylated proteins may get their molecular weight considerably reduced upon deglycosylation.

9. Perform standard immunoblot procedure according to the specifications of the material and antibodies used. We block the membrane for at least 1 h at room temperature and add the primary antibody and incubate at 4 °C overnight. We wash the membrane with washing buffer and incubate with the secondary antibody for 1 h in darkness at room temperature. We wash the membrane again and visualize the fluorescence signal on the membrane (*see* **Notes 5** and **6**).

Examples of PD-L1, PD-L2, B7-H2, B7-H3, B7-H4, B7-H5, B7-H6, and B7-H7 protein migration in a SDS-PAGE gel with and without PNGase F treatment are shown in Fig. 2. Anti-Flag antibody was used to visualize the migration of proteins containing the Flag-tag, whereas antibodies targeting B7 proteins were used to visualize proteins lacking the epitope. Figure 2a illustrates the different migration patterns of B7 family members under the removal of N-glycans. When lysates were treated with PNGase F, the range of bands shifted from a high-molecular-weight range to a lower-molecular-weight range, due to the hydrolysis of N-glycans. In some cases, such as B7-H3, PNGase F digestion rendered partially cleaved proteins (Fig. 2a). Since deglycosylation is more complete for many glycoproteins under denaturing conditions (*see*

Note 15), we tested the same protocol with denaturing reaction conditions. B7-H3 underwent a greater glycan cleavage under denaturing conditions (Fig. 2b). In some cases, native or denaturing conditions do not affect protein deglycosylation extent, but it is convenient to employ denaturing conditions when digesting a glycoprotein with PNGase F for the first time.

The *second method* included in this chapter (*see* Subheading 3.2) consists of methodology to further study the effects of N-glycosylation in protein expression by site-directed mutagenesis and subsequent monitoring by immunoblot. Using this protocol, by a simple one-step inverse PCR-based mutagenesis, we generate multiple amino acid substitutions of residues undergoing N-glycosylation [38]. Examples of this methodology are provided for single and multiple amino acid substitutions on human B7-H5 (Fig. 3). Mammalian cells were transiently transfected with cDNAs encoding B7-H5 N-glycosylation mutants to ectopically express the generated protein variants. The different migration patterns of N-glycosylation variants and their expression and stability, as inferred by their steady-state expression level, are assessed by SDS-PAGE.

3.2 Site-Directed Mutagenesis and Study of the Effect of N-Glycosylation on B7 Protein Expression

1. Identify potential N-glycosylated Asn (N) residues (N-glycosylation consensus sequence: Asn-xxx-Ser/Thr; N-X-S/T) using the Net-N-Glyc web server (https://services.healthtech.dtu.dk/services/NetNGlyc-1.0/). Potential N-glycosylated residues from B7 proteins are shown in Table 1 (*see* **Note 20**).

2. Design mutagenic primers to create B7 variants mutating the N-glycosylation sites. Here, we generated protein variants mutating Asn (N) residues to Ala (A), but Asn (N) to Gln (Q) substitutions are also commonly used. We routinely design two fully complementary forward and reverse 29-mer primers for amino acid substitution, with the mutated codon in the centre (*see* **Note 8**) [38]. See the example of primers designed for B7-H5 N49A mutagenesis in Fig. 3. Note that compound mutations need to be generated by sequential mutagenesis (*see* **Note 21**).

3. Mix the following components for PCR reaction mixture (25 μL final volume): 5 μL template plasmid (5 ng/μL), 14.5 μL H_2O, 2.5 μL buffer Pwo 10×, 0.1 μL Pwo DNA polymerase (5 U/μL), 1.25 μL dNTP mix (4 × 2.5 mM), and 1 μL of each mutagenic primer (10 μM).

4. Run the PCR at the following cycling conditions: 1 min at 95 °C, followed by 18 cycles of 50 s at 95 °C, 50 s at 60 °C, and 5 min at 68 °C, with a final 7 min extension at 68 °C.

5. Digest the PCR product with 0.15 μL of the DpnI restriction enzyme (20 U/μL) at 37 °C overnight (*see* **Notes 22** and **23**).

6. Transform competent *E. coli* bacteria with the DpnI-digested PCR mixture.

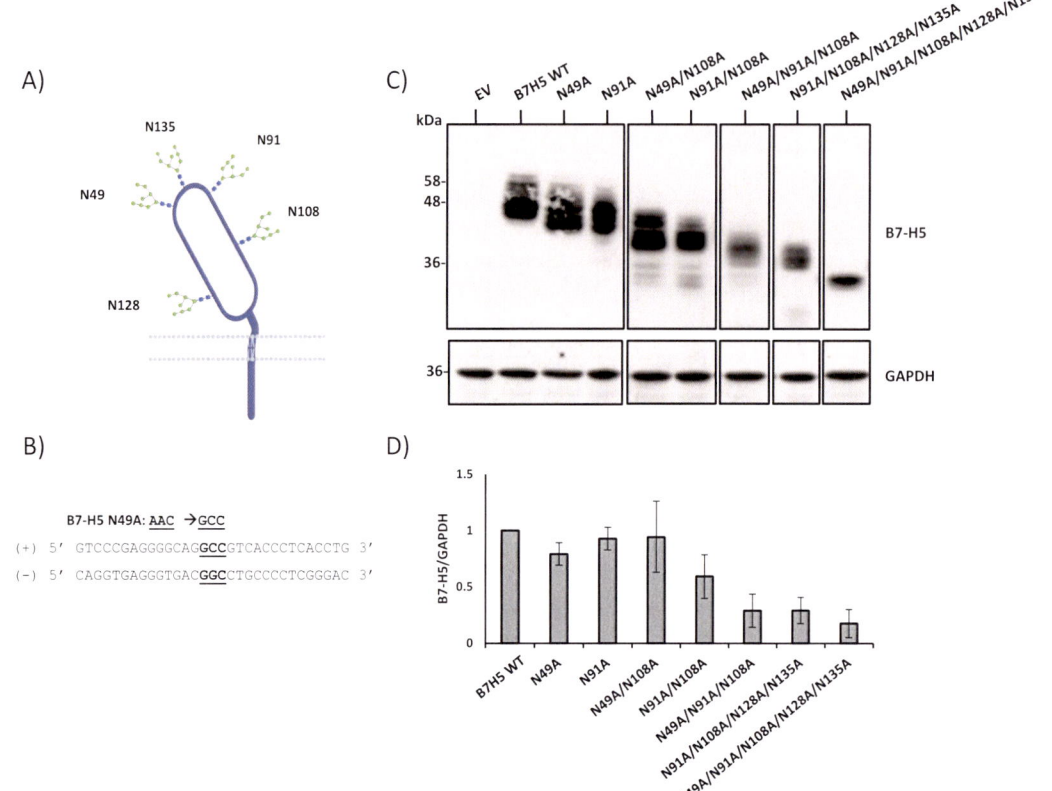

Fig. 3 N-glycosylation analysis of B7-H5. Panel A shows a schematic depiction of B7-H5 transmembrane protein indicating the five N-glycosylated Asn residues: N49, N91, N108, N128, and N135. Panel B shows an example of mutagenic complementary forward and reverse primers for B7-H5 N49A mutation (AAC to GCC). The mutated codon is underlined. Panel C shows representative immunoblots of total HEK293 cell lysates containing B7-H5 wild type (WT) or single and multiple N-glycosylation mutations (N49A, N91A, N108A, N128A, N135A). B7-H5 proteins were detected using anti-B7-H5 antibody, and GAPDH was used as a loading control and detected with anti-GAPDH antibody. Panel D shows quantification of B7-H5 protein expression across different mutations. Graph shows B7-H5 expression normalized to GAPDH band quantification from two independent experiments. Results illustrate a decrease in B7-H5 expression with increasing multiple mutations

7. Pick individual colonies to inoculate 5 mL LB-ampicillin medium and incubate under shaking at 37 °C overnight.

8. Purify plasmid DNA using a miniprep plasmid purification kit and check for the desired mutation by DNA sequencing (*see* **Note 24**).

9. To assess the migration patterns of the N-glycosylation variants obtained, perform transient transfection of mammalian cells and immunoblot analysis, as indicated in Subheading 3.1.

10. Quantify the band intensity of the N-glycosylation protein variants in comparison to the wild-type protein. Steady-state

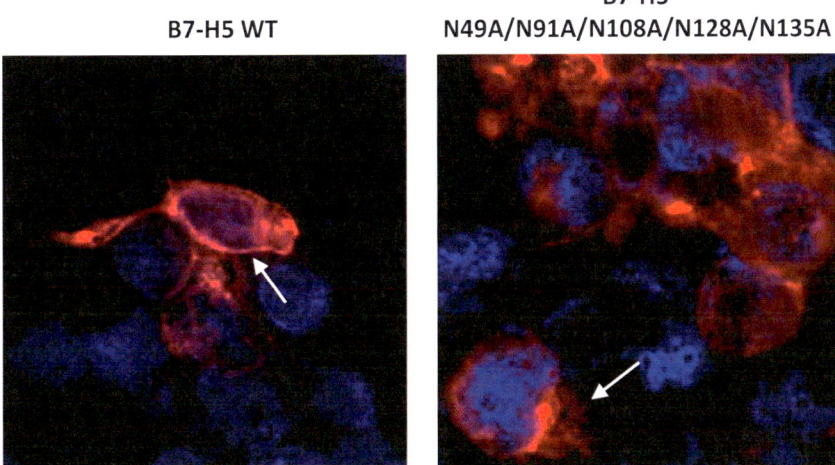

Fig. 4 Protein localization of B7-H5 wild type and B7-H5 N-glycosylation compound mutation. Confocal fluorescence microscopy images show subcellular localization of B7-H5 wild type (WT) (left panel) and N-glycosylation compound mutation (right panel) in HEK293 cells. B7-H5 is stained in red, and nuclei are stained in blue (DAPI). Arrows illustrate the major localization of the B7-H5 protein variants

protein expression can be considered an indirect indicator of protein stability (*see* **Note 25**). Protein expression can be represented in arbitrary units of band intensity normalized to a housekeeping protein expression (*see* **Notes 5** and **26**).

Experimental validation of the identity of the N-glycosylated residues is necessary. An example of validation of N-glycosylated residues in B7-H5 is shown in Fig. 3. A depiction of the glycosylated Asn residues in B7-H5 is shown in Fig. 3a. Figure 3b illustrates an example of the complementary forward and reverse primers designed for B7-H5 N49A mutation (*see* **Notes 8** and **21**). Mobility shifts of B7-H5 individual and compound N-glycosylation mutations, monitored by SDS-PAGE, confirmed glycosylation of Asn potential residues (Fig. 3c). Figure 3d illustrates the quantification of protein expression of the different B7-H5 N-glycosylation variants. Protein variant expression levels gradually decrease in a N/A residue mutation-dependent manner (Fig. 3d), suggesting that lack of N-glycosylation plays a pivotal role in B7-H5 protein expression.

The *third method* that we present in this chapter illustrates immunofluorescence methodology to visualize the role of N-glycans in protein localization (*see* Subheading 3.3). After obtaining the N-glycosylation mutants of B7-H5 (*see* Subheading 3.2), mammalian cells were transiently transfected with the plasmids to ectopically express the protein variants. Protein localization of the wild-type and N-glycosylation variant proteins was visualized by immunofluorescence detection with confocal microscopy (Fig. 4), which allows high resolution and multi-planar images.

3.3 Study of the Effect of N-Glycosylation on Protein Localization by Immunofluorescence Staining

1. Plate cells in 12-well chamber slides for immunofluorescence (1.5×10^4 cells/well) (*see* **Notes 1** and **13**).

2. Transiently transfect the cells following the procedure explained in Subheading 3.1.

3. Wash cells with PBS and fix in 200 μL methanol/well for 5 min at −20 °C.

4. Block cells with 200 μL PBS 3% BSA blocking solution overnight at 4 °C (*see* **Note 27**).

5. Incubate cells with 100 μL of the primary antibody diluted in blocking solution at 37 °C in a wet chamber for 90 min (*see* **Notes 6** and **28**).

6. Rinse 3 times with 200 μL PBS 3% BSA for 10 min and incubate with 100 μL secondary antibody for 1 h at room temperature in a wet chamber.

7. Rinse three times with 200 μL PBS for 5 min in darkness.

8. Mount the coverslip by adding three drops of mounting medium with DAPI and visualize by standard fluorescence microscope or confocal microscopy (*see* **Note 29**), or store slides in darkness at 4 °C until visualization.

Figure 4 illustrates the different localization of the B7-H5 wild-type and B7-H5 variant containing N-glycosylation sites mutated. The wild-type form of the protein was mainly distributed in the cell membrane, whereas the N-glycosylation compound mutant displayed a diffused cytoplasmic localization. These results suggest a direct impact of N-glycosylation on B7-H5 protein localization.

4 Notes

1. HEK293 cells are suitable for relatively high transfection efficiency and high overexpression level of transfected protein, but other mammalian cell lines could be used for this protocol after optimizing transfection conditions.

2. A high expression vector is recommended. For this purpose, we used the pCDNA3.1 or pCDNA6 plasmids, containing the human CMV promoter, and which works efficiently in HEK293 cells.

3. There is a wide variety of transfection reagents for adherent mammalian cells that could be used for this method. Each protocol should be optimized for each specific cell line. For HEK293 cell transfection we used the GenJet™ (SignaGen® Laboratories) transfection reagent.

4. There are several commercially available PNGase F cleavage kits that could be used for this method. Each protocol should be

optimized for each specific protein of interest. For this study, we used the PNGase F Protocol from New England BioLabs. Be aware that PNGase F itself (about 30 kDa) may cross-react with the antibodies used in the immunoblot analysis.

5. We employ the *Odyssey® CLx Imaging System* (LI-COR Biosciences) fluorescent detection system, which allows accurate protein band quantifications using the *Odyssey Image Studio™* v4.0.21 (LI-COR Biosciences) software.

6. Antibody dilution and washing conditions need to be individually tested for each antibody. Consider that the location of the epitope recognized by some antibodies might include glycosylated regions, that may not be properly recognized after cleavage of the glycans. The use of artificial epitope tags, such as Flag-tag, in the protein sequence could be helpful to visualize the deglycosylated protein forms (Fig. 2). Note that for type 1 transmembrane proteins, the tag has to be C-terminal. The addition of the epitope sequence may vary the basal protein expression levels, so this should be checked before performing the PNGase F digestion experiments.

7. Protocols using the DpnI enzyme require a methylated dsDNA template plasmid. Most of *E. coli* (*dam*+) strains used in laboratory produce Dam-methylated DNA plasmids.

8. We design primers with the minimal number of nucleotide changes in the mutated codon, which is positioned in the centre of the primer and flanked by an equal number of nucleotides on both sides (13 + 3 + 13; codon to be changed underlined, Fig. 3b). For templates difficult to amplify, mutagenic primer design may need to be further optimized [38].

9. For mutagenesis, high-fidelity thermostable polymerases are required to avoid undesired mutation incorporations. For this methodology, we use Pwo DNA polymerase, but several other high-fidelity thermostable polymerases are suitable.

10. We routinely employ DH5α *E. coli* competent bacteria generated by the CaCl$_2$ method [39]. Commercial competent bacteria are also suitable for PCR product transformation.

11. We use confocal microscopy [ZEISS LSM880 AIRYSCAN (Zeiss, Jena, Germany)] for high resolution images, but standard fluorescence microscopes could also be used for visualization of protein localization.

12. For nuclei staining, we routinely use a mounting medium containing DAPI, but staining can be performed separately with the dye of choice followed by mounting of the coverslips.

13. Optimal cell confluency may vary depending on the cell line. In our experience, HEK293 cells are optimally transfected when they are at about 50% confluency.

14. To deglycosylate a native glycoprotein, a long incubation time may be required. Conditions should be adjusted for each protein, including the amount of enzyme. Incubation time may vary between 1 and 24 h. For this study we incubated the reactions for 2 h (double the time indicated in the commercially available protocol), to ensure deglycosylation of our proteins of interest.

15. PNGase F reaction conditions can be carried out under denaturing or non-denaturing conditions. In our experience, some B7 glycoproteins undergo a higher extent of deglycosylation after denaturing (Fig. 2b). Denaturing reaction conditions should be considered when digesting a glycoprotein with PNGase F for the first time. When carrying out the digestion under denaturing conditions, it is essential to use NP-40 in the reaction mixture, as PNGase F is inhibited by SDS. Not including NP-40 in the denaturing reaction mixture might result in a loss of enzyme activity.

16. If required, the PNGase F-digested lysates can be stored at −20 °C before loading them in SDS-PAGE gels.

17. Final loading volumes depend on the size of the SDS-PAGE gel wells.

18. We routinely run 10% SDS-PAGE gels, but other percentage gels can be run, depending on the molecular weight of the protein of interest.

19. The range of bands corresponding to the glycosylated form of proteins are more easily observed when gels are run at a higher voltage. For our experimental setting, we use small gels that we run at 130 V for 1.5 h.

20. NetNGlyc web server provides all potential N-glycosylation sites of proteins. In some cases, amino acids predicted as potential glycosylation residues by the server are not finally glycosylated at the post-translational modification process of the protein. Glycosylation of the predicted residues should be verified before performing any functional studies.

21. To generate DNA plasmids containing multiple N-glycosylation site mutations, we perform site-directed mutagenesis using the previously obtained mutated DNA plasmid as the template for the next mutagenesis process. This way, we generate multiple mutants sequentially targeting N-glycosylation sites with mutagenic primers on the previously obtained variants. Simultaneous mutagenesis of several target sites can also be performed, but the efficiency of the mutation is lower [40].

22. The efficiency of the DpnI digestion can be tested with different incubation times, as the methylated parental DNA can be digested within 2–3 h. For this method we performed overnight incubation to ensure complete parental DNA digestion.

23. If desired, PCR product or DpnI-digested PCR product can be stored at 4 °C for some time or at −20 °C for a longer period before proceeding to the next step.

24. We routinely check that the amplified DNA corresponds to the template plasmid by restriction analysis before sequencing for the mutation of interest.

25. Note that analysis of protein expression upon cycloheximide cell treatment is required to determine protein stability of the variants.

26. We routinely use GAPDH as a housekeeping control for protein expression. Any other endogenous protein expressed by the cell line used for this procedure can be employed for this purpose.

27. Cells can be blocked at room temperature for 10 min or overnight at 4 °C.

28. Incubation of the primary antibody can be done at 37 °C for 1–2 h or overnight at 4 °C. Always keep the slide in a wet chamber to prevent from drying. Incubation of multiple primary antibodies can be done at the same time as long as secondary antibodies with no overlapping spectra are used. It is convenient to use antibodies raised in different species.

29. For optimal results, visualize protein localization immediately after performing immunofluorescence staining.

Acknowledgments

The work of C.E.N-X. is funded by Instituto de Salud Carlos III (grant numbers CP20/00008 and PI22/00386, Spain and cofinanced by the European Union), Biobizkaia Health Research Institute (Ayudas para el fortalecimiento de grupos emergentes, Spain), and Stiftelsen til fremme av forskning innen nyresykdommer/ Foundation for promoting research in kidney diseases (Unifor, Norway). M.E. is the recipient of a Fellowship 2023/2024 from Biobizkaia Health Research Institute, and fellowships from the Jesus Gangoiti Barrera Foundation. E.R-I. is the recipient of a predoctoral fellowship from Asociación Española Contra el Cáncer (AECC, grant number PRDVZ222375REY, Junta Provincial de Bizkaia, Spain). We would like to thank Javier Díez García (Microscope Core facility) and personnel at Genetic and Genomic Core facility for their expert assistance with microscopy and DNA sequencing, respectively, at the Biobizkaia Health Research Institute (Spain). This publication is based upon work from COST Action IMMUNO-model, CA21135, supported by COST (European Cooperation in Science and Technology).

References

1. Ni L, Dong C (2017) New B7 family checkpoints in human cancers. Mol Cancer Ther 16:1203–1211. https://doi.org/10.1158/1535-7163.MCT-16-0761

2. Chen DS, Mellman I (2013) Oncology meets immunology: the cancer-immunity cycle. Immunity 39:1–10. https://doi.org/10.1016/j.immuni.2013.07.012

3. Khan M, Arooj S, Wang H (2021) Soluble B7-CD28 family inhibitory immune checkpoint proteins and anti-cancer immunotherapy. Front Immunol 12. https://doi.org/10.3389/fimmu.2021.651634

4. Emaldi M, Nunes-Xavier CE (2022) B7-H4 immune checkpoint protein affects viability and targeted therapy of renal cancer cells. Cells 11:1448. https://doi.org/10.3390/cells11091448

5. Prasad DVR, Richards S, Mai XM, Dong C (2003) B7S1, a novel B7 family member that negatively regulates T cell activation. Immunity 18:863–873. https://doi.org/10.1016/S1074-7613(03)00147-X

6. Bolandi N, Derakhshani A, Hemmat N, Baghbanzadeh A, Asadzadeh Z, Afrashteh Nour M, Brunetti O, Bernardini R, Silvestris N, Baradaran B (2021) The positive and negative Immunoregulatory role of B7 family: promising novel targets in gastric cancer treatment. Int J Mol Sci 22:10719. https://doi.org/10.3390/ijms221910719

7. Ye G, Barrera C, Fan X, Gourley WK, Crowe SE, Ernst PB, Reyes VE (1997) Expression of B7-1 and B7-2 costimulatory molecules by human gastric epithelial cells: potential role in CD4+ T cell activation during helicobacter pylori infection. J Clin Invest 99:1628–1636. https://doi.org/10.1172/JCI119325

8. Ribas A, Hu-Lieskovan S (2016) What does PD-L1 positive or negative mean? J Exp Med 213:2835–2840. https://doi.org/10.1084/jem.20161462

9. Solinas C, Aiello M, Rozali E, Lambertini M, Willard-Gallo K, Migliori E (2020) Programmed cell death-ligand 2: a neglected but important target in the immune response to cancer? Transl Oncol 13:100811. https://doi.org/10.1016/j.tranon.2020.100811

10. Cao Y, Cao T, Zhao W, He F, Lu Y, Zhang G, Hu H, Wang Z (2018) Expression of B7-H2 on CD8+ T cells in colorectal cancer microenvironment and its clinical significance. Int Immunopharmacol 56:128–134. https://doi.org/10.1016/j.intimp.2018.01.018

11. Getu AA, Tigabu A, Zhou M, Lu J, Fodstad Ø, Tan M (2023) New frontiers in immune checkpoint B7-H3 (CD276) research and drug development. Mol Cancer 22:43. https://doi.org/10.1186/s12943-023-01751-9

12. Kryczek I, Zou L, Rodriguez P, Zhu G, Wei S, Mottram P, Brumlik M, Cheng P, Curiel T, Myers L, Lackner A, Alvarez X, Ochoa A, Chen L, Zou W (2006) B7-H4 expression identifies a novel suppressive macrophage population in human ovarian carcinoma. J Exp Med 203:871–881. https://doi.org/10.1084/jem.20050930

13. Wang J, Wu H, Chen Y, Zhu J, Sun L, Li J, Yao Z, Chen Y, Zhang X, Xia S, Chen W, Shi T (2021) B7-H5 blockade enhances CD8+ T-cell-mediated antitumor immunity in colorectal cancer. Cell Death Dis 7:248. https://doi.org/10.1038/s41420-021-00628-4

14. Cherif B, Triki H, Charfi S, Bouzidi L, Ben KW, Khanfir A, Chaabane K, Sellami-Boudawara T, Rebai A (2021) Immune checkpoint molecules B7-H6 and PD-L1 co-pattern the tumor inflammatory microenvironment in human breast cancer. Sci Rep 11:7550. https://doi.org/10.1038/s41598-021-87216-9

15. Fu Y, Ding Y, Liu J, Zheng X, Wei W, Ying Y, Wu C, Jiang J, Ju J (2020) B7-H7 is a prognostic biomarker in epithelial ovarian cancer. Transl Cancer Res 9:5360–5370. https://doi.org/10.21037/tcr-20-697

16. Flem-Karlsen K, Fodstad Ø, Tan M, Nunes-Xavier CE (2018) B7-H3 in cancer—beyond immune regulation. Trends Cancer 4:401–404. https://doi.org/10.1016/j.trecan.2018.03.010

17. Flem-Karlsen K, Fodstad Ø, Nunes-Xavier CE (2020) B7-H3 immune checkpoint protein in human cancer. Curr Med Chem 27:4062–4086. https://doi.org/10.2174/0929867326666190517115515

18. Andrews LP, Yano H, Vignali DAA (2019) Inhibitory receptors and ligands beyond PD-1, PD-L1 and CTLA-4: breakthroughs or backups. Nat Immunol 20:1425–1434. https://doi.org/10.1038/s41590-019-0512-0

19. Schjoldager KT, Narimatsu Y, Joshi HJ, Clausen H (2020) Global view of human protein glycosylation pathways and functions. Nat Rev Mol Cell Biol 21:729–749. https://doi.org/10.1038/s41580-020-00294-x

20. Lin Y, Lubman DM (2024) The role of N-glycosylation in cancer. Acta Pharm Sin B 14:1098–1110. https://doi.org/10.1016/j.apsb.2023.10.014

21. Varki A, Kornfeld S (2022) Historical background and overview. In: Essentials of Glycobiology, 4th edn. Cold Spring Harbor, New York. https://doi.org/10.1101/glycobiology.4e.1

22. Chandler KB, Costello CE (2016) Glycomics and glycoproteomics of membrane proteins and cell-surface receptors: present trends and future opportunities. Electrophoresis 37: 1407–1419. https://doi.org/10.1002/elps.201500552

23. Stowell SR, Ju T, Cummings RD (2015) Protein glycosylation in cancer. Annu Rev Pathol Mech Dis 10:473–510. https://doi.org/10.1146/annurev-pathol-012414-040438

24. Pinho SS, Reis CA (2015) Glycosylation in cancer: mechanisms and clinical implications. Nat Rev Cancer 15:540–555. https://doi.org/10.1038/nrc3982

25. da Costa V, Freire T (2022) Advances in the immunomodulatory properties of glycoantigens in cancer. Cancers (Basel) 14:1854. https://doi.org/10.3390/cancers14081854

26. Munkley J, Elliott DJ (2016) Hallmarks of glycosylation in cancer. Oncotarget 7:35478–35489. https://doi.org/10.18632/oncotarget.8155

27. Perdicchio M, Cornelissen LAM, Streng-Ouwehand I, Engels S, Verstege MI, Boon L, Geerts D, van Kooyk Y, Unger WWJ (2016) Tumor sialylation impedes T cell mediated antitumor responses while promoting tumor associated-regulatory T cells. Oncotarget 7: 8771–8782. https://doi.org/10.18632/oncotarget.6822

28. Zhao R, Chinai JM, Buhl S, Scandiuzzi L, Ray A, Jeon H, Ohaegbulam KC, Ghosh K, Zhao A, Scharff MD, Zang X (2013) HHLA2 is a member of the B7 family and inhibits human CD4 and CD8 T-cell function. Proc Natl Acad Sci 110:9879–9884. https://doi.org/10.1073/pnas.1303524110

29. Chen H, Zhang Y, Shen Y, Jiang L, Zhang G, Zhang X, Xu Y, Fu F (2023) Deficiency of N-linked glycosylation impairs immune function of B7-H6. Front Immunol 14:1255667. https://doi.org/10.3389/fimmu.2023.1255667

30. Lankipalli S, Mahadeva Swamy HS, Selvam D, Samanta D, Nair D, Ramagopal UA (2021) Cryptic association of B7 −2 molecules and its implication for clustering. Protein Sci 30:

1958–1973. https://doi.org/10.1002/pro.4151

31. Song X, Zhou Z, Li H, Xue Y, Lu X, Bahar I, Kepp O, Hung M-C, Kroemer G, Wan Y (2020) Pharmacologic suppression of B7-H4 glycosylation restores antitumor immunity in immune-cold breast cancers. Cancer Discov 10:1872–1893. https://doi.org/10.1158/2159-8290.CD-20-0402

32. Xiao L, Guan X, Xiang M, Wang Q, Long Q, Yue C, Chen L, Liu J, Liao C (2022) B7 family protein glycosylation: promising novel targets in tumor treatment. Front Immunol 13: 1088560. https://doi.org/10.3389/fimmu.2022.1088560

33. Li C-W, Lim S-O, Xia W, Lee H-H, Chan L-C, Kuo C-W, Khoo K-H, Chang S-S, Cha J-H, Kim T, Hsu JL, Wu Y, Hsu J-M, Yamaguchi H, Ding Q, Wang Y, Yao J, Lee C-C, Wu H-J, Sahin AA, Allison JP, Yu D, Hortobagyi GN, Hung M-C (2016) Glycosylation and stabilization of programmed death ligand-1 suppresses T-cell activity. Nat Commun 7:12632. https://doi.org/10.1038/ncomms12632

34. Xu Y, Gao Z, Hu R, Wang Y, Wang Y, Su Z, Zhang X, Yang J, Mei M, Ren Y, Li M, Zhou X (2021) PD-L2 glycosylation promotes immune evasion and predicts anti-EGFR efficacy. J Immunother Cancer 9:e002699. https://doi.org/10.1136/jitc-2021-002699

35. Lee H-H, Wang Y-N, Xia W, Chen C-H, Rau K-M, Ye L, Wei Y, Chou C-K, Wang S-C, Yan M, Tu C-Y, Hsia T-C, Chiang S-F, Chao KSC, Wistuba II, Hsu JL, Hortobagyi GN, Hung M-C (2019) Removal of N-linked glycosylation enhances PD-L1 detection and predicts anti-PD-1/PD-L1 therapeutic efficacy. Cancer Cell 36:168–178.e4. https://doi.org/10.1016/j.ccell.2019.06.008

36. Emaldi M, Alamillo P, Rey-Iborra E, Mosteiro L, Lecumberri D, Pulido R, López JI (2024) A functional role for glycosylated B7-H5/VISTA immune checkpoint protein in metastatic clear cell renal cell carcinoma. iScience 27:110587. https://doi.org/10.1016/j.isci.2024.110587

37. Wang T, Voglmeir J (2014) PNGases as valuable tools in glycoprotein analysis. Protein Pept Lett 21:976–985. https://doi.org/10.2174/0929866521666140626111237

38. Luna S, Mingo J, Aurtenetxe O, Blanco L, Amo L, Schepens J, Hendriks WJ, Pulido R (2016) Tailor-made protein tyrosine phosphatases: in vitro site-directed mutagenesis of PTEN and PTPRZ-B. Methods Mol Biol:79–93. https://doi.org/10.1007/978-1-4939-3746-2_5

39. Sambrook J, Russell DW (2006) Preparation and transformation of competent *E. coli* using calcium chloride. Cold Spring Harb Protoc 2006:pdb.prot3932. https://doi.org/10.1101/pdb.prot3932

40. Mingo J, Erramuzpe A, Luna S, Aurtenetxe O, Amo L, Diez I, Schepens JTG, Hendriks WJAJ, Cortés JM, Pulido R (2016) One-tube-only standardized site-directed mutagenesis: an alternative approach to generate amino acid substitution collections. PLoS One 11: e0160972. https://doi.org/10.1371/journal.pone.0160972

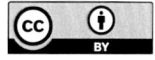

Chapter 5

Evaluation of Immune Checkpoint Inhibitors in a Jurkat-Based Transcriptional Reporter System: A Cell-Based Reporter Platform for Evaluation of Immune Checkpoint Inhibitors

Magdalena Bojko, Judith Leitner, and Peter Steinberger

Abstract

Humanity has been facing cancer since the beginning of its existence, and the number of new cancer cases grows each year. Immunotherapies based on immune checkpoint inhibition have been intensively developed over the last decade and focus on the blockade of the co-inhibitory molecule complexes such as CTLA-4 with its ligands CD80 and CD86, PD-1 with PD-L1 and PD-L2, and many more. The investigation and development of new immune checkpoints inhibitors is necessary for better cancer treatment. One way of inhibitor evaluation is to assess them in cell-based assays. In this protocol, we focus on describing the cell-based reporter platform for PD-1/PD-L1 inhibitors assessment, which is based on measuring the expression of eGFP under the transcription factor NF-κB, responsible for transcriptional program required for T-cell activation and differentiation.

Key words PD-1, PD-L1, Immune checkpoint inhibitors, Cell-based reporter platform, Inhibitors evaluation

1 Introduction

The cell-based reporter platform for the evaluation of immune checkpoint inhibitors presented in this chapter assesses the molecules targeting co-inhibitory receptors by monitoring nuclear factor κB (NF-κB) activity through measuring the expression of the fluorescent protein, enhanced green fluorescence protein (eGFP). The platform is a flexible and convenient tool that allows for the investigation of peptides, antibodies, and small molecules, among others.

The functioning of this assay is based on a two-stage mechanism of T-cell activation occurring through the connection with antigen-presenting cells (APCs). The primary signal is generated by the engagement of the major histocompatibility complex (MHC)

Sweta Rani and Lukasz Skalniak (eds.), *IMMUNO-model in Cancer: Methods and Protocols*, Methods in Molecular Biology, vol. 2959, https://doi.org/10.1007/978-1-0716-4734-9_5, © The Author(s) 2026

molecules on APC with the T-cell receptor (TCRs)/CD3 complex and coreceptors CD4 or CD8 on the T cell. These interactions lead to activation and nuclear translocation of transcription factors, namely NF-κB, nuclear factor of activated T cells (NFAT), and activator protein 1(AP-1) responsible for T-cell activation, proliferation, cytokine production, and cytolytic function [1]. The second signal is transduced by co-stimulatory and co-inhibitory receptors known as immune checkpoints. To induce a second signal the immune checkpoint receptor located on the T cell has to bind to its ligand on APC [2, 3]. The immune checkpoint receptors and their ligands are an ever-growing group of molecules, which includes CTLA-4 and CD28 and their ligands CD80 and CD86, PD-1 with PD-L1 and PD-L2, and the BTLA/HVEM complex [4–6]. The assay focuses on the second signal and abolishing its effect by application of the chosen complex's inhibitor.

The assay is based on the human leukemic T-cell line Jurkat E6.1, which has been widely employed as a model system for T-cell activation and effector function studies [7]. Transformed T-cell lines are an excellent alternative to the use of primary human T cells, which is labor-intensive and requires ethical approval. In addition, there is considerable variation between primary T cells derived from different donors and they express a plethora of co-stimulatory and co-inhibitory receptors, which could potentially interfere with studies on the pathway of interest. The conjunction of the transformed T-cell line with the genetically engineered T-cell stimulator cell line (fulfilling a function of APC) creates a platform for the evaluation of immune checkpoint inhibitors [8, 9].

Jurkat E6.1 cell line was retrovirally transduced with an NF-κB::eGFP reporter construct and with a PD-1 construct creating the reporter cell line (JE6.1-NF-κB::eGFP PD-1). The T lymphoblast cell line from mice with lymphoma BW5147 (wtBW) was used as a T-cell stimulator cell line (TCS) and was transduced to stably express membrane-bound antihuman CD3 single-chain variable fragment (scFv) (mb aCD3) anchored to the cell membrane via a human CD14 stem (CD5L-OKT3scFv-CD14). In the coculture, the mb CD3 antibody fragment induces activation via the TCR/CD3 complex, which leads to NF-κB-activation and eGFP expression (the first signal required for T-cell activation). Moreover, TCS was transduced to express PD-L1 (TCS PD-L1), enabling the formation of a complex with PD-1. The engagement of PD-1 on the reporter cells by PD-L1 on the stimulator cells attenuates NF-κB activation and thereby also eGFP expression on the reporter cells (the second signal). The inhibitory signal can be assessed by the measurement of the expression level of eGFP, whose expression is reduced when PD-1 and PD-L1 create a complex and increases when the interaction between those proteins is disrupted. The cell lines required for the validation of the platform are presented in Table 1. Reporter cell line lacking PD-1 and TCS

Table 1
Cell lines required for the assay validation and their description

Cell line name	Description of the cell line
JE6.1-NF-κB::eGFP Ctrl	Reporter cell line constructed on the Jurkat E6.1 cell line PD-1 negative
JE6.1-NF-κB::eGFP PD-1	Reporter cell line constructed on the Jurkat E6.1 cell line expressing PD-1
TCS Ctrl	T-cell stimulator cell line expressing mb aCD3 constructed on the wtBW cell line
TCS PD-L1	T-cell stimulator cell line expressing mb aCD3 and PD-L1 constructed on the wtBW cell line

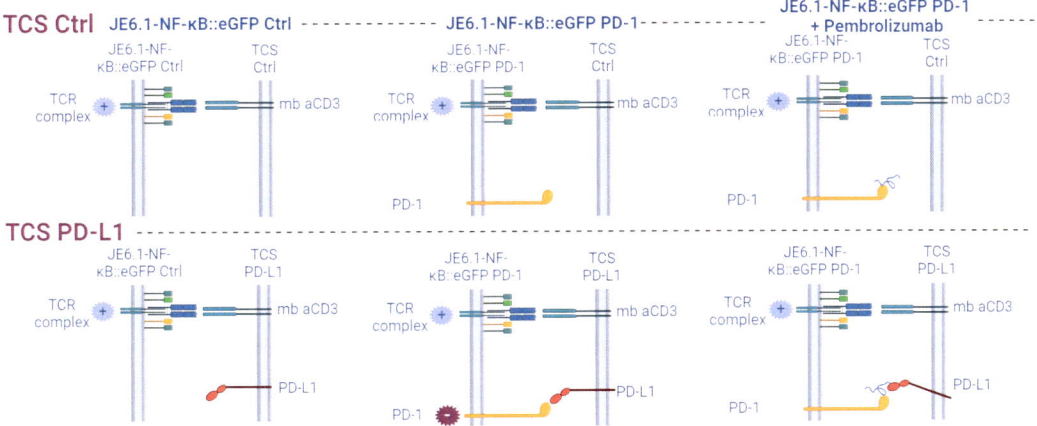

Fig. 1 Schematic representation of cell coculture. "+" - the eGFP reporter gene activated, "−" - the eGFP reporter gene inhibited

expressing mb aCD3 but lacking PD-L1 are crucial to verify the functionality of the platform.

A schematic representation of the cell coculture required for a complete assessment of PD-1 and PD-L1 interaction is shown in Fig. 1. For platform verification, it is important to test combinations of the TCS Ctrl and TCS PD-L1 with two reporter cell lines: JE6.1-NF-κB::eGFP Ctrl and JE6.1-NF-κB::eGFP PD-1. Finally, the influence of the PD-1/PD-L1 complex inhibitor should be investigated. For this purpose, the anti-PD-1 mAb pembrolizumab, or any other validated PD-1/PD-L1 complex inhibitor, may be utilized.

Platform functionality is verified by the eGFP expression measured by the flow cytometry. The reporter gene expression by the JE6.1-NF-κB::eGFP Ctrl should be on a comparable level when stimulated by the TCS Ctrl and TCS PD-L1 due to the lack of the PD-1 on reporter cells. In the case of coculture of the JE6.1-NF-κB::eGFP PD-1 reporter cells with TCS PD-L1, the eGFP

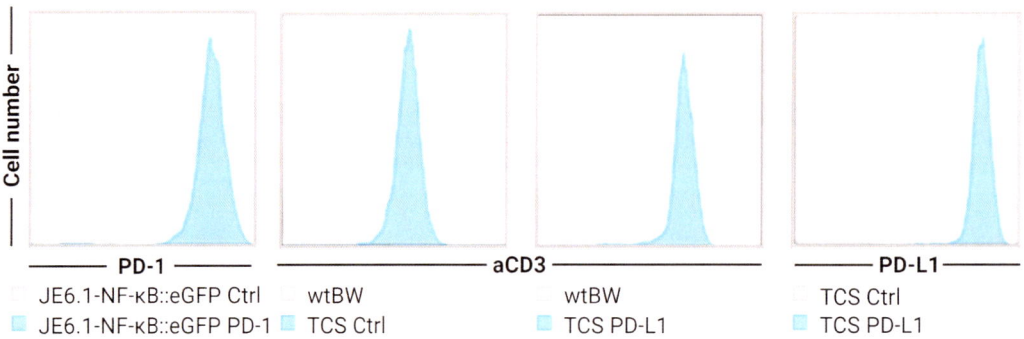

Fig. 2 Flow cytometry analysis of the molecular profile of cell lines used in the stimulation assay - JE6.1-NF-κB::eGFP reporter cells and TCS. Light gray histograms: staining of control cells. Blue histograms: staining of cells expressing the indicated molecules

expression should be diminished in comparison to the coculture of these reporter cells with TCS Ctrl, which indicates the generation of an inhibitory signal by PD-1 upon interaction with PD-L1. Adding the PD-1/PD-L1 complex inhibitor to the system should abolish the suppression of reporter gene expression.

Flow cytometry can be used to confirm the molecular profile of the Jurkat reporter cells and the TCS. Fig. 2 shows the expression of PD-1 on JE6.1-NF-κB::eGFP PD-1 cells, whereas JE6.1-NF-κB::eGFP control cells stained negative (Fig. 2 - left side). Moreover, the presence of mb aCD3 on TCS Ctrl and TCS PD-L1, and also the absence of PD-L1 on TCS Ctrl cell line have to be verified (Fig. 2 - right side). As a mb aCD3 negative cell line, wild-type BW5147 (wtBW) cell line should be used.

2   Materials

2.1   Cell Lines

1. Jurkat E6.1 (JE6.1-NF-κB::eGFP Ctrl and JE6.1-NF-κB:: eGFP PD-1) and BW5147 (TCS Ctrl and TCS PD-L1) were derived from in-house stocks, generated as previously described [8–10] (*see* **Note 1**).

2. Maintain the modified Jurkat E6.1 (reporter cell lines) and BW5147 (TCS) cell lines in Roswell Park Memorial Institute 1640 medium (RPMI 1640) supplemented with 1% of penicillin and streptomycin with the addition of 10% heat-inactivated fetal bovine serum (FBS). Grow the cell lines in a 5% CO_2 atmosphere in a humidified incubator at 37°C. Maintain cultures at a cell concentration between 1×10^5 and 1×10^6 viable cells/mL. Perform cell maintenance every 2 to 3 days. Maintain cultures by the addition of the fresh medium or replacement of the medium (centrifuge the cells at approximately $300 \times g$ for 5–10 min and resuspend them at 1×10^5 viable cells/mL).

2.2 Cell Culture and Experiment Preparation	1. Growth medium: RPMI 1640 supplemented with 1% of penicillin and streptomycin with the addition of 10% of heat-inactivated FBS.

2.2 Cell Culture and Experiment Preparation

1. Growth medium: RPMI 1640 supplemented with 1% of penicillin and streptomycin with the addition of 10% of heat-inactivated FBS.

2. 25 cm^3 and 75 cm^3 cell culture flasks for suspension cells.

3. 6-, 12-, and 96-well transparent tissue culture plates for suspension cells.

4. Equipment: standard cell culture lab equipment 37°C, 5% CO$_2$ incubator, cell counter, 37°C water bath, laminar flow hood, tube shaker, rotator, pipets, sterile plastic materials for cell culture;

5. Control antibody, anti-PD-1, or anti-PD-L1.

2.3 Flow Cytometry

1. Flow cytometer.

2. Running buffer for flow cytometry.

3. Conical tubes for flow cytometry analysis.

4. Antibodies for flow cytometry analysis (sample antibody set): APC-conjugated antihuman PD-1 Ab, PE-conjugated antihuman PD-L1 Ab, APC-conjugated anti-CD14 antibody (clone HCD14) (to detect mb aCD3), APC-conjugated anti-mouse CD45.2 Ab (reacts with murine CD45.2 expressed on TCS; is used to exclude TCS in reporter assays).

2.4 Software

1. Software for data analysis - FlowJo.

2. Software for graphic visualization, for example, GraphPad Prism.

3   Methods

3.1 Verification of the Molecular Profile of the Cells by Flow Cytometry

1. Take out the cells for staining (JE6.1-NF-κB::eGFP Ctrl, JE6.1-NF-κB::eGFP PD-1, wtBW, TCS Ctrl, and TCS PD-L1 cell lines).

2. Centrifuge the cells at 300 × g for 5 min.

3. Discard the supernatant and resuspend the pellet in 1 mL of FACS buffer (PBS with 0.5% FBS and 0.0125% NaN$_3$).

4. Determine the cell concentration and distribute 5 × 10^4 cells to conical tubes for each staining (*see* **Note 2**).

5. Stain the cells by the use of antibodies conjugated with the desired fluorochrome in concentration defined by the manufacturer or determined by titration in-house. Test JE6.1-NF-κB::eGFP Ctrl for lack of PD-1 and JE6.1-NF-κB::eGFP PD-1 for its presence. This can be done by using APC-conjugated antihuman PD-1 Ab. Verify the expression of mb aCD3 in both TCS Ctrl and TCS PD-L1 cell lines by using APC-conjugated

anti-CD14 Ab; additionally, TCS PD-L1 cells have to be PD-L1 positive, test them using PE-conjugated antihuman PD-L1 Ab.

6. Incubate the cell lines with appropriate antibodies with fluorochrome for 30 min at 4 °C.

7. Afterward, centrifuge the cells at $300 \times g$ for 5 min at 4°C.

8. Discard the supernatant and resuspend the pellet in FACS buffer.

9. Repeat **steps 7** and **8**.

10. Resuspend the cell pellet in an appropriate volume of FACS buffer for flow cytometry analysis.

11. Perform the analysis by measuring the geometric mean of the fluorescence intensity (gMFI). The flow cytometry analysis conditions should be adjusted to the equipment and antibodies used.

3.2 Investigation of Inhibitory Properties of Tested Molecules

3.2.1 Day I

1. Perform the experiment on the 96-well tissue culture-treated transparent plates.

2. Prepare at least 300 μL of starting dilutions of tested molecules (2× final concentration) using RPMI 1640 medium with 10% FBS (test medium) as a diluent (*see* **Notes 3** and **4**). Use the starting dilution to prepare serial replicate dilutions ($n = 3$) (*see* **Note 5**).

3. To receive a full spectrum of information, get prepared to set up the following cocultures:

   • JE6.1-NF-κB::eGFP Ctrl with medium control.

   • JE6.1-NF-κB::eGFP Ctrl with TCS Ctrl and medium control.

   • JE6.1-NF-κB::eGFP Ctrl with TCS PD-L1 and medium control.

   • JE6.1-NF-κB::eGFP PD-1 with medium control.

   • JE6.1-NF-κB::eGFP PD-1 with TCS Ctrl and medium control.

   • JE6.1-NF-κB::eGFP PD-1 with TCS PD-L1 and medium control.

   • JE6.1-NF-κB::eGFP PD-1 with test sample.

   • JE6.1-NF-κB::eGFP PD-1 with TCS Ctrl and test sample.

   • JE6.1-NF-κB::eGFP PD-1 with TCS PD-L1 and test sample.

4. Prepare the cells by centrifuging them at $300 \times g$ for 5–10 min, discard the supernatant, and resuspend the cell pellet in an adequate volume of test medium (*see* **Note 6**).

5. In the case of the molecules targeting PD-1, in the first place, seed reporter cells in the density of 5×10^4 cells per well in 50 μL of the test medium.

6. To each well, add either 100 μL of tested molecules' dilutions prepared in the second step or 100 μL of tested medium (vehicle control) (*see* **Note 7**).

7. Incubate cells with inhibitors for 90 min in a cell culture incubator.

8. Add TCS cells in the density of 2×10^4 cells per well in 50 μL of the test medium.

9. During the examination of molecules targeting PD-L1, in the first step, incubate TCS cells with inhibitors and afterward add reporter cells.

10. Perform the coculture for 24 h at 37°C in an atmosphere of 5% CO_2 in a humidified incubator.

3.2.2 Day II

1. Harvest the cells and transfer them to conical FACS tubes.

2. Centrifuge cell suspension at $300 \times g$ for 5 min at 4°C, afterward discard supernatant.

3. Wash the pellet twice by adding the FACS buffer (PBS with 0.5% FBS and 0.0125% NaN_3), centrifuging, and removing the supernatant.

4. Stain the cells with anti-mouse CD45.2 mAb conjugated with the desired fluorochrome in concentration defined by the manufacturer or set through in-house titration. Anti-mouse CD45.2 mAb is added to the sample to exclude TCS cells from the analysis.

5. Resuspend the cell pellet and incubate samples for 30 min at 4°C.

6. Repeat the wash step (**step 3**, Day II).

7. Resuspend the cell pellet in the appropriate volume of FACS buffer for flow cytometry analysis.

8. Perform the analysis by measuring the reporter gene expression (eGFP) by flow cytometry. The flow cytometry analysis conditions should be adjusted to the equipment and anti-mouse CD45.2 mAb used.

9. The experiment should be run at least three times.

3.3 Analysis

1. Use gMFI of the viable cell population for analysis. Determine the cell viability according to their FSC/SCC profile and by excluding CD45.2 positive TCS. Analyze the data using FlowJo software.

2. The inhibitory properties of the tested molecules are measured by reporter gene expression (NF-κB::eGFP) by the JE6.1-NF-

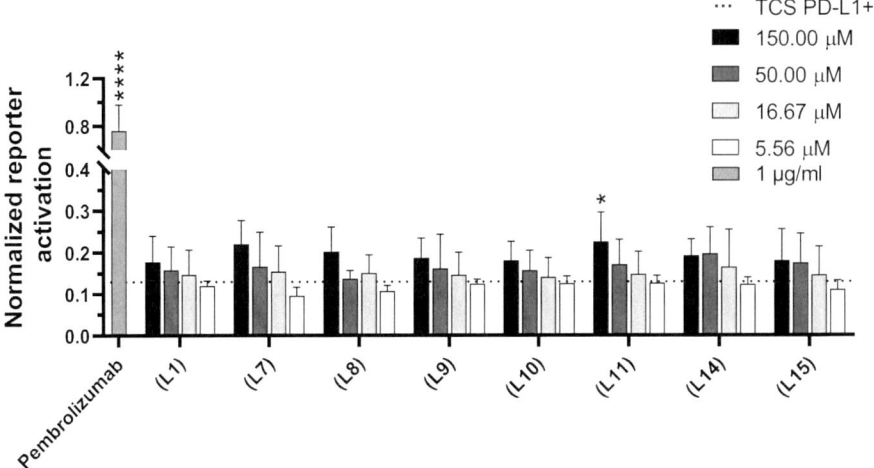

Fig. 3 Inhibitory properties of the peptides targeting PD-L1 (fragments of PD-1) and control mAb in the cell-based reporter assay. The PD-1 reporter cells were stimulated with TCS PD-L1 in the absence or presence of the peptides. The inhibitory properties of the peptides were measured based on eGFP expression by flow cytometry and normalized to gMFI eGFP obtained for the PD-1 reporter/TCS Ctrl cells treated with the peptides. The dotted line shows the normalized eGFP expression level from the coculture of the PD-1 reporter cells with TCS PD-L1 [11]

κB::eGFP PD-1 in coculture with TCS PD-L1. Normalize results to gMFI of eGFP received for the JE6.1-NF-κB:: eGFP PD-1/TCS Ctrl cells (TCS without PD-L1) treated by the tested molecules. Express results as a fold induction.

3. Plot the results using appropriate graphical software (e.g., GraphPad Prism 8).

4. When a tested molecule inhibits the PD-1/PD-L1 complex, the reporter gene expression should be restored leading to the increase of the signal from eGFP compared with the control - eGFP expression level from the coculture of the PD-1 reporter cells with TCS/PD-L1 without the peptides (Fig. 3) (*see* **Notes 8** and **9**).

4   Notes

1. The reporter and the stimulator cell lines may be shared with other institutions within a material transfer agreement (MTA). Please contact the head of the Division of Immune Receptors and T-Cell Activation at the Medical University of Vienna in this matter.

2. Some cells may be lost during centrifugation and discarding of the supernatant which is why the amount of the cell taken to the experiment should be selected with consideration.

3. The concentration of tested molecules used in the experiment should be adjusted each time to the tested molecule and their influence on cell viability has to be determined.

4. When investigating the small molecules, use of the DMSO or another dissolvent may be necessary to dissolve them. Remember that using the lowest possible dissolvent is recommended as it may influence the cells' viability. Moreover, using dissolvent requires adding the vehicle control.

5. It is recommended to perform the experiments in duplicates or triplicates. Each test should be repeated at least three times.

6. Bear in mind that the test requires a significant number of cells. While examining many inhibitors and testing different conditions, the cell expansion should be started early enough to collect the proper amount of cells. The population doubling time of the Jurkat E6.1 cell line is approximately 20 h. However, the doubling time of the transformed cell line may be extended. The BW5147 cell line doubles its population faster than Jurkat E6.1, which should be taken into consideration during experiment planning.

7. Remember to add positive and negative controls to the experiment.

8. When the results obtained for inhibitors are ambiguous due to a small difference between the increase of reporter gene expression after the use of the inhibitor and the level of reporter expression when the PD-1/PD-L1 complex is formed, it is possible to introduce a co-stimulatory signal to enlarge this difference. Jurkat E6.1 cell line (our reporter cell line) expresses on the surface CD28, which is an immune checkpoint receptor. This receptor creates a complex with its ligand CD86. Introducing CD86 expression to the TCS cell line leads to the formation of a CD28/CD86 complex contributing to a higher reporter gene expression. In the platform with additional stimulation signal, the effect of the reporter gene suppression induced by the PD-1/PD-L1 complex formation is more visible (Fig. 4). In this system, the TCS Ctrl cell line is replaced by TCS CD86 Ctrl, and the TCS PD-L1 cell line is replaced by TCS CD86/PD-L1 (Table 2).

9. When the amount of the reporter gene expression is not sufficient for the detection the number of cells taken to the experiment may require optimization. Additionally, the relation of reporter cells to the TCS cells may influence the signal intensity.

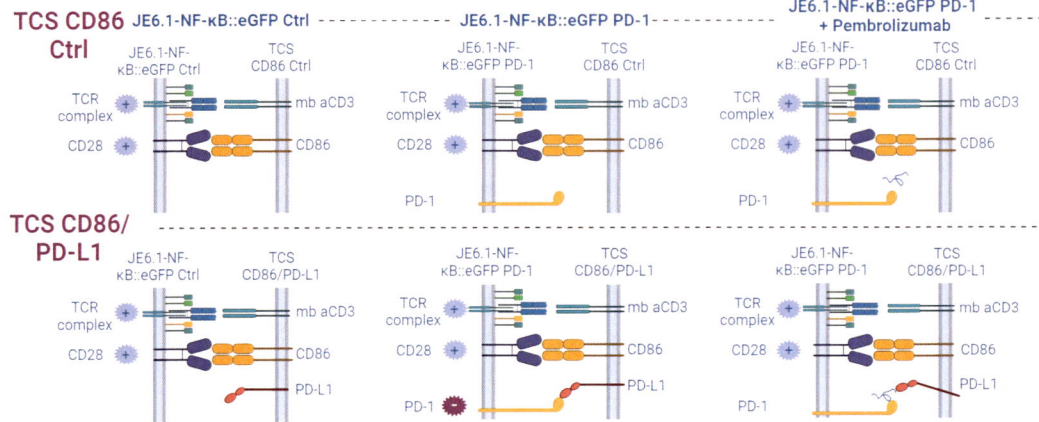

Fig. 4 Schematic representation of cell coculture. "+" - the eGFP reporter gene activated, "−" - the eGFP reporter gene inhibited

Table 2
Cell lines required for higher reporter gene expression and their description

Cell line name	Description of the cell line
JE6.1-NF-κB:: eGFP Ctrl	Reporter cell line constructed on the Jurkat E6.1 cell line expressing CD28, PD-1 negative
JE6.1-NF-κB:: eGFP PD-1	Reporter cell line constructed on the Jurkat E6.1 cell line expressingCD28 and PD-1
TCS CD86 Ctrl	T-cell stimulator cell line expressing mb aCD3 and CD86 (CD86 create a complex with CD28 expressing on the reporter cell line) constructed on the wtBW
TCS CD86/PD-L1	T-cell stimulator cell line expressing mb aCD3, CD86, and PD-L1 constructed on the wtBW cell line

Acknowledgments

This publication is based upon work from COST Action IMMUNO-model, CA21135, supported by COST (European Cooperation in Science and Technology).

References

1. Okazaki T, Honjo T (2007) PD-1 and PD-1 ligands: from discovery to clinical application. Int Immunol 19:813–824

2. Paul WE (2013) Fundamental immunology-seventh edition. Fundam Immunol 7:1312

3. Actor JK (2019) T lymphocytes: ringleaders of adaptive immune function. In: Introductory immunology. Elsevier, Amsterdam, pp 45–62

4. Chen L, Flies DB (2013) Molecular mechanisms of T cell co-stimulation and co-inhibition. Nat Rev Immunol 13:227–242

5. Ward-Kavanagh LK, Lin WW, Šedý JR et al (2016) The TNF receptor superfamily in co-stimulating and co-inhibitory responses. Immunity 44:1005–1019

6. Liu W, Zang X (2019) Structures of immune checkpoints: an overview on the CD28-B7 family. In: Advances in experimental medicine and biology. Springer, New York LLC, pp 63–78

7. Carrasco-Padilla C, Aguilar-Sopeña O, Gómez-Morón A et al (2023) T cell activation and effector function in the human Jurkat T cell model. In: Methods in cell biology, pp 25–41

8. Jutz S, Leitner J, Schmetterer K et al (2016) Assessment of costimulation and coinhibition in a triple parameter T cell reporter line: simultaneous measurement of NF-κB, NFAT and AP-1. J Immunol Methods 430:10–20

9. Jutz S, Hennig A, Paster W et al (2017) A cellular platform for the evaluation of immune checkpoint molecules. Oncotarget 8:64892–64906

10. Leitner J, Kuschei W, Grabmeier-Pfistershammer K et al (2010) T cell stimulator cells, an efficient and versatile cellular system to assess the role of costimulatory ligands in the activation of human T cells. J Immunol Methods 362:131–141

11. Bojko M, Węgrzyn K, Sikorska E et al (2024) Peptide-based inhibitors targeting the PD-1/PD-L1 axis: potential immunotherapeutics for cancer. Transl Oncol 42:101892

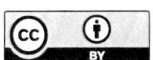

## Chapter 6

A PD-1/PD-L1-Sensitive Co-culture-Based Primary T-Cell Activation Assay

Justyna Kocik-Krol, Malgorzata Stec, Maciej Siedlar, Thanh Hoa Vo, Sweta Rani, and Lukasz Skalniak

Abstract

Programmed cell death protein 1 (PD-1) is crucial in inhibiting immune responses by modulating the activity of T cells. We present an in vitro assay that is based on a co-culture of primary immune cells represented by human peripheral blood mononuclear cells (PBMCs), isolated from healthy donors with Chinese hamster ovary-derived cell line (CHO-K1) overexpressing human PD-L1 protein (hPD-L1) and an artificial TCR-activator construct (TCRAct). CHO-K1/TCRAct/hPD-L1 cells mimic antigen-presenting cells by activating T cells via the T-cell receptor (TCR) and providing a ligand for the negative immune checkpoint (PD-L1 protein). The two components, PBMCs and CHO-K1/TCRAct/hPD-L1 cells, when in co-culture, provide a T-cell activation (TCA) assay, which may be used to test the potency of molecules targeting the PD-1/PD-L1 immune checkpoint. This method relies on monitoring the activation of helper CD4+ and cytotoxic CD8+ T cells using flow cytometry by analyzing the expression levels of early (CD69), intermediate (CD25 and HLA-DR), and late (PD-1) activation/exhaustion markers. This is the well-established in vitro co-culture assay in which primary T-cell activation via the TCR is diminished by the concurrent presence of PD-1/PD-L1 immune checkpoint, which can be blocked resulting in increased expression of T-cell surface markers.

Key words PD-1/PD-L1 immune PD-1 blockade, Co-culture model, T-cell activation, Flow cytometry, Immunotherapy

Abbreviations

aAPCs	Artificial antigen-presenting cells
BD	Becton Dickinson
BV510	Brilliant Violet 510
CBA	Cytometric bead array
FITC	Fluorescein isothiocyanate
ICB	Immune checkpoint blockade
ICIs	Immune checkpoint inhibitors
PBMCs	Peripheral blood mononuclear cells
PD-1	Programmed death receptor 1
PD-L1	Programmed death-ligand 1

Sweta Rani and Lukasz Skalniak (eds.), *IMMUNO-model in Cancer: Methods and Protocols*, Methods in Molecular Biology, vol. 2959, https://doi.org/10.1007/978-1-0716-4734-9_6, © The Author(s) 2026

PerCP   Peridinin-chlorophyll-protein
PE-Cy™7   Phycoerythrin-Cyanine 7
TCA   T-cell activation assay

1 Introduction

Immunotherapy, an innovative approach to cancer treatment, aims to restore the immune system's ability to recognize and eliminate cancer cells. In recent years, therapy targeting immune checkpoints has achieved promising results [1, 2]. Among the known immune checkpoints, the inhibition of excessive interaction between the PD-1 protein (programmed cell death protein 1) presented on the surface of immune cells and its ligand, PD-L1, utilized by cancer cells to "silence" the immune response, is under intensive investigation. The discovery of the PD-1/PD-L1 interaction, along with another checkpoint molecule, CTLA-4, and characterization of their role in evading immune system response by cancer cells, was awarded the Nobel Prize in Physiology or Medicine in 2018 to James Allison and Tasuku Honjo [3–6].

Currently, ten monoclonal antibodies (mAbs, four anti-PD-L1 antibodies, and six anti-PD-1 antibodies) are the only FDA-approved drugs as PD-1/PD-L1 interaction inhibitors used in clinical cancer therapies (www.fda.gov). Despite the numerous scientific reports on the discovery of non-mAb PD-1/PD-L1 immune checkpoint inhibitors (ICIs), there have been only two commercially available in vitro assays that enable the verification of ICIs activity. The immune checkpoint blockade (ICB) assays consist of Jurkat T cells overexpressing human PD-1 protein (*h*PD-1) and containing nuclear factor of activated T-cells response element (NFAT-RE) or β-galactosidase reporter system, co-cultured with cells overexpressing human PD-L1 protein (*h*PD-L1). In these assays, the potential effect of blocking PD-1/PD-L1 is reflected by a luminescent signal from reactivated Jurkat T/*h*PD-1 cells. In addition, in one of the researches, the PD-1/PD-L1 interaction was studied in vitro when breast cancer cell lines MDA-MB-231, MDA-MB-469, and MCF-7 were co-cultured with human PBMCs pre-stimulated using anti-CD3 and anti-CD28 antibodies [7].

In the TCA assay that we describe here, CHO-K1/TCRAct/*h*PD-L1 cells, also named artificial antigen-presenting cells (aAPCs), are in co-culture with fresh PBMCs isolated from healthy blood donors (Fig. 1) to verify the immunostimulatory activity of PD-1/PD-L1-blocking molecules, as monitored by reactivation of primary T cells. We designed an easy-to-follow flow cytometry panel based on the most commonly used fluorochromes to characterize T-cell activation by the surface expression of early (CD69), intermediate (CD25 and HLA-DR), and late (PD-1) activation/

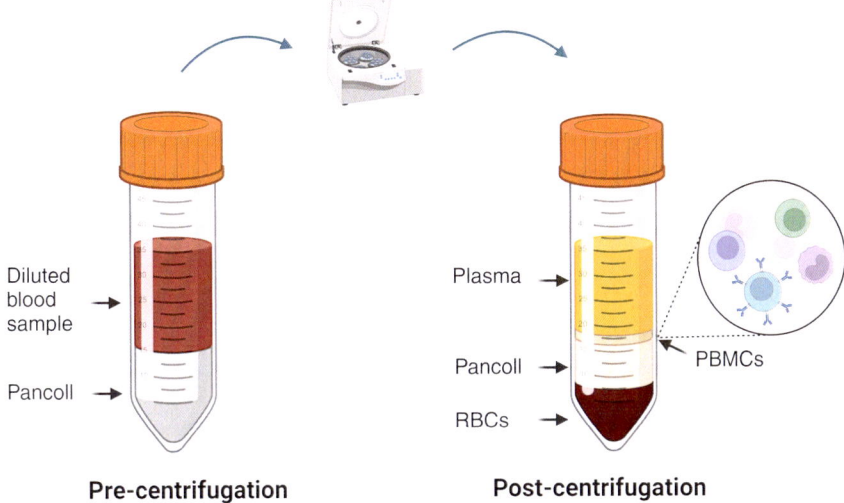

Fig. 1 Schematic representation of PBMC isolation from whole blood using density gradient centrifugation and Pancoll separating solution. After the centrifugation, four layers are observed and a layer with PBMCs is used for the next steps of the procedure described in this protocol. (The graphic was created in Biorender)

Table 1
The list of cell surface proteins selected as markers of T-cell activation

Type of marker	Characteristic	Marker	Main functions
Cell surface	Early activation	CD69	Lymphocytes proliferation and migration [8]
	Intermediate activation	CD25	Subunit of IL-2 receptor, T-cell proliferation, activation-induced cell death [9]
	Intermediate/late activation	HLA-DR	Presenting peptide antigens [10]
	Late activation/exhaustion	PD-1	Inhibiting immune response [11]

exhaustion markers (Table 1). Easy gating strategy allows for separate analysis of the activation of CD4+ and cytotoxic CD8+ T cells (Fig. 2). Flow cytometry data collected for 13 independent individuals allowed us to determine PD-1 as a marker, which, out of the four markers tested, best reflects the blockade of PD-1/PD-L1 immune checkpoint and can be used as a determinant of successful targeting of this immune checkpoint (Fig. 3).

2 Materials

2.1 Cell Culture

1. Whole blood from healthy donors, mixed with an anticoagulant, such as citrate-phosphate-dextrose adenine (CPDA-1).

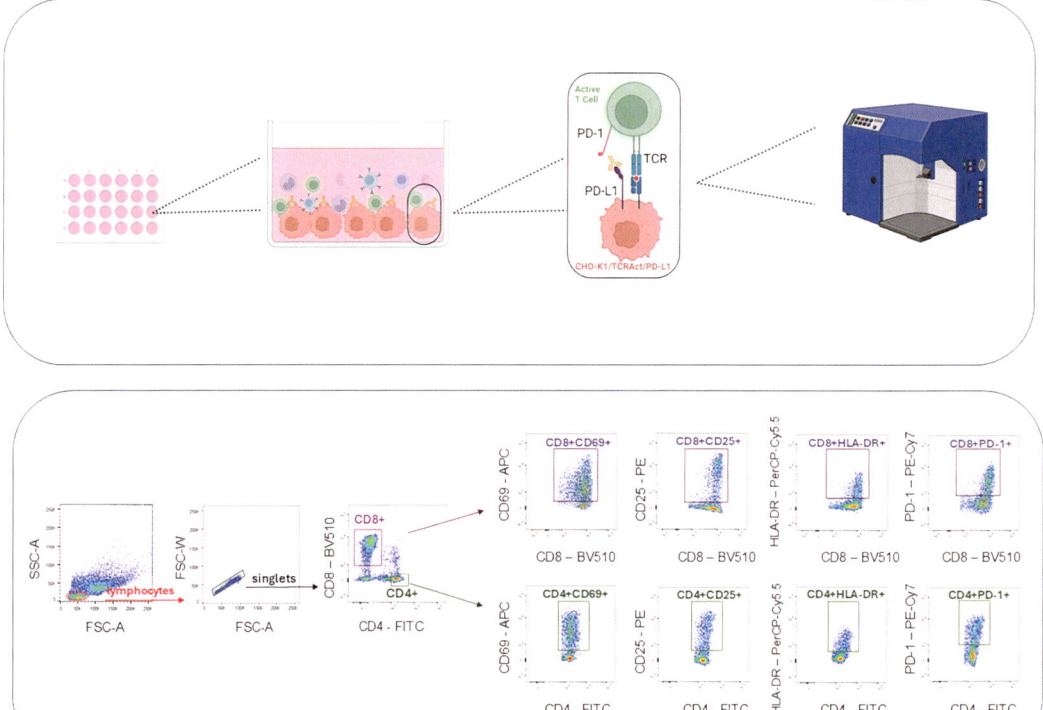

Fig. 2 Illustration of gating strategy for T-cell activation assay (TCA). After 48 h of the co-culture, without, and in the presence of PD-1/PD-L1 inhibitors, the activation of helper CD4+ and cytotoxic CD8+ T cells is analyzed using flow cytometry, where the activation of CD4+ and CD8+ lymphocytes are monitored by the expression level of early (CD69), intermediate (CD25 and HLA-DR), and late (PD-1) activation/exhaustion markers. The gating strategy scheme was created in FlowJo. (The graphic was created in Biorender)

2. Cell-culture medium: RPMI 1640, 10% volume/volume (v/v) FBS, 2 mM L-glutamine.

3. CHO-K1/TCRAct/hPD-L1 cells (such as *PD-L1 aAPC/ CHO-K1 cells* from Promega or *PD-L1/TCR Activator-CHO Recombinant Cell Line* from BPS Bioscience), cultured in a recommended cell-culture medium (such as RPMI 1640, 10% (v/v) FBS, 2 mM L-glutamine).

4. Phosphate-buffered saline (PBS) without calcium and magnesium.

5. L-Trypsin-EDTA 0.02% (v/v).

6. CO_2 cell-culture incubator.

2.2 Isolation of PBMCs from Whole Blood

1. Pancoll human, density: 1.077 g/mL solution.

2. Centrifuge with a swing-out rotor.

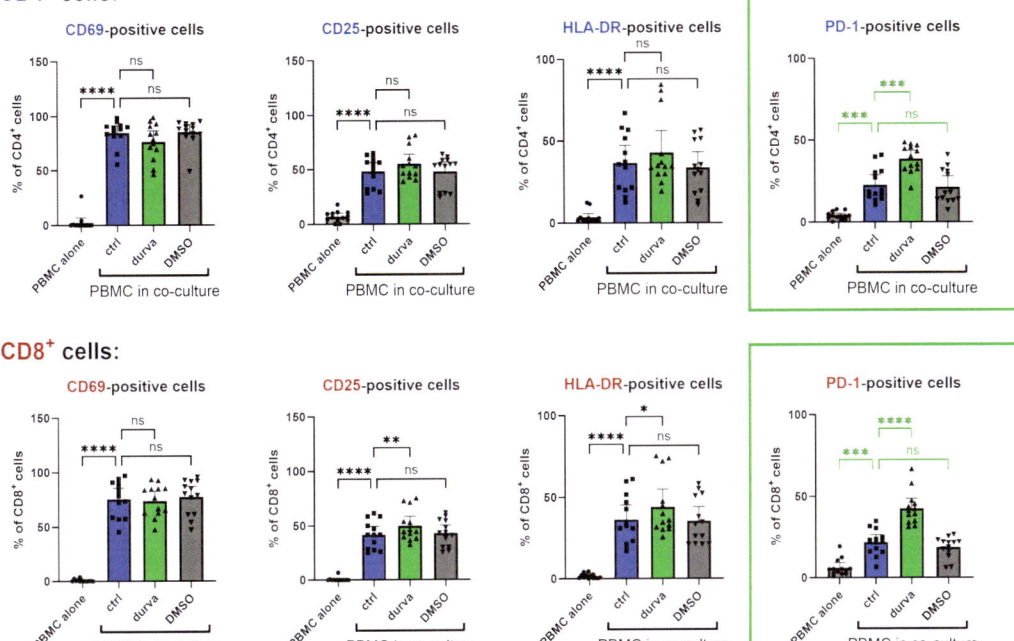

Fig. 3 Example of results. The expression of activation markers: CD69, CD25, HLA-DR, and PD-1 was assessed after 48 h of co-culture of PBMCs with CHO-K1/TCRAct/*h*PD-L1 cells in the presence of durvalumab (durva), an anti-PD-L1 antibody, at the final concentration of 5 μg/mL. DMSO-treated (DMSO) and untreated (ctrl) cells were also used as controls. The "PBMCs alone" condition represents PBMC cultured without any stimulants to detect the baseline level of expression of the analyzed markers. On the graphs, the fractions of CD69, CD25, HLA-DR, and PD-1 expressing cells (% positive cells) are shown as calculated data from 13 individual PBMC donors. The data is retrieved from our previous publications [13–16]. Statistical significance was analyzed using RM one-way ANOVA, with the Geisser-Greenhouse correction, followed by Tukey's multiple comparisons test, with individual variances computed for each comparison * $p < 0.05$, ** $p < 0.01$, *** $p < 0.001$, ****, $p < 0.0001$. The data was computed and visualized with the use of GraphPad Prism 10.3.1

2.3 Preparing Flow Cytometry Samples

1. TrypLE™ Express (Gibco, MA, USA).

2. Flow Cytometry Staining Buffer.

3. Antibodies for flow cytometry:

- Mouse anti-human CD69, clone FN50, conjugated with allophycocyanin (APC), Becton Dickinson Biosciences BD (NJ, USA), cat.no. 555533, 3 μL/sample.

- Mouse anti-human CD25, clone 2A3, conjugated with phycoerythrin (PE), BD, cat no. 341011, 3 μL/sample.

- Mouse anti-human HLA-DR, clone L243, conjugated with peridinin-chlorophyll-protein (PerCP), BD, cat no. 347402, 3 μL/sample.

- Mouse anti-human CD4, conjugated with fluorescein isothiocyanate (FITC), BD, cat no. 555346, 2 µL/sample.
- Mouse anti-human CD8, clone SK1, conjugated with, Brilliant Violet 510 (BV510), BD, cat. no. 563919, 3 µL/sample.
- Mouse anti-human PD-1, conjugated with phycoerythrin-Cyanine 7 (PE-Cy™7), BD, cat. no. 561272, 2 µL/sample.

4. UltraComp eBeads™ Compensation Beads.
5. Centrifuge.
6. Flow cytometer.

2.4 Laboratory Plastics

1. Culture flasks.
2. 24-well transparent cell-culture plates.
3. 15 mL Falcon tubes.
4. 50 mL Falcon tubes.
5. 1.5 mL Eppendorf tubes.
6. 5 mL round bottom tubes.

2.5 Other

1. PD-1/PD-L1 inhibitors to be tested, including positive controls, such as durvalumab or atezolizumab (*see* **Note 1**).

3   Methods

3.1 Seeding of the Artificial Antigen-Presenting Cells (aAPCs): 24 H Before Starting the Co-culture (DAY 1)

1. Seed CHO-K1/TCRAct/*h*PD-L1 cells at a density 60,000 cells/well, in a 24-well transparent plate in a total volume of 1 mL of culture medium per well (*see* **Note 2**).
2. Culture the cells for 24 h in a cell-culture incubator with 5% CO_2 at 37 °C in a humified atmosphere.

3.2 Isolation of PBMCs from Whole Blood: On the Day of Starting the Co-culture (DAY 2)

1. Transfer 15 mL of Pancoll into a 50 mL Falcon tube.
2. Equilibrate the vial to room temperature.
3. Dilute the blood sample with PBS (we normally dilute between one- and threefold to achieve 20 mL of the diluted blood sample) and carefully layer 20 mL of the diluted blood over the Pancoll (*see* **Note 3**).

   Do not mix the blood sample with Pancoll.
4. Centrifuge: 800 × *g*, 20 min, room temperature. Switch the brake off to avoid disturbing separated phases (*see* **Note 4**).
5. After centrifugation, slowly remove and discard the top layer of the blood sample (diluted plasma) using a pipette.
6. Transfer the PBMC-containing layer (*see* Fig. 1) into a new 50 mL Falcon tube.

7. Add three volumes of PBS to PBMCs.

8. Centrifuge: $300 \times g$, 10 min, at room temperature.

9. Remove the supernatant and add 25 mL of PBS to the PBMCs.

10. Mix by pipetting.

11. Centrifuge: $300 \times g$, 10 min, at room temperature.

12. Remove the supernatant and resuspend PBMCs in the culture medium (*see* **Note 5**).

13. Count the cells.

14. Prepare a cell suspension in a culture medium at the density of 700,000 cells per mL.

15. Keep the cells at 4 °C (*see* **Note 6**).

3.3 Preparation Dilutions of PD-1/PD-L1 Inhibitors That Will Be Tested (DAY 2)

1. Prepare 2× concentrated dilutions of PD-1/PD-L1 inhibitors in the culture medium (*see* **Note 7**).

2. Prepare the "medium-only" control sample.

3. Prepare the "medium + compound solvent" control sample (*see* **Note 7**).

3.4 Establishing a Co-culture (DAY 2)

1. Carefully remove the medium from the plates with seeded CHO-K1/TCRAct/hPD-L1 cells (aAPCs).

2. Add 0.5 mL of the 2 × concentrated dilutions of PD-1/PD-L1 inhibitors prepared in **step 1** in Subheading 3.3.

3. Remember to include medium-only and "medium + compound solvent" (such as DMSO) conditions on the plate.

4. Remember to include the positive-control condition (such as a well-known anti-PD-L1 antibody).

5. Pipette PBMCs prepared in a 50 mL Falcon tube in **step 14** in Subheading 3.2 and transfer 0.5 mL of cell suspension (350,000 cells) into each dedicated well.

6. Remember to prepare one well containing only PBMCs (no co-culture—unstimulated cells).

7. Incubate the co-culture for 48 h at 37 °C in a cell-culture incubator with 5% CO_2 in a humified atmosphere.

3.5 Performing Flow Cytometry Analysis of the T-Cell Activation Assay (DAY 4)

1. Pipette and transfer culture wells content into 5 mL round bottom tubes (to collect PBMCs) (*see* **Note 8**).

2. Add 200 μL of TrypLE™ Express Enzyme into the wells (to detach adherent aAPCs cells). Incubate for 5 min at room temperature.

3. Add 1 mL of pre-warmed culture medium into the wells, pipette carefully, and add well content into the previously used 5 mL round-bottom tubes.

4. Centrifuge (500 × g, 7 min) and remove the supernatant.

5. Add 2 mL of Flow Cytometry Staining Buffer to each sample (first wash step). Mix by pipetting (*see* **Note 9**).

6. Centrifuge (500 × g, 7 min) and remove the supernatant.

7. Add 2 mL of Flow Cytometry Staining Buffer to each sample (second wash step). Mix by pipetting (*see* **Note 9**).

8. Centrifuge (500 ×g, 7 min) and remove the supernatant. Perform **step 9** while centrifuging.

9. Prepare a working solution of antibodies used in the flow cytometry staining panel that will be used for staining (*see* **Note 10**). The total amount of antibody working solution required for one sample is 150 μL.

The amount of each antibody per sample is presented in the Subheading 2.3.

10. Add 150 μL of antibodies working solution per sample and mix well.

11. Incubate for 25 min in the dark (cover tubes with aluminum foil if needed).

12. Add 3.5 mL of Flow Cytometry Staining Buffer into each sample (first wash step). Mix well.

13. Centrifuge (500 g, 7 min) and remove the supernatant.

14. Add 3.5 mL of Flow Staining Cytometry Buffer into each sample (second wash step). Mix well.

15. Centrifuge (500 × g, 7 min) and remove the supernatant.

16. Add 150 μL of Flow Cytometry Staining Buffer into the samples. Protect from light and analyze on the flow cytometer as soon as possible (*see* **Notes 11** and **12**).

4   Notes

1. Please keep in mind that the use of either anti-PD-1 positive control antibodies (such as nivolumab) or PD-1-targeting molecules may block the binding of anti-PD-1 antibody and detection of PD-1 in a flow cytometry analysis.

2. Control cells, such as CHO-K1 (cells without hPD-L1 and TCAct) or CHO-K1/TCRAct (cells without hPD-L1), can also be used in the experimental setups, in parallel with CHO-K1/TCRAct/hPD-L1 aAPCs [12–16]. These cells either do not activate T cells (CHO-K1) or activate T cells without concomitant blockade by the PD-1/PD-L1 immune checkpoint (CHO-K1/TCRAct).

3. The protocol is optimized for 5–10 mL blood samples. In cases where a smaller amount of blood is collected, PBMC isolation can be optimized to 15 mL Falcon tubes.

4. It is important NOT TO mix the sample after centrifugation. The samples should be carefully removed from the centrifuge and the phases should be separated immediately.

5. For PBMC culture, we recommend preparing fresh culture medium (RPMI-1640, 10% FBS, 2 mM L-glutamine) on the day of the cells' isolation since the cells are sensitive to the quality of the medium.

6. In the assays, we always set up the co-culture with PBMCs within 1–2 h after the isolation from whole blood.

7. These 2×concentrated dilutions will be diluted further to final 1× concentrations at the stage of adding PBMCs in a volume ratio of 1:1. In the case when the compound stocks are prepared in DMSO, the final concentration of DMSO in the culture medium should be kept as low as possible. In our experiments, the final concentration of DMSO does not exceed 0.1% (v/v).

8. Before pipetting and detaching cells, you can collect around 100–200 μL of culture medium from each well and store it for further procedures such as the determination of the content of cytokines released to the medium. We have performed such an analysis in some of our previous works [12, 13].

9. In our hands, pipetting with an automatic pipette worked better than vortexing. During vortexing, cell aggregates appeared spontaneously.

10. When preparing the staining master mix for 40 samples, we normally prepare a 2-sample excess to compensate for any pipetting errors, bubbles of the Flow Cytometry Staining Buffer, etc. In such case, the master mix of antibodies would include the following volumes: 42 samples ×134 μL of Flow Cytometry Staining Buffer +42 samples × volume per sample of each of the antibodies (3 μL/sample for anti-human CD69, anti-human CD25, anti-human HLA-DR, anti-human CD8, 2 μL/sample for anti-human CD4, anti-human PD-1).

11. In our experiments, we worked on BD FACSCanto™ II flow cytometer (BD) and BD FACSuite™ and FlowJo™ software.

12. Compensation is the process of correcting spillover from one fluorescent channel to another. It is required to provide the compensation process before the proper experimental measurement on flow cytometry, especially when panel staining is used.

In our experiments, we used UltraComp eBeads™ Compensation Beads according to the manufacturer's protocol.

Acknowledgments

This research was funded by the National Science Centre, Poland Sonata Bis Grant number UMO-2021/42/E/NZ7/00422. J. K.-K. is supported by the Foundation for Polish Science (FNP) START scholarship awarded in 2024. This publication is based upon work from COST Action IMMUNO-model, CA21135, supported by COST (European Cooperation in Science and Technology).

References

1. Liu C, Yang M, Zhang D et al (2022) Clinical cancer immunotherapy: current progress and prospects. Front Immunol 13:1–22

2. Waldman AD, Fritz JM, Lenardo MJ (2020) A guide to cancer immunotherapy: from T cell basic science to clinical practice. Nat Rev Immunol 20:651–668

3. Leach DR, Krummel MF, Allison JP (1996) Enhancement of antitumor immunity by CTLA-4 blockade. Science 80-) 271:1734–1736

4. Huang P, Chang JW (2019) ScienceDirect news and perspectives immune checkpoint inhibitors and win the 2018 Nobel prize. Biom J 42:299–306

5. Iwai Y, Ishida M, Tanaka Y et al (2002) Involvement of PD-L1 on tumor cells in the escape from host immune system and tumor immunotherapy by PD-L1 blockade. Proc Natl Acad Sci U S A 99:12293–12297

6. Ishida Y, Agata Y, Shibahara K et al (1992) Induced expression of PD-1, a novel member of the immunoglobulin gene superfamily, upon programmed cell death. EMBO J 11:3887–3895

7. Saleh R, Toor SM, Khalaf S et al (2019) Breast cancer cells and PD-1/PD-L1 blockade upregulate the expression of PD-1, CTLA-4, TIM-3 and LAG-3 immune checkpoints in CD4+ T cells. Vaccine 7:1–13

8. Cibrián D, Sánchez-Madrid F (2017) CD69: from activation marker to metabolic gatekeeper. Eur J Immunol 47:946–953

9. Brusko TM, Wasserfall CH, Hulme MA et al (2009) Influence of membrane CD25 stability on T lymphocyte activity: implications for immunoregulation. PLoS One 4:e790

10. Chen B, Khodadoust MS, Olsson N et al (2019) Predicting HLA class II antigen presentation through integrated deep learning. Nat Biotechnol 37:1332–1343

11. Simon S, Labarriere N (2018) PD-1 expression on tumor-specific T cells: friend or foe for immunotherapy? Onco Targets Ther 7:1–7

12. Konieczny M, Musielak B, Kocik J et al (2020) Di-bromo-based small-molecule inhibitors of the PD-1/PD-L1 immune checkpoint. J Med Chem 63:11271–11285

13. Muszak D, Surmiak E, Plewka J et al (2021) Terphenyl-based small-molecule inhibitors of programmed cell Death-1/programmed death-ligand 1 protein-protein interaction. J Med Chem 64:11614–11636

14. Magiera-Mularz K, Kuska K, Skalniak L et al (2021) Macrocyclic peptide inhibitor of PD-1/ PD-L1 immune checkpoint. Adv Ther 4: 2000195

15. Zaber J, Skalniak L, Gudz GP et al (2024) N-methylmorpholine incorporation into the structure of biphenyl leads to the bioactive inhibitor of PD-1/PD-L1 interaction. Bioorg Med Chem Lett 110:1–7

16. Rodriguez I, Kocik-krol J, Skalniak L et al (2023) Structural and biological characterization of pAC65 , a macrocyclic peptide that blocks PD-L1 with equivalent potency to the FDA- approved antibodies. Mol Cancer 22: 150

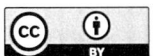

Chapter 7

In Vitro Model for Studying Interaction of Immune Cells and Cancer Cells

Thanh Hoa Vo, Amie Menton, Orla O'Donovan, Edel A. McNeela, Jai Prakash Mehta, and Sweta Rani

Abstract

The tumor microenvironment (TME) is a complex environment composed of a variety of cell types including cancer cells, endothelial cells, and immune cells. Cross talk between the cells in TME plays a central role in tumor growth, progression, metastasis, and response to therapy. Coculture is a method to study the interaction between various types of cells in vitro and provides a way to mimic the in vivo conditions. Two or more types of cells can be cultured in a way that, they are in direct contact with each other (direct coculture) or, separated while still communicating through the secretion of soluble factors (indirect coculture). In this chapter, we focus on indirect coculture, specifically studying the modulation of immune cells by breast cancer lines through paracrine signaling. Cells are grown in transwells that allow the transfer of soluble factors but prevent cell-to-cell contact. This model helps us understand the effects of soluble factors on both immune cells and cancer cells.

Key words Coculture, Indirect coculture, Paracrine signaling, Transwells, Migration, Cancer, Immune cells

1 Introduction

One of the most common cancers is breast cancer, with 1 in 7 women being diagnosed in their lifetime [1]. Breast cancer is a complex disease and is classified based on the presence or absence of various receptors. Breast cancer cells overexpressing human epidermal growth factor receptor 2 (HER2) are called HER2 positive breast cancer. HER2 is a member of the epidermal growth factor receptor (EGFR) family of receptor tyrosine kinases that also includes HER1, HER3, and HER4 proteins [2]. Triple-negative breast cancer (TNBC) lacks the three receptors—estrogen, progesterone, and HER-2. Cancer cells expressing estrogen (ER-positive) or progesterone (PR-positive) are called hormone receptor-positive breast cancer [2].

Sweta Rani and Lukasz Skalniak (eds.), *IMMUNO-model in Cancer: Methods and Protocols*, Methods in Molecular Biology, vol. 2959, https://doi.org/10.1007/978-1-0716-4734-9_7, © The Author(s) 2026

Our immune system plays a central role in identifying and eliminating foreign and abnormal cells including cancer cells. Chemokine are the soluble factors that signals the immune cells to infiltrate an infected area or tumor microenvironment (TME) [3]. The main effector cells are T cells that are activated by tumor-associated antigens (TAAs) and damage-associated molecular patterns (DAMPs). Several cytokines, including CXCL12, limit the infiltration of cytotoxic T cells, reducing their effector capacity. CXCL12 also plays a central role in recruiting regulatory T cells (Treg) and tumor-associated macrophages resulting in tumor progression and metastasis [4].

The Food and Drug Administration (FDA) passed a legislation in 2022 that newer drugs are not required to be tested on animals. Changes in the legislation was required as only 10.4% of the drug entering phase I clinical trial were approved [5]. As preclinical models are no longer required for drug approval, a lot of research is being done to develop in vitro models for testing drugs, cell-to-cell interaction, etc.

2   Materials

2.1   Cell Culturing

1. Culture THP-1 cells in RPMI-1640, supplemented with 10% fetal bovine serum (FBS), % L glutamine, and 1% penicillin-streptomycin (penstrep).

2. Grow RAW cells in Dulbecco's Modified Eagle's Medium (DMEM) supplemented with 10%FBS, % L glutamine, and 1% penstrp.

3. Grow HCC1954 cells in RPMI-1640 supplemented with 10% FBS, 1% L glutamine, and 1% penstrp.

4. Trypsin/ethylenediaminetetraacetic acid (EDTA).

5. Phosphate-buffered saline (PBS) without Ca^{2+}/Mg^{2+}.

6. Cell culture T-flask—25 $cm^{2.}$

7. Cell scraper.

8. 24-well plate.

9. Haemocytometer.

10. Ethanol.

2.2   Coculturing of Immune Cells and Cancer Cells

1. 8 μm pore size transwell chambers.

2. 1 μm pore size transwell chambers.

3. Crystal violet.

4. Acetic acid.

2.3 **Equipment**	1. Incubator at 37 °C with 5% CO_2.
	2. Inverted microscope.
	3. Centrifuge.
	4. Absorbance microplate reader.

---

3   Methods

3.1 **Subculturing of Cells**	Grow all the cell lines in the incubator at 37 °C with 5% CO_2. Subculture the cells when they reach 70–80% confluency. Visualize the cells under a microscope, checking for any contamination before subculturing them in a biosafety cabinet.

3.1.1 Culturing THP-1 Suspension Cells

1. THP-1 cells are suspension cells, so to subculture remove the cells from the T-flask using pipette and transfer them to a centrifuge tube.

2. Centrifuge the cells at 200 × *g* for 5 min.

3. After centrifugation remove the supernatant and resuspend the cell pellet in 1 mL of complete media.

4. For cell counting mix the cells with trypan blue (1 in 2 dilution) and incubate for 5 min (*see* **Note 1**).

5. In the meantime, clean the hemocytometer with 70% ethanol, fix the coverslip by pushing it in circular motions until Newtonian rings could be visualized.

6. Pipette 10 μL of the cell and trypan blue solution onto the hemocytometer.

7. Count the cells and use the following formula to calculate the concentration of cells/mL:

$$\frac{n \; x \; d \; x \; 10^4}{S}$$

8. Where.

n = total number of cells counted.

d = dilution factor.

S = number of squares counted.

3.1.2 Culturing HCC1954 Cells

1. HCC1954 cancer cells are cultured in RPMI-1640 supplemented with 10% FBS, 1% L glutamine, and 1% penstrp.

2. Remove media from the flask and wash the cells with prewarmed PBS to remove traces of media/FBS (*see* **Note 2**).

3. HCC1954 cell is an adherent cell line; detach the cells using prewarmed trypsin/EDTA solution (*see* **Note 3**).

4. Incubate the cells at 37 °C for 5 min or till they are detached (*see* **Note 4**).

5. Deactivate trypsin by adding equal volume of prewarmed medium and transfer the content to a centrifuge tube.

6. Centrifuge the cells at $125 \times g$ for 5 min.

7. After centrifugation decant the supernatant and resuspend the cell pellet in 1 mL of media.

8. Count the cells and use the formula in Subheading 3.1.1, **step 7** for determining the cell number.

3.1.3 Culturing RAW 264.7

1. RAW cells are grown in Dulbecco's Modified Eagle's Medium (DMEM) supplemented with 10%FBS, 1% L glutamine, and 1% penstrp.

2. Remove media from the flask and wash the cells using prewarmed PBS.

3. Use cell scraper to detach the cells, add media to collect all the cells, and transfer the cells to a centrifuge tube.

4. Follow the protocol of centrifugation and cell counting as in Subheading 3.1.2, **steps 6–8**.

3.2 Coculturing of HCC1954 Cells with THP-1 Cells

To determine the effect of immune cells and cytokines on cancer cells, THP-1 cells and HCC1954 cells can be cocultured using transwell method.

1. Seed THP-1 cells in a 1 μm transwell at the concentration of 5×10^5 cells/transwell in 200 μL of complete medium (*see* **Note 5**).

2. In a 24-well plate seed HCC1954 cells at a concentration of 1×10^5 cells/well in 200 μL of complete medium.

3. Allow the cells to grow for 72 h at 37 °C incubator with 5% CO_2.

4. After 72 h, cells in the transwell, and 24-well plate can be washed, trypsinized, and stored appropriately.

5. Media conditioned by these cells can be centrifuged, filtered using 0.45 μm filter, and stored appropriately for further analysis like secreted cytokines.

3.3 Migration of Immune Cells Toward Cancer Cells

Migration of cancer cells and immune cells are highly regulated by paracrine signaling via secretion of cytokines and chemokines. This model can be used to study pathways associated with tumor progression and identify new biomarker for metastasis. Migration of THP-1 cells toward HCC1954 breast cancer cells and HER-targeted drug-resistant variant is being assessed here using this method.

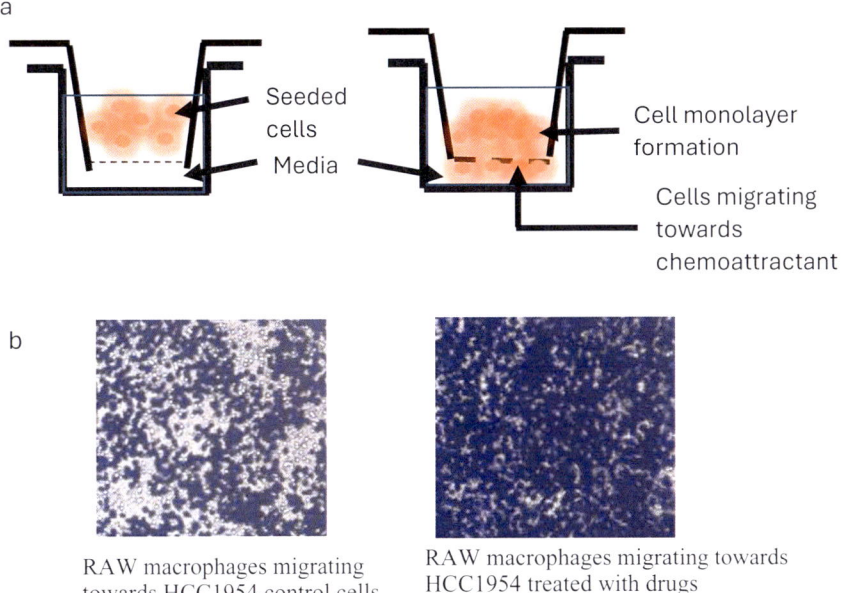

RAW macrophages migrating towards HCC1954 control cells

RAW macrophages migrating towards HCC1954 treated with drugs

Fig. 1 (**a**) Migration assay setup using transwell in a multi-well plate; (**b**) Migration of raw macrophages toward HCC1954 under different conditions

1. For migration assay, 8 μm pore size transwell is used.

2. Seed HCC1954 untreated control cells (1×10^5 cells/well) in a 24-well plate and seed the drug-resistant variant in another well.

3. Place the transwells in the 24-well plate (Fig. 1a).

4. Seed RAW 264.7 cells (5×10^4 cells/transwells) in the transwell.

5. Allow the cells to migrate for 24 h by growing them in an incubator at 37 °C with 5% CO_2 (*see* **Note 6**).

6. After 24 h, remove the cells from the transwell that failed to migrate.

7. Cells can be removed from the transwells using Q-Tip (*see* **Note 7**).

8. Wash the inside of the transwells by submerging it in PBS.

9. Stain the migrated cells using 25% crystal violet (*see* **Note 8**).

10. Pipette 500 μL of crystal violet in a new 24-well plate and place the transwells to stain (*see* **Note 9**).

11. Incubate it at room temperature on a shaker for 15 min.

12. After incubation wash the transwells at least three times with PBS (*see* **Note 10**).

13. Label the transwells and leave them to dry at room temperature.

14. Once the transwells are dry they can be photographed (Fig. 1b).

15. After photographing solubilize the crystal violet stain using 33% acetic acid.

16. Incubate the plate for 15 min on a shaker or till all the color from the transwells is solubilized.

17. Remove the transwells and measure the absorbance at 595 nm.

18. To graph this, take the reading from RAW cells exposed to HCC1954 control cells as 100%.

19. Calculate the % migration of RAW cells in the presence of drug-resistant variant compared to control.

4   Notes

1. Trypan blue exclusion test is used to determine viable cells in a cell suspension.

2. Cell-culture medium consists of FBS that might interfere with the activity of trypsin. Washing with PBS will remove traces of FBS and facilitate trypsinization.

3. EDTA is a chelating agent that increases the ability of trypsin to dissociate the cells. Volume of trypsin used depends on the surface of the cell culture vessel.

4. Trypsin is an enzyme that digest proteins to dissociate the adherent cells. Prolonged incubation of cells in trypsin should be avoided as it might damage the cell membrane proteins.

5. Height and compatibility of the transwells with the multi-well plate must be checked before purchasing.

6. Migration of cells through the transwells depends on the invasive property of the cell lines. Optimization might require when using any different cell lines.

7. Avoid using too much pressure when removing the cells from inside of the transwells. Cells are attached to the other side of the transwells, too much pressure might lead to detaching of the cells that have migrated through the transwell.

8. Crystal violet should be filtered before use as it might crystalise when stored for long duration.

9. Avoid any air bubble between the stain and the transwells as it will prevent the staining of the cells.

10. Transwells should be washed till the PBS is clear and no more violet color is released from the transwells.

Acknowledgments

This work is supported by funds from South East Technological University (WD-2022-14-WSCH) and Research Connexions 2024. This publication is based upon work from COST Action IMMUNO-model, CA21135, supported by COST (European Cooperation in Science and Technology).

References

1. https://www.breastcancerireland.com/education-awareness/facts-and-figures/

2. Zhang X (2023) Molecular classification of breast cancer: relevance and challenges. Arch Pathol Lab Med 147:46

3. Kohli K, Pillarisetty VG, Kim TS (2022) Key chemokines direct migration of immune cells in solid tumors. Cancer Gene Ther 29:10

4. Ryan AT, Kim M, Lim K (2024) Immune cell migration to cancer. Cells 13:10

5. Zushin PH, Mukherjee S, Wu JC (2023) FDA modernization act 2.0: transitioning beyond animal models with human cells, organoids, and AI/ML-based approaches. J Clin Invest 133(21)

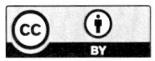

Chapter 8

In Vitro Coculture Model of Immune and Tumor Cells for Immunotherapy Studies of High Mutational Load Tumors

Piroska Virág, Ioana Brie, and Maria Perde-Schrepler

Abstract

To obtain a better tumor cell killing mediated by cytotoxic T lymphocytes (CTLs), several strategies were developed that might prime tumor-specific T-cell responses. One such strategy is combining the immune checkpoint inhibitors (CPI) blockade with radiotherapy (RT), considering the synergy between these two types of therapies. Here, we present an in vitro experimental model of cocultures of human tumor cell lines (A549 lung carcinoma and SK-Mel-1 melanoma) and immune cells (CTLs), in which CTLs activation is attempted by irradiation of the tumor cells with ionizing radiations and by the treatment of CTLs with an anti-programmed death-1 (anti-PD-1) drug. This model is suitable for studying cellular death, inflammatory responses, molecule expression, and immunotherapy.

Key words Immunogenicity, High mutational load tumors, Immune checkpoint inhibitors, Programmed cell death protein, Cocultures, Cytotoxicity, Cellular death, Inflammatory responses, Immunotherapy

1 Introduction

Cancer immunogenicity, the ability of tumors to induce an immune response that can regulate their growth [1], increases with the rate of mutations, since tumor antigens can trigger the immune response. Several studies have shown that cancers bearing the highest rate of mutations are non-small cell lung cancers (NCSLC) and malignant melanoma (MM) [2, 3]; hence, they have higher immunogenicity. Besides the classical therapies (chemo- and radiotherapy), immunotherapy (IT) holds great promise for increasing cure rates for these highly immunogenic and poor prognostic cancers. Immune checkpoint inhibitors (CPI) through the blockade of some checkpoint proteins, such as programmed cell death protein 1 (PD-1) and its ligand (PDL-1), may lead to the reactivation of T cells [4]. Despite the clinical efficacy of CPI blockade, they are far from being perfect predictive biomarkers and that there is much room for improvement. Combining CPI blockade with strategies

Sweta Rani and Lukasz Skalniak (eds.), *IMMUNO-model in Cancer: Methods and Protocols*, Methods in Molecular Biology, vol. 2959, https://doi.org/10.1007/978-1-0716-4734-9_8, © The Author(s) 2026

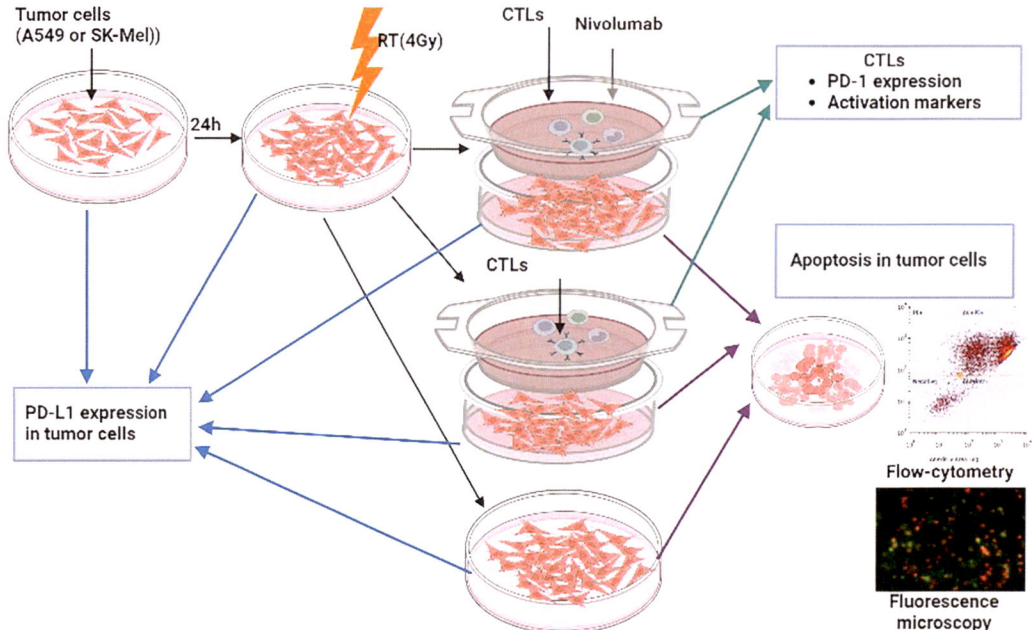

Fig. 1 An in vitro experimental model of cocultures of human tumor cell lines (A549 lung carcinoma and SK-Mel-1 melanoma) and immune cells (CTLs) separated from peripheral blood mononuclear cells (PBMCs). (Made with Biorender)

that prime tumor-specific T-cell responses is an attractive and synergistic approach. Preclinical and clinical data also point toward a strong synergy between radiotherapy (RT) and IT, with a possible systemic effect of RT ("abscopal effect") [5]. RT induces release of antigens and pro-inflammatory factors, which are able to trigger tumor-specific T cells. If successful, it may result not only in the rejection of the irradiated tumor but also in the rejection of the systemic disease [6].

Here in, we present an in vitro experimental model of cocultures of human tumor cell lines (A549 lung carcinoma and SK-Mel-1 melanoma) and immune cells (CD8+ cytotoxic T cells (CTLs) separated from peripheral blood mononuclear cells (PBMCs)), suitable for cellular death, inflammatory responses, molecule expression, and IT studies. In this model, in attempt to enhance the ability of CTLs to kill tumor cells, we propose ionizing radiations and an anti-PD-1 drug (Nivolumab) (Fig. 1).

2   Materials

2.1   Equipment

1. Laminar airflow hood—all the procedures involving cell cultures are performed under laminar airflow to ensure sterility.

2. CO_2 incubator at 37 °C, 5% CO_2, 85% humidity.

3. Swing-out centrifuge, with adjustable rcf and temperature.

4. Optical and fluorescence microscope equipped with a highly sensitive camera and software.

5. Inverted phase microscope.

6. Flow cytometer equipped with a blue 488 nm, 20 mW solid-state laser, and a red 633 nm 17 mW HeNe laser.

7. ELISA plate-reader.

8. Automated plate washer.

9. Electronic cell counter (optional).

2.2 Preparing Cell-Culture Media and Other Reagents for the Tumor Cell Lines and Blood Cells

Prepare all solutions using ultrapure water (prepared by purifying deionized water). Use ready-to-use cell liquid, sterile-filtered, commercially available cell-culture media, supplements, and reagents whenever available. Alternatively, prepare them from solid powder, according to the manufacturer's indications. Keep all cell-culture media, supplements, and reagents at refrigerator (-20 °C or 4–8 °C, according to the manufacturer's indications), and bring them to room temperature before usage (unless indicated otherwise). Follow all waste disposal regulations when disposing waste materials.

2.2.1 The Cell-Culture Media and Other Reagents for the Tumor Cell Lines (A549 and SK-Mel-1)

1. Nutrient mixture F-12 (for A549) and RPMI-1640 (for SK-Mel-1), (with both L-glutamine and sodium bicarbonate), as liquid, sterile-filtered solutions, suitable for cell cultures, supplemented with 20% fetal calf serum (FCS) for cells' thawing and with 10% FCS for further cells' cultivation; 1% penicillin-streptomycin; 1% amphotericin B (for SK-Mel-1).

2. 0.25% Trypsin/0.02% EDTA solution.

3. Trypan-blue dye.

2.2.2 Reagents for the PBMCs and CTLs Preparation, Cultivation, and Treatment

1. Phosphate-buffered saline (PBS), without calcium chloride and magnesium chloride, liquid, sterile-filtered, suitable for cell culture.

2. Ficoll-Paque/Histopaque (density 1.077).

3. Hank's balanced salt solution (HBSS), as liquid, sterile-filtered solutions, suitable for cell cultures.

4. RPMI-1640 medium (with L-glutamine and sodium bicarbonate), as liquid, sterile-filtered solution, suitable for cell cultures, supplemented with 20% FCS, 1% nonessential aminoacids (NEA), 1% beta-mercaptoethanol, 1% HEPES, and 1% sodium pyruvate.

5. Anti-PD-1 drug (Nivolumab).

2.3 Reagents for the Immunomagnetic Separation of CTLs Population from PBMCs

1. Colloidal super-paramagnetic microbeads conjugated to monoclonal mouse antihuman CD8 antibody.

2. Buffer: PBS supplemented with 0.5% bovine serum albumin (BSA) and 2 mM ethylenediaminetetraacetic acid (EDTA), pH 7.2.

3. Release reagent (available in magnetic cell sorting kits).

4. Stop reagent (available in magnetic cell sorting kits).

2.4 Reagents for Cellular Death Evaluation by Flow Cytometry and Fluorescence Microscopy

1. Cold PBS.

2. Annexin V/propidium iodide (PI) kit suitable for flow cytometry containing binding buffer (50 mM HEPES, 700 mM NaCl, 12.5 mM $CaCl_2$, pH 7.4), annexin V (solution in 25 mM HEPES, 140 mM NaCl, 1 mM EDTA, pH 7.4, 0.1% bovine BSA), and propidium iodide (1 mg/mL (1.5 mM) solution in deionized water) fluorescent microparticles.

2.5 Reagents for Enzyme-Linked Immunosorbent Assay (ELISA)

1. ELISA kit containing 96-well microplate pre-coated with the appropriate antibody.

2. Horseradish peroxidase-conjugated detection antibody.

3. Calibrated immunoassay standard, assay diluent.

4. Calibrator diluent.

5. Wash buffer.

6. Color reagents A and B.

7. Stop solution.

(All the reagents required to this method are available in ELISA kits).

2.6 Reagents for the Flow-Cytometric Analysis of Tumor Cells and CTLs

1. Cold PBS.

2. Cell-staining buffer (PBS supplemented with 0.5% FCS).

3. Antibodies conjugated with either of the fluorochromes: phycoerythrin (PE), fluorescein isothiocyanate (FITC), allophycocyanin (APC): CD274/PE (B7-H1, PDL-1), PD-1/FITC, CD40/PE, CD95/APC, Ox40/FITC, PDL-1/PE, KRGL/APC, CD25/ FITC, GITR/ PE, CTLA-4/APC.

2.7 Reagents for Analysis of Tumor Cells by Immunocytochemistry

1. 4% paraformaldehyde.

2. PBS.

3. 10% BSA (in PBS).

4. Primary monoclonal antibodies: antihuman CD279 (PD-1) antibody, unlabeled; antihuman CD274 (B7-H1, PDL-1) antibody labeled with PE.

5. Secondary antibodies: Goat-anti-mouse IgG FITC; anti-PDL-1 antibody labeled with PE.

6. Mounting medium with 4',6-diamidino-2-phenylindole (DAPI).

2.8 Consumables

1. Centrifuge tubes (11, 14 mL).

2. 25 cm^2 cell-culture flasks

3. 6-well plates, chamber slides

4. Cell-culture inserts (with 0.4 µm porosity and diameter suitable for 6 well-plates).

5. Flow-cytometry tubes.

6. Test tubes for the standard dilutions.

7. Eppendorf tubes.

8. Cryotubes.

9. Bürker-Türck cell-counting chambers.

10. Microscopy slides.

11. Vacutainers with LiHeparine.

12. Magnetic cell separators.

13. Positive selection columns (type MS+/RS+).

14. Plate sealers.

3 Methods

3.1 Preparation of Tumor Cell Lines (A549 and SK-Mel-1)

1. Thaw the cell lines in 4 mL of the appropriate cell culture media prepared in a 11 mL polypropylene centrifuge tube at room temperature (20–21 °C).

2. Centrifuge the cells at 157 rcf, 5 min, at 20–21 C, and discard the supernatants.

3. Resuspend the cells in 1 mL of the appropriate cell-culture media.

4. Proceed to cell count and viability verification as follows: mix together equal amounts of the cell suspensions and Trypan-blue dye (i.e., 10: 10 µL) in an Eppendorf tube. Count the cells using an optical microscope (at 20× magnitude) or an electronic cell counter, then establish their viability (the Trypan-blue dye's exclusion rate). Cells can be considered for further experiments if their viabilities reach at least 85%.

5. Seed the cells in 25 cm^2 cell-culture flasks, at cells' population density of 1×10^6 cells/mL.

6. When cells reach confluence, seed them in 6-well plates at a cell's population density of 3×10^5 cells/well and incubate for 24 h to settle. A second set of 6-well plates will be used for the

microscopic assessment of PDL-1 expression and cell death evaluation of tumor cells by immunocytochemistry.

7. For both cell lines, one plate will be considered as control (unirradiated) and another one will be prepared for irradiation (with gamma radiation, irradiation dose: 4 Gy, based on previous determinations).

8. A second set of 6-well plates, treated similarly, will be used for the microscopic assessment of cell death and PDL-1 expression in tumor cells by immunocytochemistry.

3.2 Preparation of the Peripheral Blood Mononuclear Cells (PBMCs)

PBMCs will be prepared from peripheral blood collected from a healthy donor, as follows:

1. Collect 6 mL of blood by venipuncture on anticoagulant (LiHeparine).

2. Dilute the blood in 1:2 ratio with PBS in a 14 mL centrifuge tube.

3. Overlay the resulted suspension on Ficoll-Paque/Histopaque (density 1.077), in 3:1 ratio, in a 11 mL tube and centrifuge for 20 min at 225 rcf, at room temperature (20–21 °C), speed 5, spin 0.

4. Remove the supernatant and aspirate the layer of PBMCs.

5. Transfer PBMCs to a 11 mL polypropylene tube, add 6 mL of HBSS, and wash for 10 min at 225 rcf, at room temperature (20–21 °C).

6. Remove the supernatant and resuspend the pellet in 1 mL RPMI-1640 medium.

7. Determine the total number of cells, and then proceed to the immunomagnetic separation in order to obtain CTLs (CD8+ cytotoxic T-cell population).

3.3 Immuno-magnetic Separation of CTLs

The separation of CTLs from PBMCs by immunomagnetic method is based on the presence of CD8 differentiation cluster on CTLs and on the use of monoclonal mouse antihuman CD8 antibody, coupled with super-paramagnetic microbeads. During incubation with the PBMCs, the antibody/microbeads complex binds to the cells expressing the corresponding epitope (CD8). When the cell suspension is placed into a magnetic field, magnetically labeled cells are retained, while unlabeled cells can be removed. To recover the labeled cells, the sample is removed from the magnetic field. The method can be performed following the steps below:

1. Resuspend PBMCs pellet in 80 μL of 0.5% BSA/2 mM EDTA PBS buffer per 10^7 total cells.

2. Label cells by adding 20 µL microbeads conjugated to monoclonal mouse antihuman CD8 antibody per 10^7 cells, mix well, and incubate for 15 min in refrigerator at 6–12 °C.

3. Wash cells with the 0.5% BSA/2 mM EDTA PBS buffer [5 min at 225 rcf, at room temperature (20–21 °C)], discard the supernatant, and resuspend the pellet in appropriate amount of 0.5% BSA/2 mM EDTA PBS buffer (500–1000 µL).

4. Choose a positive selection column (type MS+/RS+) and place it in the separator.

5. Prepare the column by washing it with appropriate amount of the 0.5% BSA/2 mM EDTA PBS buffer (500 µL).

6. Apply the cell suspension to the column (500–1000 µL) and let the negative cells pass through, then rinse with the 0.5% BSA/2 mM EDTA PBS buffer solution (3 × 500 µL).

7. Remove the column from separator and place it on a suitable collection tube, then pipette an appropriate amount of the 0.5% BSA/2 mM EDTA PBS buffer (1000 µL) to the column and flush the positive fraction using the plunger and collect the positive cells (CTLs) in a 11 mL polypropylene centrifuge tube.

8. In order to remove the microbeads, incubate the selected CTLs with 20 µL release reagent per mL cell suspension for 10 min in refrigerator (at 6–12 °C).

9. Wash cells from the released fraction (5 min at 225 rcf, at room temperature [20–21 °C]), remove supernatant completely, and resuspend cell pellet in the 0.5% BSA/2 mM EDTA PBS buffer to a final volume of 50 µL per 10^7 cells.

10. Add 30 µL of stop reagent, mix well, then cells are suitable for further experiments.

3.4 Treatment of the CTLs in Cell-Culture Inserts

1. Seed the CTLs in inserts, at a cell's population density of 6×10^5 cells/insert in RPMI-1640 cell-culture medium.

2. Set for 1 h, then proceed to the treatment with Nivolumab (100 µM /insert).

3. Place the inserts in cocultures with the tumor cells, previously irradiated then incubate for 4 and 24 h, respectively, at 37 °C, 5% CO_2.

4. Tumor cells (A549 and Sk-Mel-1), irradiated in vitro with 4 Gy using a source of ionizing radiations.

5. The cocultures are prepared by placing the inserts containing the treated/nontreated CTLs in the wells with the irradiated/nonirradiated tumor cells.

3.5 Sampling of Supernatants, Tumor Cells, and CTLs for Further Determination

1. After 4 or 24 h of cocultivation of the tumor cells and CTLs, collect the supernatants and the cells and proceed to determinations or alternatively, store both at −80 °C until further determinations (see the next paragraphs).

2. Centrifuge the supernatants 5 min at 157 rcf, at room temperature, proceed to proinflammatory cytokines (IL2, IL10, TNFα, etc.) determination or freeze at −80 °C for the subsequent determination.

3. Detach tumor cells by trypsinization: add 0.5 mL 0.25% Trypsin/0.02% EDTA for 5 min.

4. Then inhibit trypsinization by the addition of 3 mL complete medium, centrifuge 5 min at 1000 rpm, then resuspend the cell pellet and use as follows: one part to evaluate cellular death and the other part to determine the expression of transmembrane protein PDL-1 by flow cytometry.

5. Collect CTLs from the inserts to determine the expression of PD-1 and of some activation molecules (CTLA-4, CD40, CD95, OX40, CD25, GITR, KRLG, CD69 etc.) by flow cytometry.

6. The tumor cells from the second set of 6-well plates, treated as described and designated for the microscopic assessment of PDL-1 expression and cell death of tumor cells by immunocytochemistry will be used without detachment.

7. Alternatively, store the tumor cells and CTLs at −80 °C using the following freezing mix: cells at $2–3 \times 10^6$ cell population density, resuspended in total volume of 1800 μL of the appropriate cell-culture media (for the tumor cell lines) and RPMI-1640 (for the CTLs), both supplemented with 50% FCS and 10% DMSO.

3.6 Evaluation of the Cellular Death of Tumor Cells (A549 and SK-Mel-1)

3.6.1 Flow Cytometry

Flow cytometry is a laser-based technique with multiple applications, from cell counting, cell sorting, biomarker detection, and DNA studies. The principle involves suspending cells in a fluid stream and passing them through an electronic detection apparatus. A flow cytometer allows the simultaneous multiparametric analysis of cell size and granularity, of the physical and chemical characteristics of up to thousands of particles per second along with the detection of up to 6 colors (fluorescence).

In early-stage apoptosis, the plasma membrane undergoes structural changes resulting in the translocation of phosphatidylserine (PS) from the inner cytoplasmic side to the exterior of the cell. Annexin V conjugates bind to the exposed PS residues staining the apoptotic cells. In these early stages of apoptosis, the cell membrane being intact, PI cannot enter the cells and stain the nuclei. In later stages of apoptosis, when the cellular membrane loses its integrity, both Annexin V and PI can enter in the cell (double staining).

1. Centrifuge tumor cells (A549 and SK-Mel-1) treated and trypsinized as previously described, 5 min at 157 rcf, then resuspend the cell pellet in cold PBS.

2. Centrifuge tumor cells for 5 min at 157 rcf, then resuspend in 100 μL binding buffer containing 5 μL annexin V dye and 1 μL propidium iodide (100 μg/mL), and incubate for 15 min at room temperature (20–21 °C).

3. The following controls are used: unstained, stained with annexin V only: 100 μL binding buffer 1× containing 5 μL annexin V, stained with PI only: 100 μL binding buffer 1× containing 1 μL propidium iodide (100 μg/mL) and stained with both annexin V and PI.

4. Add 400 μL binding buffer to the samples and keep on ice until reading on the flow cytometer.

5. Proceed to the calibration and compensation of the fluorescence spectra of the flow cytometer.

6. Cells then are analyzed for annexin V and/or propidium iodide binding using FL1 channel (530/30 BP filter) for annexin V and FL3 channel (670 LP filter) for propidium iodide.

7. Through this protocol, 4 categories of cells will be identified: unmarked (viable), marked with annexin V only (green, apoptotic cells), marked with both annexin V and propidium iodide (double stained, cells in late apoptosis), respectively, stained with propidium iodide only (red, cells in necrosis).

8. The data obtained are analyzed with the flow cytometer and expressed as graphs and/or histograms, along with the appropriate statistical analysis.

3.6.2 Fluorescence Microscopy

1. Aspirate the cell culture media from the 6-well plates containing tumor cells (A549 and SK-Mel-1).

2. Wash the cells three times with cold PBS.

3. Add to each well 200 μL binding buffer containing 10 μL annexin V and 5 μL propidium iodide, and incubate for 15 min at room temperature (20–21 °C).

4. Incubate for 30 min in the dark at room temperature.

5. Wash the cells three times with binding buffer, and then proceed to the microscopic examination.

6. The slides are examined under an inverted fluorescence microscope at an excitation wavelength 488 nm, detection 515 nm for annexin V, and excitation at 568 nm with detection at 590 nm for propidium iodide.

7. Annexin V binds to the phosphatidylserine (PS) residues exposed on the extracellular side of the plasma membranes in the first stages of apoptosis (inaccessible to annexin V binding in living cells). They will appear with a significant marking of the membrane with annexin V (green). Living cells show only a weak staining of the cell membrane. Cells in the late phase of apoptosis with important membrane damage show fluorescent labeling of the membrane with annexin V (green), as well as nuclear labeling with propidium iodide (red); necrotic cells will show only red fluorescence (propidium iodide).

8. 200 cells/sample will be counted, and the percentage of each cell category will be calculated.

3.7 Evaluation of Inflammatory Cytokines by Enzyme-Linked Immunosorbent Assay (ELISA)

The method is based on the sandwich-type immunoenzymatic quantitative determination of inflammatory cytokines (IL-2, IL-10, TNFα, etc.) with the help of specific monoclonal antibodies immobilized on a solid support (96-well plastic plates). The cytokines that constitute the antigen in the standards and test samples bind specifically to the immobilized reactant (antibody). After washing the samples, to remove all traces of unbound substances, a polyclonal antibody bound to an enzyme support is added to the wells. Visualization of the reaction between the enzyme reactant and the antigen-antibody complex is achieved by adding a substrate corresponding to the enzyme used. The color developed indicates the presence or absence of the tested molecules in the sample. For quantitative determination, the color intensity is read on the ELISA plate reader, which is directly proportional to the amount of cytokine in the sample.

1. Use the supernatants collected earlier or thaw the stored ones.

2. Prepare the standard samples, through successive dilutions as indicated in the manufacturer's protocol.

3. The primary antibody is immobilized on the support of the plastic plates.

4. The dilution solution (assay diluent) is added to each well containing the specific antibodies immobilized on the solid support (96-well plate).

5. The test samples (supernatants) are added in the corresponding wells.

6. The plates are incubated at room temperature for the time interval mentioned in the protocol.

7. The wells are washed with the wash buffer using automated plate washer, volume and number of cycles being indicated in the manufacturer's protocol.

8. The conjugates (the corresponding polyclonal antibody) are added to the wells and the samples are incubated at room temperature for the time interval mentioned in the protocol.

9. The wells are washed with the wash buffer using automated plate washer, volume and number of cycles being indicated in the manufacturer's protocol.

10. The substrate solution is added, followed by incubation at room temperature, protected from light, for the time mentioned in the protocol.

11. The stop solution which stops the enzymatic reaction is added, followed by a change of color.

12. The optical density of the samples is assessed using the ELISA plate reader at the specific wavelength for each molecule (usually 450 nm) within 30 min.

3.8 Evaluation of PDL-1 Expression of Tumor Cells (A549 and SK-Mel-1)

The transmembrane protein PDL-1, also called CD274, is expressed on the surface of the tumor cell membranes (of A549 and SK-Mel-1 cell lines) and can be highlighted using fluorescent markers detected by flow cytometry as follows:

3.8.1 Flow Cytometry

1. The tumor cells detached by trypsinization (as described above) are washed with PBS resuspended in cell staining buffer and labeled with anti-PDL-1 antibody combined with the fluorescent dye PE), in concentrations and cell population densities according to the manufacturer.

2. The samples are vortexed and incubated in the dark, on ice, for 20 min.

3. The next steps are two washes with 2 mL of cold staining buffer each (0.5% FCS containing PBS).

4. The cells are resuspended in 500 μL of buffer (0.5% FCS containing PBS) and subjected to flow-cytometry measurements.

5. A number of 10^4 cells are analyzed for each individual sample.

6. The histograms provided by the analysis software show data on the intensity and polarization of the fluorescence emitted by each individual cell and provide quantitative data on the number of PDL-1 positive cells.

3.8.2 Immuno-cytochemistry

1. Fix the tumor cells in 6-well plates with 4% paraformaldehyde for 20 min at room temperature (20–21 °C).

2. Wash the cells three times with PBS.

3. Block the nonspecific binding of the antibodies with 10% BSA (solution in PBS).

4. Wash the cells three times with PBS.

5. Incubate cells with PDL-1 antibody at concentration and incubation time recommended by the manufacturer.

6. Wash the cells three times with PBS.

7. Add the secondary antibody—anti-PDL-1 labeled with PE—and incubate for another 30 min at room temperature.

8. Wash the cells three times with PBS.

9. Mount the wells with DAPI medium and visualize in fluorescence, with an inverted microscope, using the filters 546 nm for PE and 346 nm for DAPI.

10. Images are taken with a color camera and analyzed with an imaging software.

11. Perform statistical analysis with an appropriate software.

3.9 Flow-Cytometry Analysis of CTLs

The CTLs from the cocultures with tumor cells are analyzed for the expression of PD-1 and activation markers expression as follows:

1. The antibodies conjugated with fluorochromes (FITC, PE, and APC) are placed in flow-cytometry tubes (5–20 μL, depending on the type of the antibody, according to the manufacturer's recommendations). The following combinations are used:

   • PD-1 FITC/CD40 PE/CD 95APC.

   • Ox40 FITC/PDL-1 PE/KRGL APC.

   • CD25 FITC/ GITR PE/ CTLA-4.

2. Add the cell suspension (10^5 cells/sample) and incubate for 30 min, at 4 °C.

3. The next steps are two washes with cold PBS through centrifugation (5 min at 157 rcf).

4. The analysis is performed on a flow-cytometer with 6 colors and appropriate software.

5. The histograms provided by the analysis software show data on the intensity and polarization of the fluorescence emitted by each individual cell and provide quantitative data on the number of PD-1 positive and activated CTLs.

4   Notes

1. Irradiation of the cells.

   – In order to deliver a homogeneous dose to all cells, the parameters of irradiation (energy, field, source-cell distance, depth, and time) should be chosen in accordance with the irradiation machine, the type of radiation (photons/electrons), the energy of the radiation beam, the dimensions of the cell container used, and the thickness of the layer of liquid (medium) that covers the cells.

– If the container is not completely filled with liquid, an adjustment for the built-up region is necessary by using a bolus (a material that has properties equivalent to tissue when irradiated, i.e., polylactic acid, polystyrene, or silica gel). The thickness of bolus applied is dependent on the cell dose required and on the angle of incidence of the radiation beams.

2. Magnetic cell sorting.

– Keep cells and all solutions cold, where indicated; higher temperatures may lead to unspecific cell labeling.

– Adapt the buffer volume to the cells number: larger numbers of cells require larger buffer volume; the maximum cell concentration is 10^8 cells/500 µL of buffer solution.

– To increase purity of the positive fraction, cells can be separated a second time over a new positive selection column.

3. Fluorescent microscopy.

– Perform gentle trypsinization or other detachment method in order to avoid the damage to the cell membranes leading to false positive results.

– For the evaluation of the cellular death of tumor cells use the pellet resulted from the centrifugation of the supernatant as well.

– Keep cells and all solutions cold, where indicated; higher temperatures may lead to unspecific cell labeling.

– Proceed to analyze the stained cells as soon as possible.

– High positivity in untreated controls can occur due to the fact that most cell populations have a low percentage of cells that are positive for apoptosis even without apoptosis inducting treatments. This basal level should be subtracted from the values read for the treated cells to obtain the percentage of cells induced to undergo apoptosis by the treatment.

4. Flow cytometry.

– Keep cells and all solutions cold, where indicated; higher temperatures may lead to unspecific cell labeling.

– Make sure to use the proper settings for the flow cytometer.

– *No or low signal* can be caused by degraded or expired antibodies. Make sure they are properly stored and not expired; avoid the fading of fluorescence by keeping the antibodies away from light; use the proper antibody concentrations for your experiment; the target antigen expression may be too low, thus the use of a positive control is needed; surface antigens can be internalized if not performing the experiment with the right technique using ice cold reagents; bleaching can be avoided by reading the samples immediately after staining or by fixation with paraformaldehyde; use bright fluorochromes and make sure the secondary antibody is specific against the species of the primary antibody.

– *Excess signal* may occur as a result of too high antibody concentrations—use positive and negative controls; unbound antibodies may remain if not washing properly; high expressing antigen paired with a bright fluorochrome.

– *High background (nonspecific staining)*—requires proper washing after every incubation step; avoiding the staining of non-specific cells by blocking Fc receptors with Fc blockers (BSA, FBS) before the primary antibody.

5. ELISA.

– *Weak or no signal*—store the reagents as indicated by the producer, check the expiration dates. Allow the reagents to reach room temperature at the start of the assay. Follow the protocol provided with the kit. Use the recommended wavelength.

– *Excess signal*—can be caused by insufficient washing, or longer incubation times than recommended.

Acknowledgments

This publication is based upon work from COST Action IMMUNO-model, CA21135, supported by COST (European Cooperation in Science and Technology).

References

1. Blankenstein T, Coulie PG et al (2012) The determinants of tumor immunogenicity. Nat Rev Cancer 12(4):307–313

2. Berger MF, Hodis E et al (2012) Melanoma genome sequencing reveals frequent PREX2 mutations. Nature 485:502–506

3. Lawrence MS, Stojanov P et al (2013) Mutational heterogeneity in cancer and the search for new cancer-associated genes. Nature 499: 214–218

4. Reynders K, Illidge T (2015) The abscopal effect of local radiotherapy using immunotherapy to make a rare event clinically relevant. Cancer Treat Rev 41(6):503–510

5. Belardelli F, Ferrantini M (2002) Cytokines as a link between innate and adaptive antitumor immunity. Trends Immunol 23:201–208

6. Demaria S, Golden EB, Formenti SC (2015) Role of local radiation therapy in cancer immunotherapy. JAMA Oncol 1(9):1325–1332

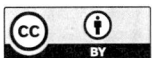

Chapter 9

Implementing Photodynamic Therapy to Activate the IFN-1 Pathway in Melanoma Cells: A Protocol for Inducing Immunogenic Cell Death and Enhancing Dendritic Cell Maturation

Fátima María Mentucci, Agustina Ercole, Natalia Belén Rumie Vittar, and María Julia Lamberti

Abstract

This chapter outlines a detailed protocol for employing photodynamic therapy (PDT) to induce immunogenic cell death (ICD) in melanoma cells, specifically targeting the type-I-interferons (IFN-1) signaling pathway. Recent studies have highlighted the role of IFN-1 in the immune response against cancer, acting as novel damage-associated molecular patterns (DAMPs) that bridge innate and adaptive immunity. Our approach utilizes methyl-aminolevulinate (Me-ALA) to induce the production of endogenous photosensitizer protoporphyrin IX (PpIX), which preferentially accumulates in the endoplasmic reticulum (ER). Activation of PpIX through visible light irradiation triggers oxidative stress-induced apoptotic cell death. This chapter provides a step-by-step guide to replicate these conditions, which have been shown to significantly upregulate IFN-α/β transcripts in B16-OVA melanoma cells, leading to enhanced expression of GMP-AMP synthase (cGAS) and interferon-stimulated genes (ISGs) like CXCL10, MX1, and ISG15. We further discuss the consequential IFN-1-dependent-phenotypic maturation of monocyte-derived dendritic cells (DCs), evidenced by increased expression of co-stimulatory molecules such as CD80 and MHC-II and enhanced tumor-directed chemotaxis. By detailing the protocol for this novel application of PDT, this chapter aims to facilitate its integration into immunotherapy regimens, providing a comprehensive toolkit for researchers and clinicians aiming to harness the antitumor potential of the IFN-1 pathway.

Key words IFNAR, Tumor immunology, Cancer, Immunotherapy, Me-ALA

1 Introduction

Melanoma is a highly aggressive form of skin cancer characterized by its rapid progression and high metastatic potential [1]. Despite advances in conventional treatments such as surgery, chemotherapy, and radiotherapy, the prognosis for advanced melanoma remains poor [1]. Over the past decade, immunotherapy has emerged as a promising strategy for melanoma treatment,

Sweta Rani and Lukasz Skalniak (eds.), *IMMUNO-model in Cancer: Methods and Protocols*, Methods in Molecular Biology, vol. 2959, https://doi.org/10.1007/978-1-0716-4734-9_9, © The Author(s) 2026

harnessing the body's immune system to target and eliminate cancer cells [2]. Melanoma is particularly suitable for immunotherapy due to its high immunogenicity, largely attributed to its significant antigen burden [3, 4]. Notable among these therapies are immune checkpoint inhibitors, which have significantly improved survival rates in melanoma patients. However, a substantial proportion of patients do not respond to these treatments, highlighting the need for novel therapeutic strategies [5, 6].

One promising approach is the induction of ICD, a form of cell death that stimulates an immune response against tumor cells. ICD is characterized by the release of DAMPs [7–9]. These DAMPs can be classified into constitutively expressed DAMPs (cDAMPs) like calreticulin (CRT), ATP, and HMGB1, and inducible DAMPs (iDAMPs) [10]. The dendritic cell (DC) population, whose function is to process and present antigens to activate the immune response, is the most stimulated by the DAMPs released during ICD [8].

Not long ago, the IFN-1 pathway was identified as a crucial inducible DAMP in the context of ICD, playing a key role in antitumor immunity [11, 12]. It aids in the recruitment of immune effector cells, enhances antigen presentation, and promotes the development of long-lasting immune memory. IFN-1 production is triggered by various stimuli, including viral infections and nucleic acid ligands, involving the activation of pattern recognition receptors (PRRs) and cytoplasmic sensors like cGAS. This cascade leads to the activation of transcription factors, such as IRFs and NF-κB, and their downstream signaling via IFNAR1/2 receptors, culminating in the production of IFN-α and IFN-β, and other ISGs [11, 13–15]. Upon induction by ICD, IFN-1 mediates antitumor immunity by promoting the recruitment of immune effector cells, enhancing antigen presentation, and establishing lasting immune memory [10].

In our previous study, we investigated the potential of PDT to induce ICD in melanoma cells [16]. PDT is a minimally invasive treatment that uses photosensitizing agents and visible light to produce reactive oxygen species (ROS), leading to cell death [17, 18]. We utilized Me-ALA to induce the production of the endogenous photosensitizer PpIX, which accumulated preferentially in the ER of B16-OVA murine melanoma cells [16]. ICD inducers can be classified into two categories: type I or II. Type I inducers, such as doxorubicin and mitoxantrone, induce ICD-associated immunogenicity through secondary ER stress effects. In contrast, type II inducers, like hypericin-mediated PDT, selectively target the ER, causing ER-focused ROS formation, loss of ER homeostasis, and rapid activation of danger signaling pathways that elicit DAMPs. Type II inducers are generally more effective at inducing ICD and generating a robust antitumor

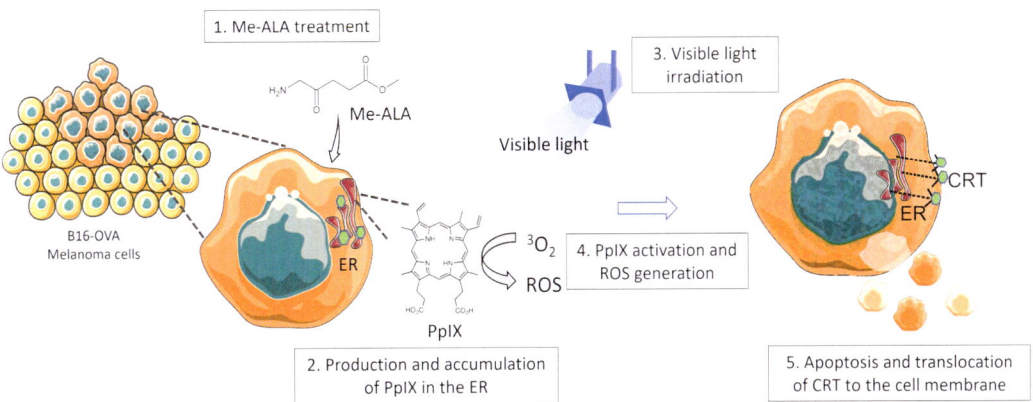

Fig. 1 Experimental workflow for photodynamic therapy-induced immunogenic cell death in melanoma. Cell culture and treatment protocol: B16-OVA melanoma cells were cultured and treated with methyl-aminolevulinate (Me-ALA) to induce the production of protoporphyrin IX (PpIX), which preferentially accumulates in the endoplasmic reticulum (ER). Cells were then exposed to visible light to activate PpIX and generate reactive oxygen species (ROS), leading to oxidative stress, apoptotic cell death, and translocation of CRT to the cell membrane

immune response, making them valuable tools in cancer immunotherapy [19]. Given that the photosensitizer we studied localizes in the ER, it can be proposed as a type II ICD inducer.

Upon activation with visible light, PpIX generates ROS, causing oxidative stress and apoptotic cell death linked to CRT translocation to the surface (Fig. 1).

Our findings demonstrated for the first time a significant upregulation of IFN-1 signaling in B16-OVA melanoma cells, marked by increased transcription of IFN-α/β, cGAS, and ISGs such as CXCL10, MX1, and ISG15 [16]. This chapter builds on these findings by providing a detailed protocol for employing PDT to activate the IFN-1 pathway and induce ICD in melanoma cells (Fig. 2). To investigate the role of the IFN-1 pathway, we utilized C57BL/6 mice, syngeneic for B16-OVA, including wild-type (WT) and IFNAR$^{-/-}$ mice, to elucidate the implications of the IFN-1 pathway. DCs were derived from hematopoietic stem cells obtained from the bone marrow (BM) of these mice through granulocyte-macrophage colony-stimulating factor (GM-CSF) stimulation. We describe methods for assessing the phenotypic maturation of BM-derived WT and IFNAR$^{-/-}$ DCs, including the evaluation of co-stimulatory molecules and tumor-directed chemotaxis [16] (Fig. 3).

By presenting this comprehensive protocol outlining the step-by-step procedures, we aim to facilitate the integration of PDT-induced ICD into immunotherapy regimens, offering researchers and clinicians a powerful tool to enhance antitumor immunity.

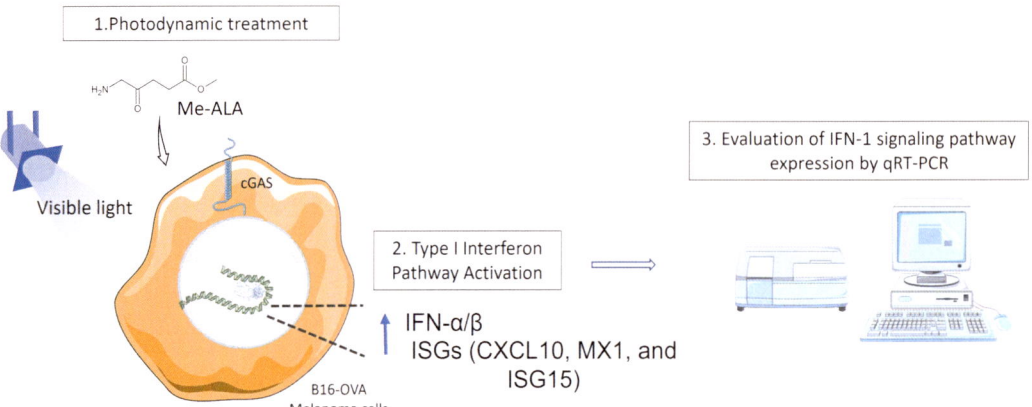

Fig. 2 Experimental workflow for evaluating type I interferon pathway activation. Post-PDT treatment, the expression levels of IFN-α/β, cGAS, and interferon-stimulated genes (ISGs), such as CXCL10, MX1, and ISG15, were quantified using qRT-PCR to evaluate the activation of the IFN-1 signaling pathway

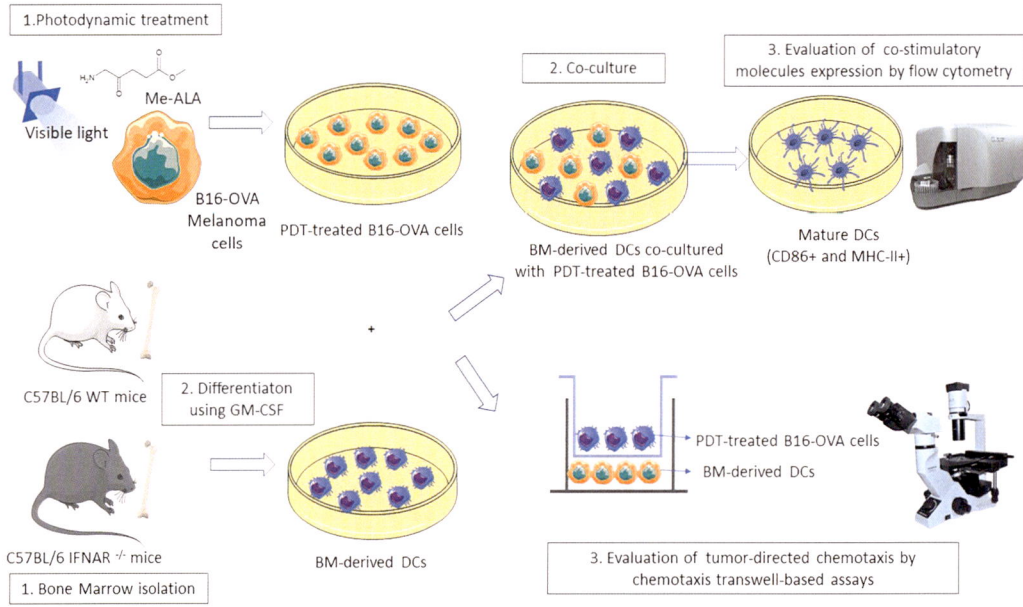

Fig. 3 Experimental workflow for IFN-1-mediated dendritic cell maturation. BM-derived dendritic cells (DCs) were isolated from C57BL/6 WT and IFNAR$^{-/-}$ mice, differentiated by GM-CSF and cocultured with PDT-treated B16-OVA cells to assess phenotypic maturation. The expression of co-stimulatory molecules (CD80 and MHC-II) and tumor-directed chemotaxis were analyzed by flow cytometry and chemotaxis transwell-based assays, respectively

2   Materials

2.1   Cell Culture

1. B16-OVA mouse melanoma cell line [20].

2. 1× phosphate-buffered saline (PBS): 10 g/L ClNa, 0.25 g/L KCl, 0.76 g/L Na_2HPO_4, 0.25 g/L KH_2PO_4. Adjust the pH to 7.2.

3. Trypsin.

4. Growth medium: DMEM (1X Dulbecco's modified Eagle medium high glucose), supplemented with 10% v/v fetal bovine serum (FBS), 1% v/v glutamine (100× GlutaMAX™), 1% v/v antibiotic (10,000 units/ml penicillin–10,000 μg/mL streptomycin), and 1% v/v of 100 mM sodium pyruvate. Adjust the pH to 7.3.

5. Minimal medium (for drug incubation): growth medium without FBS.

2.2   Intracellular Localization Analysis of the Photosensitizer PpIX

1. 24-well plate.

2. FuGENE® HD transfection reagent (Roche Applied Science).

3. pEYFP-Mito plasmid [21], pEYFP-C1-KDEL-GFP plasmid [22] provided by Dr. Sergio Grinstein (University of Toronto, Canada).

4. Photosensitizer prodrug: Me-ALA.

5. 4% Paraformaldehyde (PAF).

6. Hoechst (HÖ) nuclear stain.

7. Confocal microscope.

8. Software: ImageJ 1.42q.

2.3   Photodynamic Treatment (PDT)

1. 96-well plate.

2. Photosensitizer prodrug: Me-ALA (Sigma Aldrich).

3. MultiLED irradiation system [20].

2.4   Cell Viability Assessment Using MTT Assay

1. MTT (1-(4,5-dimethylthiazol-2-yl)-3,5-diphenylformazan) powder dissolved in DMSO.

2. Dimethyl sulfoxide (DMSO).

3. ELISA reader (Thermo Scientific, Multiskan FC) [23].

4. GraphPad Prism software.

5. Evaluation of oxidative stress protocol: N-acetylcysteine (NAC).

6. Evaluation of ER stress-associated cell death protocol: BAPTA-AM.

2.5 Assessment of Cell Death Type Using Annexin V/PI Assay by Flow Cytometry

1. FITC Annexin V Apoptosis Detection Kit II (BD Pharmingen™).
2. Flow cytometer.
3. FlowJo VX 10.0.7 software.

2.6 Calreticulin Localization Assay

1. 24-well plates.
2. pCRT-EGFP (Green fluorescent protein-tagged calreticulin) plasmid [24] kindly provided by Dra. Marta Hallak (CIQUIBIC, Argentina).
3. FuGENE® HD transfection reagent (Roche Applied Science) [25].
4. PDT reagents.
5. Fluorescence microscope (Carl Zeiss) coupled to a high-resolution monochromatic digital camera.
6. Software: ImageJ 1.42q software.

2.7 Analysis of IFN-1 Pathway Expression Using RT-qPCR

1. 60 mm plate.
2. Cell scrapers.
3. 1.5 Eppendorf tubes.
4. RNA extraction: trizol reagent, chloroform, isopropanol, 80% ethanol, nuclease-free sterile water.
5. NanoDrop™ One/OneC Microvolume UV-Vis spectrophotometer.
6. Reverse transcription: M-MLV Reverse Transcriptase kit.
7. Real-time PCR: SYBR Green PCR Master Mix [26].
8. Thermocycler Stratagene MX3000Pro.
9. Real-time PCR primers: The sequences of used primers are specified in Table 1. The specificity of the primers was confirmed using the free platform Primer-BLAST—NCBI-NIH.

2.8 Isolation and Differentiation of Hematopoietic Cells from Bone Marrow of C57BL/6 Mice

1. WT and IFNAR$^{-/-}$ C57BL/6 mice aged 4–6 weeks. WT mice were purchased from Universidad Nacional de La Plata (Buenos Aires, Argentina) and IFNAR$^{-/-}$ were kindly provided by CIBICI-UNC (Cordoba, Argentina, purchased from Jackson Laboratory) [27].
2. Induction chamber for anesthesia: SCIENTIFIC-Estación de Anestesia. Sistemas de Anestesia de No Reinhalación MOD. VITAL-VEN [28, 29].
3. Isoflurane: INELTANO VET Isoflurano USP. RICHMOND VET PHARMA [29].
4. Needles and disinfected surfaces (Styrofoam) for securing mice [30].

Table 1
Primer sequences used for real-time RT-qPCR

Gene	Primer sequence (5′-3′)
GAPDH	Fw: TGCACCACCAACTGCTTAG Rv: GGATGCAGGGATGATGTTC
IFN-α	Fw: TCTGATGCAGCAGGTGGG Rv: AGGGCTCTCCAGACTTCTGCTCTG
IFN-β	Fw: GCACTGGGTGGAATGAGACT Rv: AGTGGAGAGCAGTTGAGGACA
RIG1	Fw: AAGAGCCAGAGTGTCAGAATCT Rv: AGCTCCAGTTGGTAATTTCTTGG
TLR3	Fw: GTGAGATACAACGTAGCTGAACT Rv: TCCTGCATCCAAGATAGCAAGT
MDA5	Fw: AGATCAACACCTGTGGTAACACC Rv: CTCTAGGGCCTCCACGAACA
cGAS	Fw: GAGGCGCGGAAAGTCGTAA Rv: TTGTCCGGTTCCTTCCTGGA
ISG15	Fw: GGTGTCCGTGACTAACTCCAT Rv: TGGAAAGGGTAAGACCGTCCT
CXCL10	Fw: AGTGCTGCCGTCATTTTCTG Rv: ATTCTCACTGGCCCGTCAT
MX1	Fw: AGACTTGCTCTTTCTGAAAAGCC Rv: GACCATAGGGGTCTTGACCAA

5. 50 mL conical tubes.

6. Sterile forceps and scissors.

7. Ethanol (70%).

8. 23G needle.

9. 10 mL syringe.

10. Cell strainer (70 μm nylon membrane).

11. Red blood cell lysis buffer: 0.16 M NH_4Cl, 10 mM $KHCO_3$, and 0.13 mM EDTA, dissolved in sterile H_2O and stored at 4 °C.

12. 10 cm plates.

13. 60 mm plates.

14. Differentiation medium: RPMI medium supplemented with 10% FBS, 1% v/v glutamine (100× GlutaMAXTM), 1% v/v antibiotic (10,000 units/mL penicillin–10,000 μg/mL streptomycin), 1% v/v of 100 mM sodium pyruvate, and GM-CSF (10% v/v J558-conditioned medium) [31].

15. Flow cytometry reagents.

Table 2
Antibodies used in flow cytometry analyses

Antibody	Dilution
Anti-CD11c-APC	1/2000
Anti-MHC-II-PerCP-Cy5.5	1/500
Anti-CD86-PeCy5	1/5000

16. Photosensitized B16-OVA cells.

17. 100 ng/mL Lipopolysaccharide (LPS), from Escherichia coli serotype 0127:B8.

18. FACS buffer (1× PBS, 2% FBS).

19. Centrifuge.

20. The antibodies used are specified in the Table 2.

2.9 Study of the Chemotactic Capacity of Photosensitized Tumor Cells on DCs Using Transwell Cell Migration Assay

1. Differentiated WT and IFNAR$^{-/-}$ DCs, photosensitized B16-OVA cells.

2. Transwell inserts (5 μm pore size).

3. Inverted fluorescence microscope.

3 Methods

3.1 Intracellular Localization Analysis of the Photosensitizer PpIX

1. Plate B16-OVA cells (2×10^4 cells/well) into 24-well plates and allow them to grow overnight until they reach 70–80% confluence.

2. Prepare the transfection mix following the manufacturer's instructions, using a transfection reagent ratio of 2:1 for both the pEYFP-Mito plasmid (mitochondria marker) and the pEYFP-C1-KDEL-GFP (ER marker), depending on the desired organelle marker.

3. Gently homogenize the transfection mixture and incubate at 37 °C for 15 min.

4. Add the transfection mixture dropwise onto the cells in each well.

5. Incubate the transfected cells overnight at 37 °C under culture conditions (5% CO_2).

6. The next day, wash the cells with 1× PBS and replace the growth medium with minimal medium containing 1 mM Me-ALA.

7. Incubate the cells for 4 h at 37 °C, 5% CO_2.

8. Fix the cells by adding 4% PAF and incubate for 20 min at room temperature.

9. Wash the cells with 1X PBS to remove the fixative.

10. Stain the cell nuclei by adding 1 μg/mL HÖ and incubate for 20 min at 37 °C.

11. Perform additional washes with 1× PBS to remove excess HÖ.

12. Acquire images of the fixed and stained cells using confocal microscope.

13. Configure the microscope to observe fluorescence in the following channels: GFP (green), corresponding to mitochondria and ER markers; PpIX (red), corresponding to the photosensitizer; and Hoechst (blue), corresponding to nuclear staining. Colocalization is evidenced in yellow.

14. Import the acquired images into ImageJ 1.42q software. Use the Coloc 2 plugin to perform co-localization analysis.

15. Calculate the Pearson correlation coefficient (R^2) to evaluate the co-localization of PpIX with mitochondria and ER (*see* **Note 1**).

3.2 Photodynamic Treatment (PDT)

1. Plate B16-OVA cells (5×10^5 cells/mL) in 96-well plates.

2. After 24 h, wash with 1× PBS and incubate the cells with increasing concentrations of the prodrug Me-ALA (0–0.3 mM) in a medium supplemented without FBS for 4 h to allow the formation of PpIX, an endogenous photosensitizer, and its accumulation in the ER.

3. Expose the cells to visible light irradiation (λ: 635 nm ± 17 nm, light dose: 0.5 J/cm^2).

4. Replace the medium with a growth medium.

3.3 Cell Viability Assessment Using MTT Assay

1. Add 10 μL of MTT solution (5 mg/mL in 1× PBS) to each well and incubate at 37 °C for 3 h in the dark.

2. Aspirate the media gently from the wells to avoid disturbing the cells or the formazan crystals.

3. Add 100 μL of DMSO to lyse the cells and solubilize the formazan product.

4. Measure absorbance using an ELISA reader at a wavelength of 540 nm. Absorbance is considered directly proportional to the percentage of living cells.

5. Create dose-response curves by applying nonlinear regression to the data using GraphPad Prism software (*see* **Note 2**).

3.4 Evaluation of Oxidative Stress

1. Incubate B16-OVA cells with Me-ALA (0.1, 0.2, and 0.3 mM) in the presence or absence of NAC (5 mM) for 4 h.

2. Expose the cells to irradiation at a dose of 0.5 J/cm^2.

3. Evaluate the effect of this treatment on cell viability as described in Subheading 3.3 (*see* **Note 3**).

3.5 Evaluation of ER Stress-Associated Cell Death

1. Incubate B16-OVA cells with Me-ALA (0.3 mM) in the presence or absence of BAPTA-AM (1 μM) for 4 h.

2. Expose the cells to irradiation at a dose of 0.5 J/cm^2.

3. The effect of this treatment on cell viability was assessed as described in Subheading 3.3 (*see* **Note 3**).

3.6 Assessment of Type of Cell Death Using Annexin V/PI Assay by Flow Cytometry

1. At 24 h post-PDT, detach the cells by trypsinization.

2. Wash with 1× PBS and centrifuge at 2000 × *g* at 4 °C for 10 min.

3. Incubate the pellet with 5 μg/mL annexin V-FITC, 5 μg/m propidium iodide (PI) and binding buffer for 15 min at room temperature in the dark.

4. Quantify annexin V and PI fluorescence using a flow cytometer. The identification of different cellular populations is conducted using the following criteria: viable cells (annexin V−/PI−), early apoptotic cells (annexin V+/PI−), and late apoptotic or secondarily necrotic cells (annexin V+/PI+).

5. Analyze the data using FlowJo VX 10.0.7 software (*see* **Note 4**).

3.7 Calreticulin Localization Assay

1. Plate B16-OVA cells (5 × 10^5 cells/mL) in 24-well plates.

2. After 24 h, transfect the cells with the following transfection-mix: pCRT-EGFP [24] and FuGENE® HD, according to the manufacturer's instructions.

3. The next day, wash twice with 1× PBS and perform the photodynamic treatment with the following conditions: 0.3 mM Me-ALA for 4 h and irradiation with a light dose of 0.5 J/cm^2 (*see* **Note 5**).

4. Observe CRT localization using an inverted fluorescence microscope.

5. Analyze the images using the free software ImageJ 1.42q (*see* **Note 6**).

3.8 Analysis of IFN-1 Pathway Expression Using RT-qPCR

1. Plate the tumor cells (5 × 10^5 cells) in 60 mm diameter dishes.

2. The next day, subject the cells to lethal photosensitization conditions (0.3 mM Me-ALA + light dose: 0.5 J/cm^2) (*see* **Note 5**).

3. At 1-, 5-, and 14-h posttreatment, wash with 1X PBS and proceed with RNA extraction.

4. Add 100 μL of Trizol and scrape the monolayer with a spatula. Collect the contents in a 1.5 mL tube.

5. Incubate for 15 min at room temperature to allow digestion.

6. Add 40 μL of chloroform, gently shake, and incubate for 10 min at room temperature.

7. Centrifuge at 17,000 × g at 4 °C for 20 min.

8. Transfer the aqueous phase to a new tube.

9. Add 200 μL of isopropanol, invert the tube to mix, and incubate at room temperature for 5 min.

10. Centrifuge at 17,000 × g at 4 °C for 20 min. Discard the supernatant.

11. Wash the pellet with 300 μL of 80% ethanol.

12. Centrifuge at 17,000 × g at 4 °C for 5 min. Discard the supernatant.

13. Allow the RNA pellet to air-dry for 5–10 min at room temperature.

14. Dissolve the RNA in nuclease-free sterile water.

15. Quantify the extracted RNA using NanoDrop.

16. Proceed with reverse transcription using the M-MLV reverse transcriptase kit (200 U/L). Prepare the following mix: 1 μg RNA, 2 μL buffer, 0.8 μL dNTP, 2 μL random primers, 1 μL MMLV, and the necessary amount of nuclease-free water.

17. Prepare the mix for the real-time PCR reaction according to the iTaq Universal SYBR Green Supermix kit protocol: 5 μL SYBR, 0.2 μL of each primer (20 μM), nuclease-free water (to a final volume of 10 μL), 0.15 μL Rox, and 1 μL cDNA. The primers for IFN-1α, IFN-1β, receptors MDA-5, TLR3, RIG-1, and cGAS, and the IFN-stimulated genes CXCL10, ISG15, and MX1 are specified in Subheading 2.

18. Perform the real-time PCR reaction using the Stratagene MX3000Pro thermocycler.

19. Calculate the change in gene expression using the $2^{-\Delta\Delta Ct}$ method. Normalize mRNA levels to the expression of the housekeeping gene GAPDH (*see* **Note** 7).

3.9 Isolation and Differentiation of Hematopoietic Cells from Bone Marrow of C57BL/6 Mice

For the protocol, WT and IFNAR$^{-/-}$ C57BL/6 (lacks type I IFN receptor function) mice, male or female, aged 4–6 weeks, weighing 120–200 g are used. Male mice are preferred due to their larger bones, which yield a higher number of progenitor cells [32]. Euthanasia techniques involve cervical dislocation following the anesthesia and euthanasia guidelines recommended by COEDI-UNRC [33].

3.9.1 Euthanizing Mice and Extracting Bones [30]

Note: These steps can be performed outside a laminar flow hood, as the sterility of bone marrow is maintained.

1. Anesthetize the mice with 3% isoflurane in 99.9% O_2 at 1 L/min in an induction chamber [29].

2. Euthanize mice using cervical dislocation.

3. Sterilize the abdomen by spraying with 70% ethanol and secure the animal on a disinfected surface (e.g., Styrofoam) by its limbs using needles.

4. Open the abdominal cavity with sterile scissors and remove the muscles from both hind limbs to expose the hip joints.

5. Cut the hind legs above the hip joint using sharp, sterile scissors and hold the limb by the tibia with forceps.

6. To extract the tibia, cut below the tibia-metatarsal joint. To extract the femur, cut below the knee joint. Remove muscles from the bones and place the cleaned bones in sterile 1× PBS.

7. Transfer to the cell culture room for sample manipulation in a biosafety cabinet.

3.9.2 Bone Marrow Extraction [30]

Note: This section must be conducted under sterile conditions within a laminar flow hood, using sterile items that can be dipped in 70% ethanol to maintain sterility.

1. Immerse bones in 70% ethanol for 2 min.

2. Cut off both ends (epiphyses) of the tibias and femurs.

3. For bone marrow extraction, use a 23-gauge needle and a 10-mL syringe filled with cold 1× PBS. Insert the needle into the bone marrow cavity and flush out with cold 1X PBS to wash thoroughly.

4. Pass the suspension through a 70 μm nylon membrane cell strainer into a collection tube. Note: If cell recovery yield is significantly low, for example, $<1 \times 10^7$ cells, scrape the inner surface of bones with the needle and rinse with an additional 5 mL of 1× PBS.

5. Pass the bone marrow through the cell strainer filter using the syringe plunger and 5 mL of 1× PBS. Wash the strainer with another ~5 mL of 1× PBS.

6. Resuspend the cell pellet with red blood cell lysis buffer (1 mL per mouse).

7. Incubate for 5 min at room temperature or 2 min at 37 °C. Neutralize the lysis buffer by adding 5 mL of FBS.

3.9.3 Differentiation of Bone Marrow-Derived DCs

1. Centrifuge cells at 1500 rpm for 7 min at 4 °C. Discard the supernatant and resuspend in growth medium.

2. Count viable cells using a Neubauer chamber and seed at a density of 3×10^6 cells per 10 cm plate in a complete differentiation medium in the presence of different concentrations (10% and 30%) of J558 cell-conditioned medium [31]. These cells produce granulocyte-macrophage colony-stimulating factor (GM-CSF) required for differentiation of bone marrow-derived hematopoietic stem cells into BMDCs.

3. Add 10 mL of the corresponding differentiation medium 72 h after cell isolation. Replace 10 mL of medium 72 h later.

4. After 24 h, collect adherent and nonadherent DCs with warm 1× PBS using scrapers.

5. Determine the percentage of differentiated DCs by flow cytometry through the analysis of the CD11c marker.

6. Analyze the data using FlowJo VX 10.0.7 software (*see* **Note 8**).

3.10 Maturation of DCs by Pulsing with Photosensitized Tumor Cells

1. Seed B16-OVA cells (5×10^5 cells) in 60 mm plates. Simultaneously, seed BMDCs cells (5×10^5 cells) derived from WT C57BL/6 in nonadherent 24-well plates in differentiation medium (as described in Subheading 2.8.14).

2. The next day, perform the photodynamic treatment on B16-OVA: incubate with 0.3 mM Me-ALA for 4 h and then irradiate with visible light (λ: 635 nm ± 17 nm, light dose: 0.5 J/cm^2).

3. Immediately after PDT, detach the photosensitized tumor cells using trypsin. Place the cell pellet into the wells of a 24-well plate where BMDCs are growing in their medium. Coculture both populations at different ratios (1:1, 1:3, and 1:5 DCs: B16-OVA for 24 h. Use 1 µg/mL of LPS for 24 h as a positive control for DC maturation.

4. After 24 h, collect cells in a 1.5 mL tube and centrifuge at 2000 rpm at 4 °C for 5 min.

5. Wash twice with 1× PBS.

6. Perform surface staining of DCs using standard protocols. To determine the percentage of differentiated DCs, use CD11c marker analysis. To assess DCs maturation by analyzing the percentage expressing the activation marker CD86 and its intensity of fluorescence by flow cytometry. Add the appropriate amount of antibody to each tube as recommended by the manufacturer in FACS buffer.

7. Incubate tubes on ice for 20 min, protected from light.

8. Add 200 µL of FACS buffer (1× PBS, 2% FBS).

9. Centrifuge at 2000 rpm at 4 °C for 5 min.

10. Resuspend the pellet in 200 µL of FACS buffer.

11. Determine the percentage of differentiated CD11c + DCs by flow cytometry. Within the CD11c + population, determine the percentage of mature/activated DCs using CD86 maturation marker and its fluorescence intensity.

12. Analyze the data using FlowJo VX 10.0.7 software (*see* **Note 8**).

3.11   Evaluation of the Implication of the IFN-1 Pathway in DC Phenotypic Maturation

1. Coculture photosensitized tumor cells with WT BMDCs or IFNAR$^{-/-}$ BMDCs at a 1:1 ratio, following the procedure described in Subheading 3.10.

2. After 24 h, collect cells in a 1.5 mL tube and centrifuge at 2000 rpm at 4 °C for 5 min.

3. Wash twice with 1× PBS.

4. Perform surface staining of DCs using standard protocols. To determine the percentage of differentiated DCs, use CD11c marker analysis. To assess DCs' maturation by analyzing the percentage expressing the activation markers CD86 and MHC-II, and their intensity of fluorescence by flow cytometry.

5. Add the appropriate amount of antibody to each tube as recommended by the manufacturer in FACS buffer. Incubate tubes on ice for 20 min, protected from light.

6. Add 200 μL of FACS buffer (1× PBS, 2% FBS).

7. Centrifuge at 2000 rpm at 4 °C for 5 min.

8. Resuspend the pellet in 200 μL of FACS buffer.

9. Determine the percentage of differentiated CD11c + DCs by flow cytometry. Within the CD11c + population, determine the percentage of mature/activated DCs using CD86 and MHC-II maturation marker and its fluorescence intensity.

10. Analyze the data using FlowJo VX 10.0.7 software (*see* **Note 9**).

3.12   Study of the Chemotactic Capacity of Photosensitized Tumor Cells on DCs Using Transwell Cell Migration Assay

1. Seed B16-OVA cells (3×10^4 cells/well) into 24-well plates. Consider three conditions:

   (a) Control: No cells were seeded.

   (b) Tumor cells: Cells without photodynamic treatment.

   (c) PDT tumor cells: Cells with photodynamic treatment.

2. The next day, perform photodynamic treatment by incubating cells with 0.3 mM Me-ALA for 4 h, followed by irradiation with visible light (λ: 635 nm ± 17 nm, light dose: 0.5 J/cm^2).

3. Immediately after the photodynamic treatment, place 5 μm pore transwells in each well.

4. Seed 2×10^5 WT or IFNAR$^{-/-}$ DCs in the upper chamber of each transwell. Incubate for 16 h.

5. Fix the DCs that migrated through the membrane with 4% PAF for 15 min at 37 °C.

6. Wash the cells with 1× PBS to remove the fixative.

7. Stain the nuclei with HÖ 1 µg/mL for 1 h at 37 °C.

8. Perform additional washes with 1× PBS to remove excess HÖ.

9. Take fluorescence microscope images and perform DCs counting based on the images.

10. Import the acquired images into ImageJ 1.42q software. Migrating cells were counted in different fields of view (*see* **Note 10**).

4 Notes

1. PpIX preferentially accumulated in the ER after 4 h of incubation with Me-ALA. Using Pearson's correlation coefficient (R^2) to measure the degree of co-localization, we found a higher accumulation of PpIX in the ER ($R^2 = 0.934$) compared to mitochondria ($R^2 = 0.643$). The localization of PpIX in the ER suggests that cell damage may initiate and concentrate in this organelle following irradiation. These preliminary results indicate that Me-ALA PDT could potentially induce type II ICD.

2. PDT reduced the viability of murine melanoma cells. The dose-response curve showed a proportional decrease in cell viability with increasing doses of Me-ALA, indicating photodynamic activity and cellular sensitivity. Since PDT specificity relies on the combined action of three components (PS, light, and O_2), damage caused by any single component negates its potential application, as each must be harmless alone. Consequently, significant inhibition of tumor cell proliferation occurred only when cells were incubated with Me-ALA and then irradiated. The lethal dose 50 (LD50), defined as the concentration of the substance required to kill 50% of the cell population, was 1.54 ± 0.01 mM.

3. PDT triggered ER stress-associated cell death. The antioxidant NAC reversed PDT's cytotoxic effect at high doses, indicating oxidative stress-induced cell death. Moreover, preincubation of melanoma cells with the calcium chelator BAPTA-AM inhibited PDT-induced cell death, highlighting ER stress linked to the photodynamic effect.

4. PDT induced apoptosis in murine melanoma cells. Results showed that 24 h posttreatment, the percentage of apoptotic cells increased proportionally with the concentration of Me-ALA. Correspondingly, the percentage of viable cells decreased as the concentration of this prodrug increased.

5. Recent advances in apoptotic cell death have shifted understanding away from the belief that apoptotic cells undergo silent demise via rapid phagocytosis without an immune response. Instead, the emergence of ICD highlights that dying apoptotic cells actively release DAMPs, crucial in cancer therapy by engaging the immune system. Photodynamic therapy's efficacy varies based on photosensitizer type, cellular localization, cell type, oxygen levels, and PDT dosage, potentially inducing apoptosis or necrosis. Both outcomes lead to the release of tumor antigens recognized by DCs, and PDT triggers an immediate inflammatory response with proinflammatory cytokines. Recent studies suggest using lethal conditions to induce high apoptotic cell death rates, enhancing immunogenic responses during photodynamic therapy. Therefore, we chose lethal conditions: 0.3 mM Me-ALA and a light dose of 0.5 J/cm^2, aiming for over 80% cell death within 24 h posttreatment, aligning with these insights and experimental protocols.

6. Significant translocation of CRT from the ER to the plasma membrane was observed. Specifically, 72.3% of photosensitized melanoma cells exhibited typical "patches" of CRT intracellular anterograde transport, suggesting PDT's influence on CRT mobilization.

7. Photodynamic therapy induced IFN-1α, IFN-1β, cGAS, CXCL10, ISG15, and MX1 expression in murine melanoma cells. A statistically significant increase in these gene expressions was observed at 5 h posttreatment, highlighting for the first time the autocrine induction of the IFN-1 pathway by PDT. The involvement of cGAS in the modulation of the IFN-1 pathway was later corroborated in a subsequent study using the specific inhibitor H151 [34].

8. Hematopoietic stem cells derived from bone marrow were incubated with two concentrations of conditioned medium from J558 cells (10% and 30%). Both the adhered and non-adhered populations were evaluated. The adhered cells incubated with 10% of J558 CM exhibited a high percentage of CD11c marker expression, confirming their identity as DCs. These conditions were used to obtain DCs for subsequent assays. Coincubation of tumor cells and DCs at a 1:1 ratio significantly enhanced DC maturation, as indicated by increased CD86+ cell percentages and elevated CD86 expression (geometric mean of fluorescence intensity). These results conclusively demonstrated the potent capability of photosensitized B16-OVA cells to induce efficient DC maturation.

9. DC maturation induced by photosensitized tumor cells was dependent on IFN-1 signaling. The absence of IFNAR

partially attenuated maturation induced by both LPS and photosensitized tumor cells, underscoring the pivotal role of the IFN-1 pathway in the immunogenic activation of this immune cell population.

10. Migration of DCs induced by photosensitized tumor cells depended on IFN-1 signaling. A statistically significant increase in migratory WT DCs towards the photosensitized tumor stimulus compared to IFNAR$^{-/-}$ counterparts was observed. This highlights the impact of IFN-1 release from photodynamic treatment on the chemotactic ability of melanoma cells.

Acknowledgments

This publication is based upon work from COST Action IMMUNO-model, CA21135, supported by COST (European Cooperation in Science and Technology). This work was supported by the Florencio Fiorini para Investigación en Ciencias Biomédicas grant, PICT-2021-GRFTI-00393, PICTO CBA 00034/2022, PIBAA-CONICET, Jóvenes en Ciencia—MinCyT-Cba grants, and COST Action IMMUNO-model CA21135.

References

1. Long GV, Swetter SM, Menzies AM et al (2023) Cutaneous melanoma. Lancet 402: 485–502. https://doi.org/10.1016/S0140-6736(23)00821-8

2. Huang AC, Zappasodi R (2022) A decade of checkpoint blockade immunotherapy in melanoma: understanding the molecular basis for immune sensitivity and resistance. Nat Immunol 23:660–670. https://doi.org/10.1038/S41590-022-01141-1

3. Chalmers ZR, Connelly CF, Fabrizio D et al (2017) Analysis of 100,000 human cancer genomes reveals the landscape of tumor mutational burden. Genome Med 9:1–14. https://doi.org/10.1186/s13073-017-0424-2

4. Mahumud RA, Shahjalal M (2022) The emerging burden of genetic instability and mutation in melanoma: role of molecular mechanisms. Cancers (Basel) 14. https://doi.org/10.3390/CANCERS14246202

5. An Q, Liu Z (2019) Comparative efficacy and safety of combination therapies for advanced melanoma: a network meta-analysis. BMC Cancer 19:43. https://doi.org/10.1186/S12885-018-5259-8

6. Tong J, Kartolo A, Yeung C et al (2022) Long-term toxicities of immune checkpoint inhibitor (ICI) in melanoma patients. Curr Oncol 29: 7953–7963. https://doi.org/10.3390/curroncol29100629

7. Galluzzi L, Agostinis P, Vitale I et al (2020) Consensus guidelines for the definition, detection and interpretation of immunogenic cell death. J Immunother Cancer 8:e000337. https://doi.org/10.1136/jitc-2019-000337

8. Lamberti M, Nigro A, Mentucci F et al (2020) Dendritic cells and immunogenic cancer cell death: a combination for improving antitumor immunity. Pharmaceutics 256:3

9. Galluzzi L, Kepp O, Hett E et al (2023) Immunogenic cell death in cancer: concept and therapeutic implications. J Transl Med 21:162. https://doi.org/10.1186/S12967-023-04017-6

10. Yatim N, Cullen S, Albert M (2017) Dying cells actively regulate adaptive immune responses. Nat Rev Immunol 17:262–275. https://doi.org/10.1038/nri.2017.9

11. Musella M, Manic G, de Maria R et al (2017) Type-I-interferons in infection and cancer: unanticipated dynamics with therapeutic implications. Onco Targets Ther 6:e1314424. https://doi.org/10.1080/2162402X.2017.1314424

12. Sistigu A, Yamazaki T, Vacchelli E et al (2014) Cancer cell-autonomous contribution of type I interferon signaling to the efficacy of chemotherapy. Nat Med 20:1301–1309

13. Zitvogel L, Galluzzi L, Kepp O et al (2015) Type I interferons in anticancer immunity. Nat Rev Immunol 15:405–414. https://doi.org/10.1038/nri3845

14. Vacchelli E, Sistigu A, Yamazaki T et al (2015) Autocrine signaling of type 1 interferons in successful anticancer chemotherapy. Onco Targets Ther 4:e988042

15. Ivashkiv L, Donlin L (2014) Regulation of type I interferon responses. Nat Rev Immunol 14: 36–49

16. Lamberti M, Mentucci F, Roselli E et al (2019) Photodynamic modulation of type 1 interferon pathway on melanoma cells promotes dendritic cell activation. Front Immunol 10:2614. https://doi.org/10.3389/fimmu.2019.02614

17. Milla Sanabria L, Rodríguez MEM, Cogno ISI et al (2013) Direct and indirect photodynamic therapy effects on the cellular and molecular components of the tumor microenvironment. Biochim Biophys Acta 1835:36–45. https://doi.org/10.1016/j.bbcan.2012.10.001

18. Rumie Vittar N, Lamberti M, Pansa M et al (2013) Ecological photodynamic therapy: new trend to disrupt the intricate networks within tumor ecosystem. Biochim Biophys Acta 1835: 86–89

19. Krysko D, Garg A, Kaczmarek A et al (2012) Immunogenic cell death and DAMPs in cancer therapy. Nat Rev Cancer 12:860–875

20. Lamberti MJ, Pansa MF, Vera RE et al (2017) Transcriptional activation of HIF-1 by a ROS-ERK axis underlies the resistance to photodynamic therapy. PLoS One 12:e0177801. https://doi.org/10.1371/journal.pone.0177801

21. Duarte A, Poderoso C, Cooke M et al (2012) Mitochondrial fusion is essential for steroid biosynthesis. PLoS One 7:e45829. https://doi.org/10.1371/journal.pone.0045829

22. Fairn GD, Schieber NL, Ariotti N et al (2011) High-resolution mapping reveals topologically distinct cellular pools of phosphatidylserine. J Cell Biol 194:257–275. https://doi.org/10.1083/jcb.201012028

23. Lamberti M, Rumie Vittar N, de Carvalho da Silva F et al (2013) Synergistic enhancement of antitumor effect of β-Lapachone by photodynamic induction of quinone oxidoreductase (NQO1). Phytomedicine 20:1007–1012

24. Goitea VE, Hallak ME (2015) Calreticulin and Arginylated Calreticulin have different susceptibilities to proteasomal degradation. J Biol Chem 290:16403–16414. https://doi.org/10.1074/jbc.M114.626127

25. Cogno IS, Vittar NBR, Lamberti MJ, Rivarola VA (2011) Optimization of photodynamic therapy response by survivin gene knockdown in human metastatic breast cancer T47D cells. J Photochem Photobiol B 104:434–443. https://doi.org/10.1016/j.jphotobiol.2011.05.001

26. Lamberti MJ, Morales Vasconsuelo AB, Chiaramello M et al (2018) NQO1 induction mediated by photodynamic therapy synergizes with β-Lapachone-halogenated derivative against melanoma. Biomed Pharmacother 108:1553–1564

27. Gatti G, Nuñez NG, Nocera DA et al (2013) Direct effect of ds <scp>RNA</scp> mimetics on cancer cells induces endogenous <scp>IFN</scp> −β production capable of improving dendritic cell function. Eur J Immunol 43:1849–1861. https://doi.org/10.1002/eji.201242902

28. https://www.herlam.com.ar/es#products

29. Caverzán MD, Oliveda PM, Beaugé L et al (2023) Metronomic photodynamic therapy with conjugated polymer nanoparticles in glioblastoma tumor microenvironment. Cells 12: 1541. https://doi.org/10.3390/cells12111541

30. Liu X, Quan N (2015) Immune cell isolation from mouse femur bone marrow. Bio Protoc 5: e1631. https://doi.org/10.21769/BioProtoc.1631

31. Lamberti MJ, Mentucci FM, Roselli E et al (2019) Photodynamic modulation of type 1 interferon pathway on melanoma cells promotes dendritic cell activation. Front Immunol 10:2614. https://doi.org/10.3389/fimmu.2019.02614

32. Inaba K, Swiggard WJ, Steinman RM et al (2009) Isolation of dendritic cells. Curr Protoc Immunol 86. https://doi.org/10.1002/0471142735.im0307s86

33. https://www.unrc.edu.ar/unrc/coedi/docs/guia-anestesia-eutanasia.pdf

34. Mentucci FM, Romero Nuñez EA, Ercole A et al (2024) Impact of genomic mutation on melanoma immune microenvironment and IFN-1 pathway-driven therapeutic responses. Cancers (Basel) 16:2568. https://doi.org/10.3390/cancers16142568

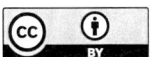

Chapter 10

3D Spheroids to Study the Impact of Immune Checkpoint Proteins in Solid Tumors

Esther Rey-Iborra, Maite Emaldi, Maider Madariaga, Rafael Pulido, and Caroline E. Nunes-Xavier

Abstract

In vitro 3D cultures are commonly used in cancer research, as they mimic the in vivo tumor growth better than conventional 2D monolayer cultures. Among the various 3D culture models, spheroids are suitable for experimental cancer research due to their simplicity and capacity to reproduce the organization and microenvironment of the tumor. The liquid overlay technique (LOT), based on the use of culture plates with non-adherent surfaces, is a low-cost and easy-handling method, commonly used to generate spheroids in the laboratory. LOT is a reliable technique in terms of reproducibility and high yield, representing a relevant 3D model for drug response screening studies in cancer research. B7-family proteins are immune checkpoint molecules involved in the regulation of antitumor immune responses. Some B7 proteins are highly expressed in different types of tumors, which often correlates with cancer progression and poor prognosis. Thus, B7 proteins are relevant immunotherapeutic targets for cancer treatment. In this chapter, we show the methodology to generate spheroids from different cancer cell lines by LOT. We illustrate the application of this technique to study the functional properties of B7 proteins.

Key words Liquid overlay technique, 3D spheroids, Cell viability, B7 immune checkpoint proteins

1 Introduction

Two-dimensional (2D) cell cultures remain the most commonly used preclinical research method in the biomedical area, due to their simplicity, reproducibility, and low cost. However, in cancer research, 2D monolayer cultures face certain limitations, as they do not faithfully recreate the tumor microenvironment and all the essential cellular organization and interactions that occur in vivo. In this regard, the development of three-dimensional (3D) cultures has been a breakthrough in the field, providing a model of intermediate complexity between the conventional monolayer cultures and animal in vivo systems [1–3]. 3D cell cultures allow to closely mimic the morphology of the tumor and to preserve some of the biological features of original tumors that may be lost in 2D culture

Sweta Rani and Lukasz Skalniak (eds.), *IMMUNO-model in Cancer: Methods and Protocols*, Methods in Molecular Biology, vol. 2959, https://doi.org/10.1007/978-1-0716-4734-9_10, © The Author(s) 2026

models, such as the cellular growth in conditions of hypoxia and low nutrient levels or the cell-cell and cell-extracellular matrix interactions [4–6].

Several 3D cell-culture models have been developed, including tissue explants, organoids, and spheroids [1]. Spheroids are one of the most suitable 3D models for cancer study due to their simplicity and capacity to reproduce the in vivo organization and microenvironment of the tumor. They consist of spherical aggregates of cells forming a multicellular mass [7]. The process of spheroid formation initiates with the spontaneous aggregation of single cells to form loosely adhesive cell spheroids. In this step, cell surface integrins bind to the long-chain extracellular matrix fibers promoting a rapid preliminary aggregation. After the first cell contact, cells upregulate E-cadherin, which accumulates on the cell surface and promotes strong adhesion of initial cell aggregate by creating a homophilic binding between cadherins of adjacent cells. Thus, the spheroid becomes a spherical compact structure where the cells show an organization and properties similar to those of the in vivo tumor [8–10].

Based on the tumor cell sources, different spheroid models have been described, including multicellular tumor spheroids (MCTS), tumor-derived spheroids, and organotypic multicellular tumor spheroids. The two last are obtained from mechanical or enzymatic dissociation of tumor tissue, whereas MCTS are typically established from cancer cell lines [1, 5].

Despite limited histological resemblance to the primary cancer, cells in MCTS mimic the metabolic and proliferative gradients of in vivo tumors and show clinically relevant multicellular chemoresistance. These properties make MCTS an appropriate tool for cancer research [5, 11].

MCTS exhibit a concentration gradient of biological factors similar to tumor cells due to the restricted diffusion of nutrients, oxygen, and growth factors. This diffusion gradient depends on the size of the spheroid; the larger the spheroid, the more difficult it becomes for the medium to reach the core [8]. Consequently, a proliferation gradient is observed in spheroids, with proliferating tumor cells located at the periphery, cell-cycle arrested cells at larger distances from the surface, and necrotic cells in the core of spheroids larger than 500 nm [9, 11, 12].

Among the various techniques available to generate spheroids, the liquid overlay technique (LOT) is the simplest and therefore one of the most widely used (Fig. 1) [7]. It is based on the use of non-adherent culture plates that prevent cells from attaching to the surface. Since the attachments are inhibited, the cells begin to adhere to each other, forming aggregates and finally spheroids. In addition to being a simple and economical method, LOT is a reliable technique in terms of reproducibility and high yield. LOT enables rapid aggregation of cells into spheroids with repeatable

Spheroid formation by LOT:

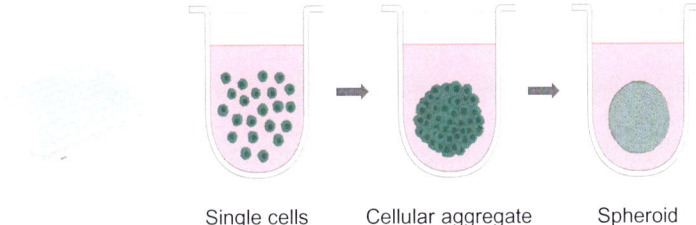

Single cells   Cellular aggregate   Spheroid

Fig. 1 Diagram illustrating spheroid formation by the liquid overlay technique (LOT). The process begins with a multiwell plate containing single cell suspension in growth medium. The cells aggregate into a cluster, forming a cellular aggregate, and eventually develop into a spheroid. Arrows indicate the progression from single cells to cellular aggregate to spheroid

morphologies that can be easily assessed by microscopy. LOT can be used for different applications in cancer research, including anticancer drug discovery, analyses of gene expression profile and gene function, studies of cancer cell invasion and migration, or studies of cell-cell interactions by coculturing the tumor spheroids with other types of cells. Due to these properties, LOT represents a relevant 3D model in cancer research [13–15].

B7 family proteins are immune checkpoint molecules, which belong to the immunoglobulin superfamily of type I membrane proteins. They are mainly expressed in the plasma membrane of antigen presenting cells as well as on tumor cells, and play important roles in the regulation of the adaptive immune system [16, 17]. To date, ten family members have been identified: B7–1 (*CD80*), B7–2 (*CD86*), B7-H1/PD-L1 (*CD274*), B7-DC/PD-L2 (*PDCD1LG2*), B7-H2 (*ICOSLG*), B7-H3 (*CD276*), B7-H4 (*VTCN1*), B7-H5/VISTA (*VSIR*), B7-H6 (*NCR3LG1*), and B7-H7 (*HHLA2*) [17, 18]. All of them are transmembrane proteins containing an extracellular region with an N-terminal region containing immunoglobulin variable (IgV) and immunoglobulin constant (IgC) domains, a transmembrane region, and, except for B7-H4, a C-terminal cytoplasmic region [18–21].

Through the extracellular region, B7 proteins interact with specific receptors on T- and NK-cells, mediating immune-modulatory functions. The different B7 proteins are considered as co-stimulatory, co-inhibitory, or dually costimulatory and co-inhibitory, depending on the type of receptor to which they bind and the functional effect they induce on immune cells [21, 22].

B7 proteins play a significant role in the immune escape of tumor cells, by binding to inhibitory receptors and reducing T-/NK-cell proliferation and the production of cytokines. In addition, B7 proteins can also promote tumorigenesis independently of the immune system, as they are involved in the regulation of several cell mechanisms, including cell growth, tumor progression, invasion, metastasis, and resistance to chemotherapy [19, 22–25]. Several members of the B7 family are highly expressed in various types of solid tumors, in association with more aggressive phenotypes of the disease and poor prognosis. Thus, the different B7 proteins have emerged as promising targets for cancer immunotherapy.

In this chapter, we show methodologies to generate multicellular tumor spheroids from different cancer cell lines using the liquid overlay technique. Additionally, we show the application of this technique to perform functional studies on B7 proteins.

2   Materials

2.1   2D Cell Cultures and 3D Spheroid Cell Cultures

2.1.1   2D Cell Cultures

- Tissue culture plates.
- Appropriate mammalian cell lines. We have used human neuro-blastoma IMR-32 and SH-SY5Y cell lines, human clear cell renal cell carcinoma (ccRCC) 786-O and Caki-1 cell lines, and human prostate cancer DU-145 and LNCaP cell lines (*see* **Note 1**).
- Cell culture medium. We have used RPMI 1640 medium for IMR-32, 786-O and LNCaP cells, Dulbecco's Modified Eagle Medium (DMEM) for SH-SY5Y cells, McCoy's 5A medium for Caki-1 cells, and EMEM for DU-145 cells. All media are supplemented with 10% heat-inactivated FBS (fetal bovine serum), 1% L-glutamine, and 1% penicillin/streptomycin (P/S). For neuroblastoma cells, media are also supplemented with 1% non-essential amino acids (NEAA). All tissue culture reagents were from Gibco.
- Trypsin-EDTA solution.

2.1.2   3D Spheroid Cell Cultures

- Round U-Bottom BIOFLAT 96-well plate (FaCellitate, F202003) and 96-well Clear Round Bottom Ultra-Low Attachment Microplate (Corning, 7007) (*see* **Notes 2**, **3**, and **4**).
- For neuroblastoma cells, we used DMEM and RPMI serum-free supplemented with epidermal growth factor (EGF) 40 ng/mL, fibroblast growth factor (FGF) 80 ng/mL, 2% B-27 supplement (Gibco), 1% L-glutamine, 1% P/S, and 1% NEAA (*see* **Note 5**). For renal and prostate cancer cells, we used the same cell-culture medium as for 2D cultures.

2.2   Effect of B7 Proteins on Cancer Cell Viability of 3D Spheroids

- PepMute siRNA Transfection Reagent (SignaGen).
- Non-specific siRNA (siNS) and siRNA for the B7 gene of interest.
- CellTiter-Glo 3D Cell Viability Assay (Promega).

- 96-Well Solid White Polystyrene Microplates (Corning, 3912).
- Microplate luminometer, Infinite M plex (TECAN).

2.3 Microscopic Measurement of Spheroid Size

- ZEN Microscopy software (ZEISS).
- FIJI software (ImageJ2).

---

3 Methods

Spheroids represent a relevant in vitro model to better understand tumor biology and to advance in cancer research. The *first method* described in this chapter (*see* Subheading 3.1) shows the methodology to generate multicellular tumor spheroids from IMR-32 and SH-SY5Y neuroblastoma cell lines, 786-O and Caki-1 renal cancer cell lines, and DU-145 and LNCaP prostate cancer cell lines, using the liquid overlay technique (Fig. 1). We present different variables that affect the capacity of the different cell lines to generate spheroids by LOT, such as the use of different types of low-attachment cell-culture plates (Figs. 2 and 3), and seeding cells at different concentrations (Fig. 4). We also show the effect of DMSO (commonly used solvent for chemicals) in spheroid formation (Fig. 5). When added at high concentrations, DMSO hinders the formation of spheroids in IMR-32 and SH-SY5Y cell lines. Daily monitoring of spheroids by microscopy is useful to assess the morphological changes the spheroids undergo under control conditions or after being exposed to a treatment. These changes can be quantified with appropriate image analysis software.

3.1 Generation of 3D Spheroids

1. Maintain the cell lines as adherent monolayers in 10 cm tissue culture plates with their specific culture media.
2. When the culture plate reaches 90% of confluence, recover the cells by using Trypsin-EDTA solution.
3. Stain the cells with Trypan Blue and count them using a hemocytometer.
4. Plate the desired number of cells in low-attachment 96-well plates with appropriate medium, for a final volume of 100 μL/well (*see* **Notes 5, 6**, and **7**).
5. Incubate the plates at 37 °C in a 5% CO_2 humidified atmosphere (*see* **Notes 8** and **9**).
6. Monitor spheroid evolution on a daily basis. Note that if the experiment involves treatment with chemical compounds, the solvent can potentially affect the formation of the spheroids (*see* **Note 10**).

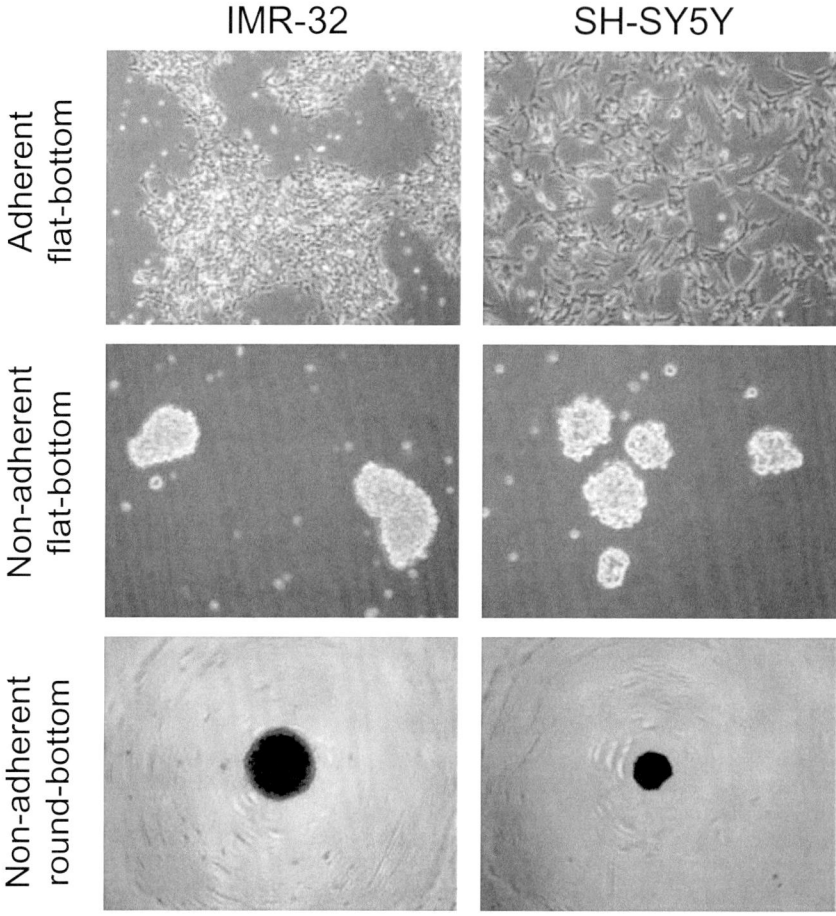

Fig. 2 Cell growth of IMR-32 and SH-SY5Y neuroblastoma cell lines on different cell culture plates. The top row displays microscopic images of cells growing as 2D monolayers when seeded in adherent flat-bottom culture plates. The middle row shows the cells forming multiple elongated or disorganized cellular aggregates when seeded in non-adherent flat-bottom culture plates. The bottom row shows cells aggregating into single and compact spheroids when seeded in non-adherent round-bottom culture plates

As shown in Figs. 2, 3, 4 and 5, optimization in the use of tissue culture media, solvents, plates, and cell density is required for each different cell line.

The *second method* (*see* Subheading 3.2) shows the application of 3D cultures to study the functional properties of immune checkpoint proteins, using B7-H5 as an example. For this purpose, we transiently silenced the expression of B7-H5 with siRNAs and monitored the changes in the growth of spheroids (Fig. 6a) and measured cell viability using a luminescent cell viability assay (Fig. 6b).

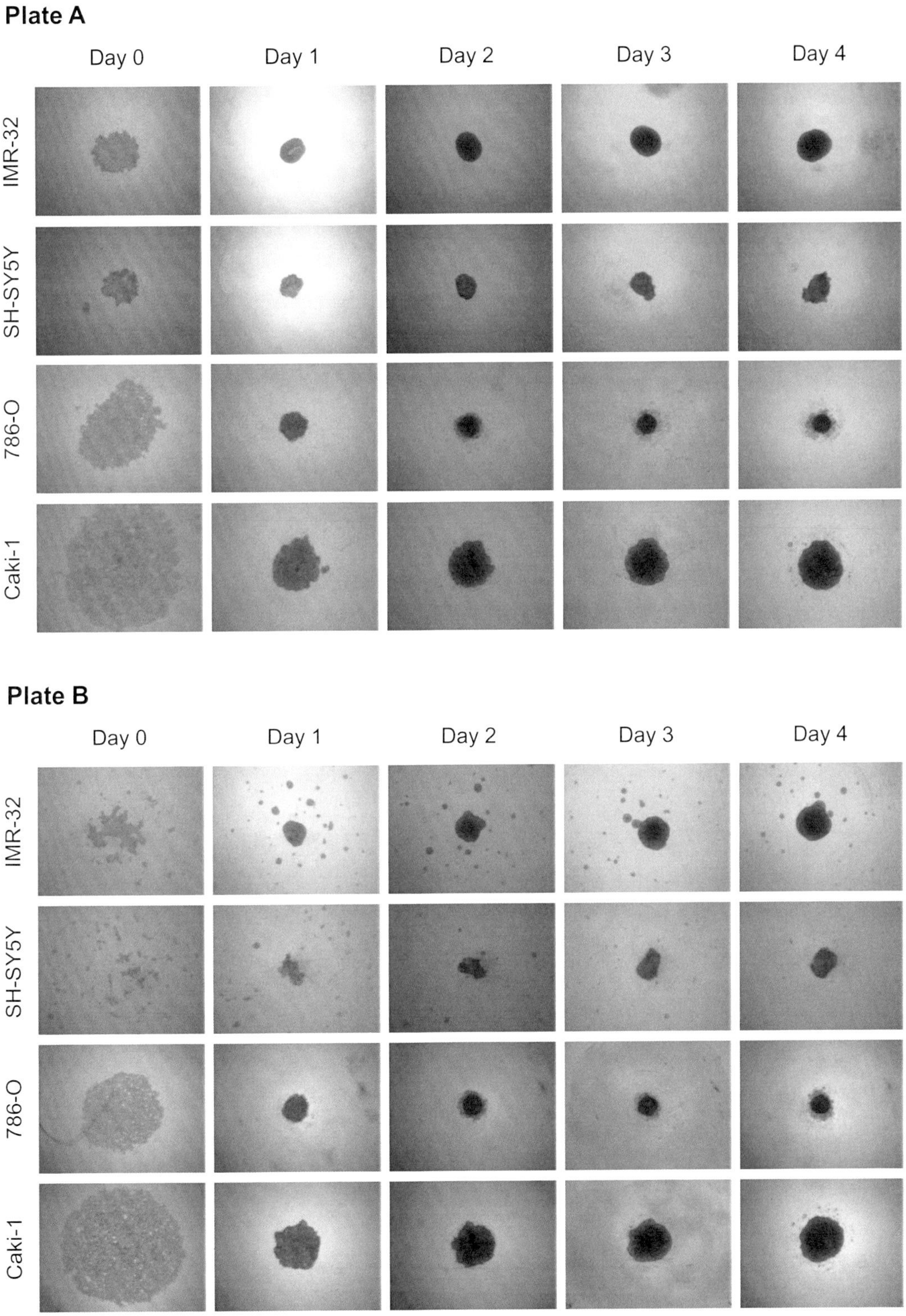

Plate A

Fig. 3 Monitoring the spheroid cell growth of IMR-32, SH-SY5Y, 786-O, and Caki-1 cell lines on different non-adherent cell culture plates. Cell lines were seeded in low-attachment round-bottom 96-well plates from FaCellitate (Plate A) or from Corning (Plate B), and the spheroid formation was monitored by microscopy on a daily basis. The microscopic images illustrate changes in cell aggregation and morphology over time. In

3.2 Effect of B7 Proteins on Cancer Cell Viability of 3D Spheroids

1. After seeding in low-attachment 96-well plates, transfect the seeded cells by adding PepMute Transfection Buffer, PepMute Reagent, and siNS or siRNA at the concentrations indicated in the PepMute siRNA Transfection Reagent (SignaGen) protocol.

2. Incubate the plates at 37 °C and 5% CO_2. Monitor spheroid evolution on a daily basis (Fig. 6a).

3. 72 h after transfection, perform the spheroid viability assay following the CellTiter-Glo 3D Cell Viability Assay protocol (*see* **Note 11**).

4. Before starting the protocol, equilibrate the plate to room temperature for 30 min.

5. Add the same volume of CellTiter-Glo 3D Reagent as the volume of culture medium present in each well (*see* **Notes 12** and **13**).

6. Shake the plate for 5 min at 300–400 rpm and 25 °C.

7. Incubate the plate for 25 min at room temperature in darkness.

8. Transfer the content of the plate to a 96-well white solid polystyrene microplate compatible with the luminometer used.

9. Record luminescence (*see* **Note 14**).

As illustrated in Fig. 6, the viability of spheroids transfected with siRNA B7-H5 was decreased, which suggests that the B7-H5 protein plays a role in maintaining the 3D viability of renal cancer cells.

The *third method* (*see* Subheading 3.3) shows an example of quantification of spheroid size variation on 786-O and Caki-1 renal cancer cells upon silencing of B7-H5 immune checkpoint protein. For this purpose, we photographed the spheroids and analyzed the size variations using appropriate image analysis software (Fig. 7).

3.3 Microscopic Measurement of Spheroid Size

1. Take pictures of the spheroids using a microscope coupled to microscopy software such as ZEN Microscopy software (ZEISS). At least one of the images has to include a scale bar.

2. Calibrate the scale of the image using the scale bar (Fig. 7a, left panel):
   - Open the image that includes the scale bar in FIJI software.
   - Use the "Straight Line" tool to draw a line the same length as the scale bar.

Fig. 3 (continued) neuroblastoma cells, the plate from FaCellitate promoted the formation of single, spherical shaped and compact spheroids, while with the Corning plates, the cells aggregated into a spheroid with multiple satellites or into a non-spherical aggregate. In renal cancer cells, the results were similar with both types of plates

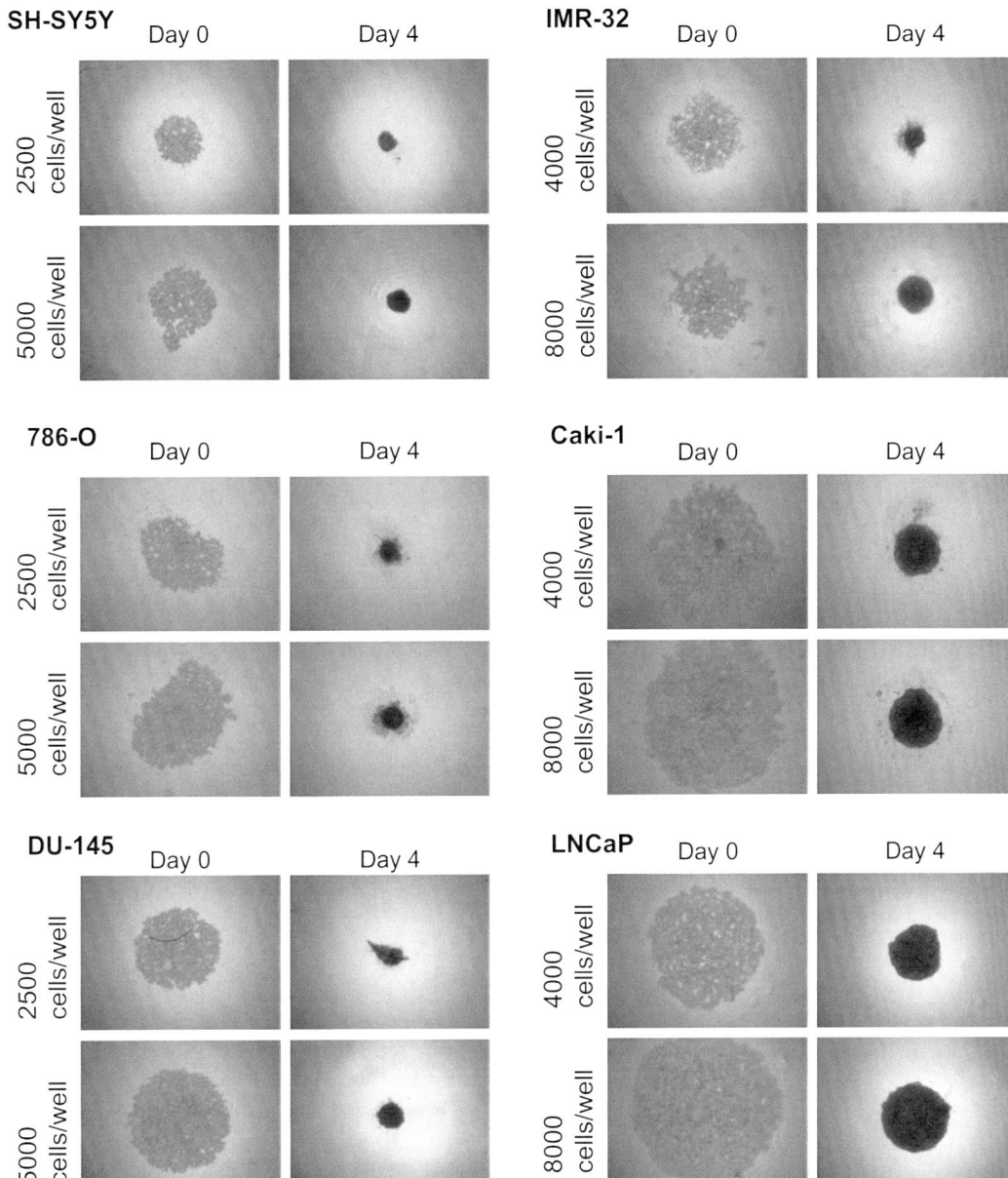

Fig. 4 Monitoring spheroid cell growth upon seeding different cell concentrations in low-attachment round-bottom 96-well plates. SH-SY5Y, 786-O and DU-145 cell lines were seeded with initial confluences of 2500 cells/well and 5000 cells/well. IMR-32, Caki-1 and LNCaP cell lines were seeded with initial confluences of 4000 cells/well and 8000 cells/well. The microscopic images illustrate changes in cell aggregation and morphology over time. Microscopy images were taken on day 0 and day 4. In all cases, larger diameters and more compact spheroids were obtained when a higher number of cells were initially seeded

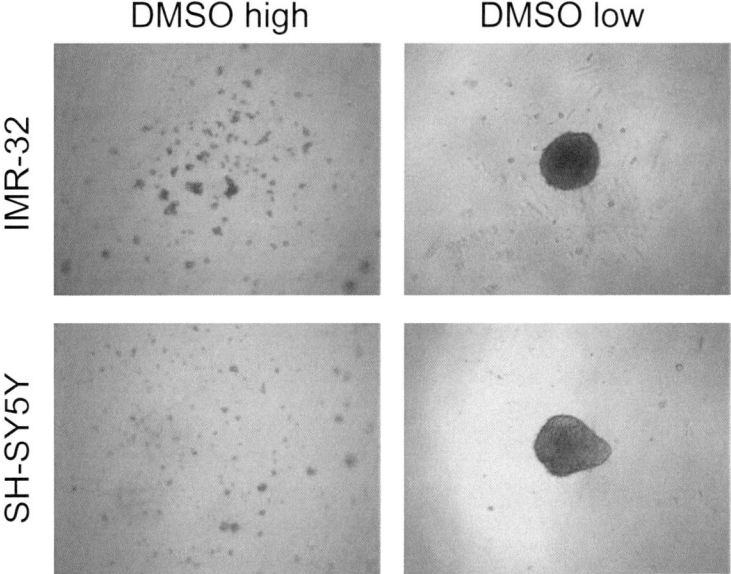

Fig. 5 Monitoring spheroid formation in the presence of DMSO. IMR-32 and SH-SY5Y neuroblastoma cell lines were seeded in 96-well non-adherent flat-bottom culture plates with high (1:50) or low levels (1:1000) of DMSO, as indicated. Microscopic images were taken at day 4. High concentrations of DMSO prevent spheroid formation in neuroblastoma cell lines (left images), while low concentrations of this solvent do not alter the ability of cells to form compact spheroids (right images)

- Click Analyze > Set Scale and change the parameter "Known distance" to the micrometers of the scale bar, the parameter "Unit of length" to "μM" and select the "Global" option.
- Press OK.

3. Measure the area of the spheroid (Fig. 7a, right panel):
   - Open the image to analyze in FIJI software.
   - Click Image > Type and select "8 bit" to convert the image to grayscale.
   - Click Image > Adjust > Threshold to detect the edges. This converts the grayscale to binary so that the values below the cutoff are detected as black and the values above are detected as white.
   - Select the spheroid by clicking on it with the "Wand tool," which allows surrounding an area with a perimeter in high contrast images.
   - Click Analyze > Measure.

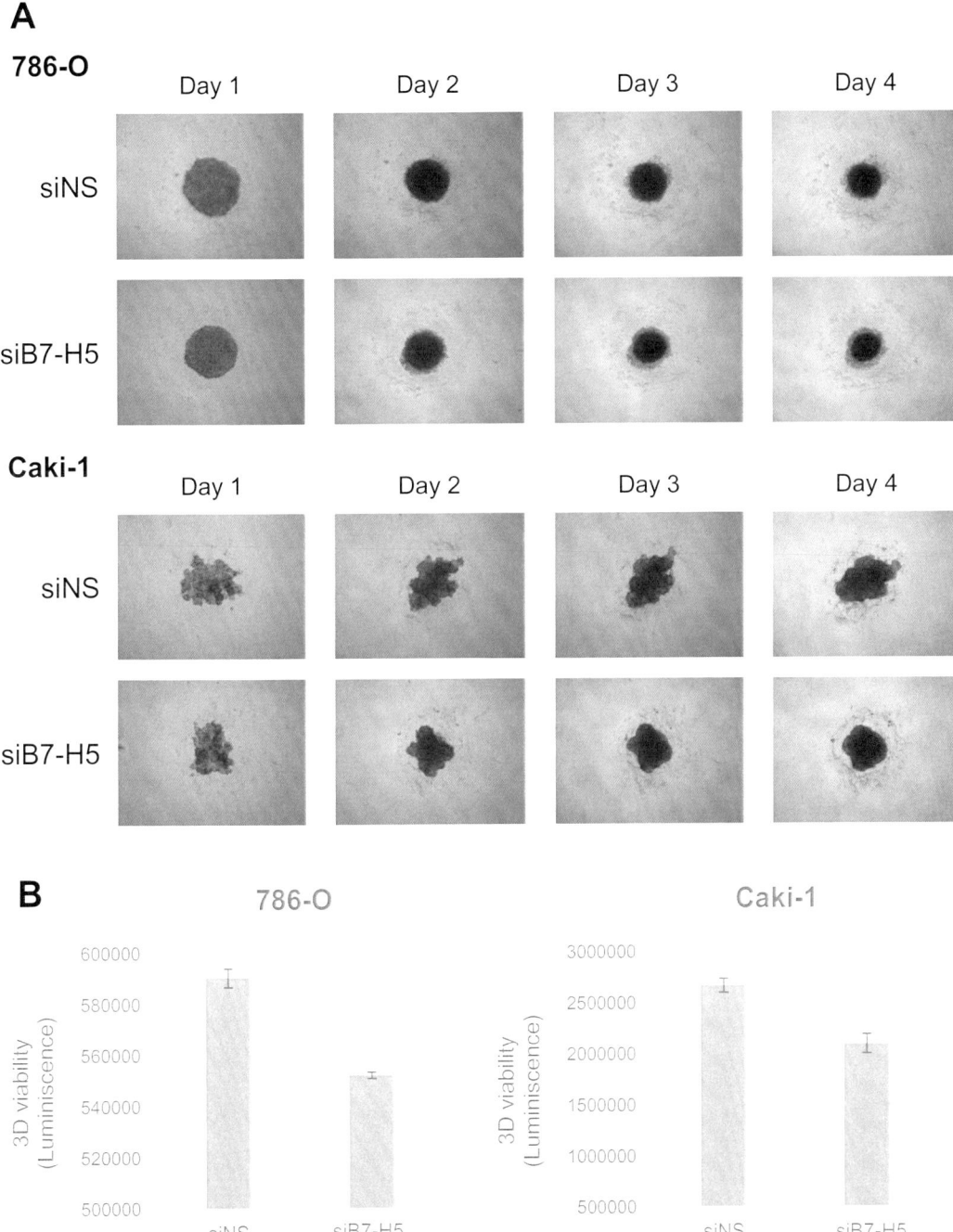

Fig. 6 Monitoring spheroid formation and viability upon silencing of B7-H5. Panel A displays microscopic images of spheroids upon silencing B7-H5 by siRNA B7-H5 transfection (siB7-H5) in 786-O and Caki-1 renal cancer cell lines. Spheroid evolution was monitored by microscopy on a daily basis (siNS, non-specific silencing). Panel B shows bar graphs of 3D cell viability of the spheroids measured by luminescence. The decrease in viability of spheroids transfected with siRNA B7-H5 suggests that B7-H5 protein plays an important role in maintaining the 3D viability of renal cancer cells

A

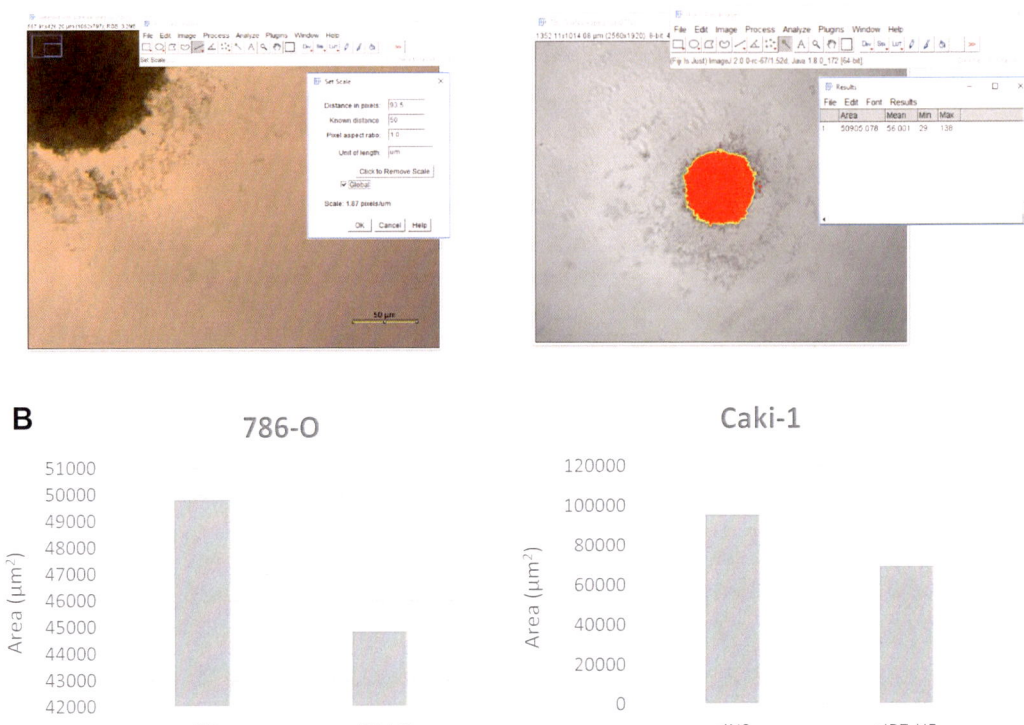

Fig. 7 Quantification of spheroid size using FIJI software. Panel A shows calibration of the microscopic image scale using a known distance of 50 μm (left image) and measurement of the spheroid area (right image). Panel B shows variations in the size of 786-O and Caki-1 renal cancer cell spheroids upon silencing B7-H5 by siRNA B7-H5 transfection (siB7-H5) (siNS, non-specific silencing). Results are shown as an area in square micro-meters (μm^2)

- A new "Results" window automatically opens where all the measurements are recorded. Use the "Area" value to assess the size variations of the spheroids (Fig. 7b).

This technique allows quantification (in terms of "area") of the size variation of the spheroids. As illustrated in Fig. 7b, size of renal cancer spheroids decreased upon silencing of B7-H5.

4   Notes

1. The capacity of different cell types to form spheroids by LOT is variable. Some cell types are unable to form spheroids or they only manage to form disorganized, non-spherical aggregates [26]. In our experience, IMR-32, SH-SY5Y, 786-O, Caki-1, DU-145, and LNCaP cell lines are able to form spheroids by LOT when using round-bottom non-adherent surface plates.

2. None or very few cellular aggregates with spherical shape are obtained by LOT when flat non-adherent surfaces are used [27]. In our experiments, neuroblastoma cancer cells seeded on flat-bottom non-adherent culture plates were only able to form elongated or disorganized cellular aggregates (Fig. 2).

3. The non-adherent properties of the plates are achieved by coating the surface of the wells with biomaterials that prevent cell adhesion. Standard cell-culture plates can be manually pre-coated in the laboratory with solutions of agar or agarose dissolved in water or serum-free medium, which are added to the bottom of the wells. However, it is important to note that storing plates coated with agar or agarose solutions for several days results in water evaporation and, consequently, in coating disruption. Moreover, the storage of the remaining agar and agarose solutions is not recommended, since these have to be heated before each application and such a process may compromise the stability of the biomaterials [14, 27, 28].

4. There are several types of non-adherent plates on the market specifically designed for the production of spheroids. In our experiments, we used round-bottom 96-well plates from FaCellitate and Corning. As shown in Fig. 3, the 96-well plate from FaCellitate promoted, in neuroblastoma cell lines, a faster formation of spheroids with a single, more compact, and spherical structure without satellites. In renal cancer cells, the results were similar with both types of plates. This indicates that distinct cell lines show differences in their ability to form spheroids depending on the low-attachment plate used. It is advisable to test different types of plates to select the most suitable one for the cell line being used.

5. For some cell lines it is difficult to establish the strong interactions needed to form spheroids, and the addition of supplements to the culture medium may be helpful for enhancing the spheroids formation [28]. Following the methodology used by Ognibene and colleges [29], when plating neuroblastoma cells for spheroid formation, we supplemented the culture media with EGF, FGF, and B-27, to facilitate the formation of spheroids.

6. Spheroids size can be optimized by modulating the initial number of cells seeded on the non-adherent surfaces [28, 30], and examples are shown in Fig. 4. After 2 days of culture, we noticed that larger diameters and more compact spheroids were obtained when a higher number of cells were initially seeded. Based on these results, we recommend a confluence of 8000 cells/well (for 96-well plates; about 2.7×10^4 cells/cm^3) for the cell lines we have tested.

7. Once the cell solution is added to a well, it cannot be aspirated and replated. This process disrupts the spheroid formation.

8. Some cell lines may require centrifuging the plate before incubation to allow cells to aggregate more rapidly [31].

9. For the majority of cell lines, cells aggregate leading to the formation of spheroids in 1–3 days [32]. Nevertheless, it is recommended to monitor by microscopy the spheroid formation on a daily basis.

10. Since dimethyl sulfoxide (DMSO) is commonly used to dissolve drugs and as a vehicle in drug-response assays, it is important to note that it may hinder spheroid formation. Based on our observations (Fig. 5), we recommend diluting treatments in culture medium rather than in DMSO. If it is necessary to use DMSO, we advise using the minimum possible volume.

11. From this step onward, maintaining sterility is no longer necessary, so the subsequent steps can be performed outside the tissue culture hood.

12. For a 96-well plate, we recommend removing the volume necessary to leave 50 µL of cell-culture medium per well (taking care not to aspirate the spheroid) and then adding 50 µL of CellTiter-Glo 3D Reagent. These volumes can be adjusted, but the 1:1 ratio should always be maintained.

13. CellTiter-Glo 3D Reagent is light-sensitive, so it is important to avoid direct exposure to light and, whenever possible, to keep the plate in the dark.

14. The instrument settings for luminescence detection vary depending on the manufacturer. If using the Infinite M plex (TECAN), set the integration time to 1000 ms and the settling time to 0 ms.

Acknowledgments

The work of C.E.N-X. is funded by Instituto de Salud Carlos III (CP20/00008 and PI22/00386, Spain and cofinanced by European Union), Biobizkaia Health Research Institute (Ayudas para el fortalecimiento de grupos emergentes, Spain), and Stiftelsen til fremme av forskning innen nyresykdommer/Foundation for promoting research in kidney diseases (Unifor, Norway). This work was also partially funded by Instituto de Salud Carlos III (PI23/00959, Spain and cofinanced by the European Union), BIOEF (BIO20/CI/004, EITB Maratoia, Basque Country, Spain), and Asociación NEN (Spain). E.R-I. is the recipient of a predoctoral fellowship from Asociación Española Contra el Cáncer (AECC, PRDVZ222375REY, Junta Provincial de Bizkaia, Spain).

M.E. is the recipient of a Fellowship 2023/2024 from Biobizkaia Health Research Institute, and fellowships from the Jesus Gangoiti Barrera Foundation. This chapter is based upon work from COST Action IMMUNO-model, CA21135, supported by COST (European Cooperation in Science and Technology).

Competing Interest Statement

The authors have no conflicts of interest to declare that are relevant to the content of this chapter.

References

1. Gunti S, Hoke ATK, Vu KP, London NR Jr (2021) Organoid and spheroid tumor models: techniques and applications. Cancers (Basel) 13(4):874

2. Pampaloni F, Reynaud EG, Stelzer EH (2007) The third dimension bridges the gap between cell culture and live tissue. Nat Rev Mol Cell Biol 8(10):839–845

3. Kim JB (2005) Three-dimensional tissue culture models in cancer biology. Semin Cancer Biol 15(5):365–377

4. Fontana F, Marzagalli M, Sommariva M, Gagliano N, Limonta P (2021) In vitro 3D cultures to model the tumor microenvironment. Cancers (Basel) 13(12):2970

5. Ishiguro T, Ohata H, Sato A, Yamawaki K, Enomoto T, Okamoto K (2017) Tumor-derived spheroids: relevance to cancer stem cells and clinical applications. Cancer Sci 108(3):283–289

6. Achilli TM, Meyer J, Morgan JR (2012) Advances in the formation, use and understanding of multi-cellular spheroids. Expert Opin Biol Ther 12(10):1347–1360

7. Jubelin C, Muñoz-Garcia J, Griscom L, Cochonneau D, Ollivier E, Heymann MF, Vallette FM, Oliver L, Heymann D (2022) Three-dimensional in vitro culture models in oncology research. Cell Biosci 12(1):155

8. Ryu NE, Lee SH, Park H (2019) Spheroid culture system methods and applications for mesenchymal stem cells. Cells 8(12):1620

9. Lin RZ, Chang HY (2008) Recent advances in three-dimensional multicellular spheroid culture for biomedical research. Biotechnol J 3(9–10):1172–1184

10. Lin RZ, Chou LF, Chien CC, Chang HY (2006) Dynamic analysis of hepatoma spheroid formation: roles of E-cadherin and beta1-integrin. Cell Tissue Res 324(3):411–422

11. Kunz-Schughart LA, Freyer JP, Hofstaedter F, Ebner R (2004) The use of 3-D cultures for high-throughput screening: the multicellular spheroid model. J Biomol Screen 9(4):273–285

12. Nath S, Devi GR (2016) Three-dimensional culture systems in cancer research: Focus on tumor spheroid model. Pharmacol Ther 163:94–108

13. Pinto B, Henriques AC, Silva PMA, Bousbaa H (2020) Three-dimensional spheroids as in vitro preclinical models for cancer research. Pharmaceutics 12(12):1186

14. Metzger W, Sossong D, Bächle A, Pütz N, Wennemuth G, Pohlemann T, Oberringer M (2011) The liquid overlay technique is the key to formation of co-culture spheroids consisting of primary osteoblasts, fibroblasts and endothelial cells. Cytotherapy 13(8):1000–1012

15. Jubelin C, Muñoz-Garcia J, Cochonneau D, Ollivier E, Vallette F, Heymann MF, Oliver L, Heymann D (2023) Technical report: liquid overlay technique allows the generation of homogeneous osteosarcoma, glioblastoma, lung and prostate adenocarcinoma spheroids that can be used for drug cytotoxicity measurements. Front Bioeng Biotechnol 11:1260049

16. Banu N, Riera-Leal A, Haramati J, Ortiz-Lazareno PC, Panikar SS, Bastidas-Ramirez BE, Gutierrez-Silerio GY, Solorzano-Ibarra F, Tellez-Bañuelos MC, Gutierrez-Franco J, Bueno-Topete MR, Pereira-Suarez AL, Del Toro-Arreola S (2020) B7-H6, an immunoligand for the natural killer cell activating receptor NKp30, reveals inhibitory effects on cell proliferation and migration, but not apoptosis, in cervical cancer derived-cell lines. BMC Cancer 20(1):1083

17. Seliger B, Quandt D (2012) The expression, function, and clinical relevance of B7 family

members in cancer. Cancer Immunol Immunother 61(8):1327–1341

18. Wang Y, Li M, Wang G, Wu H (2023) Role of B7 family members in glioma: promising new targets for tumor immunotherapy. Front Oncol 12:1091383

19. Mohammadi A, Najafi S, Amini M, Mansoori B, Baghbanzadeh A, Hoheisel JD, Baradaran B (2022) The potential of B7-H6 as a therapeutic target in cancer immunotherapy. Life Sci 304:120709

20. Flem-Karlsen K, Fodstad Ø, Nunes-Xavier CE (2020) B7-H3 immune checkpoint protein in human cancer. Curr Med Chem 27(24):4062–4086

21. Ni L, Dong C (2017) New B7 family checkpoints in human cancers. Mol Cancer Ther 16(7):1203–1211

22. Flem-Karlsen K, Fodstad Ø, Tan M, Nunes-Xavier CE (2018) B7-H3 in cancer—beyond immune regulation. Trends Cancer 4(6):401–404

23. Nunes-Xavier CE, Karlsen KF, Tekle C, Pedersen C, Øyjord T, Hongisto V, Nesland JM, Tan M, Sahlberg KK, Fodstad Ø (2016) Decreased expression of B7-H3 reduces the glycolytic capacity and sensitizes breast cancer cells to AKT/mTOR inhibitors. Oncotarget 7(6):6891–6901

24. Emaldi M, Alamillo P, Rey-Iborra E, Mosteiro L, Lecumberri D, Pulido R, López JI, Nunes-Xavier CE (2024) A functional role for glycosylated B7-H5/VISTA immune checkpoint protein in metastatic clear cell renal cell carcinoma. iScience 27(9):110587

25. Emaldi M, Rey-Iborra E, Marín Á, Mosteiro L, Lecumberri D, Øyjord T, Roncier N, Mælandsmo GM, Ángulo JC, Errarte P, Larrinaga G, Pulido R, López JI, Nunes-Xavier CE (2024) Impact of B7-H3 expression on

metastasis, immune exhaustion and JAK/STAT and PI3K/AKT pathways in clear cell renal cell carcinoma. Oncoimmunology 13(1):2419686

26. Carlsson J, Nilsson K, Westermark B, Pontén J, Sundström C, Larsson E, Bergh J, Påhlman S, Busch C, Collins VP (1983) Formation and growth of multicellular spheroids of human origin. Int J Cancer 31(5):523–533

27. Costa EC, Gaspar VM, Coutinho P, Correia IJ (2014) Optimization of liquid overlay technique to formulate heterogenic 3D co-cultures models. Biotechnol Bioeng 111(8):1672–1685

28. Costa EC, de Melo-Diogo D, Moreira AF, Carvalho MP, Correia IJ (2018) Spheroids formation on non-adhesive surfaces by liquid overlay technique: considerations and practical approaches. Biotechnol J 13(1)

29. Ognibene M, Pezzolo A (2020) Roniciclib down-regulates stemness and inhibits cell growth by inducing nucleolar stress in neuroblastoma. Sci Rep 10(1):12902

30. Ma HL, Jiang Q, Han S, Wu Y, Cui Tomshine J, Wang D, Gan Y, Zou G, Liang XJ (2012) Multicellular tumor spheroids as an in vivo-like tumor model for three-dimensional imaging of chemotherapeutic and nano material cellular penetration. Mol Imaging 11(6):487–498

31. Carroll LJ, Tiwari B, Curtin JF, Wanigasekara J (2021) U-251 MG Spheroid generation using low attachment plate method protocol. https://doi.org/10.17504/protocols.io.bszmnf46

32. do Amaral JB, Rezende-Teixeira P, Freitas VM, Machado-Santelli GM (2011) MCF-7 cells as a three-dimensional model for the study of human breast cancer. Tissue Eng Part C Methods 17(11)1097–1107

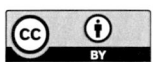

Chapter 11

A 3D Co-Culture Model of Endometrial Carcinoma Cells with Peripheral Blood Immune Cells (PBMCs) to Study the Activity of Immune Checkpoint Inhibitors

Justyna Kocik-Krol and Marcin Krzykawski

Abstract

The 3D co-culture model we describe was developed to study the potency of immune checkpoint inhibitors. In the assay, the first step is to provide 3D cell growth of endometrial carcinoma RL95-2 cells on a hydrogel, LifeGel®, and then to co-culture cancer cells with PBMCs isolated from healthy blood donors. After 5 days of the co-culture, in the presence of anti-PD-1/PD-L1 or anti-VISTA immune checkpoint inhibitors, the cancer cells' viability is measured using a colorimetric assay and fluorescence readout.

The key features of the presented model are (1) a direct 3D co-culture model that involves cancer cells and immune cells represented by PBMCs, (2) the use of LifeGel® hydrogel, where cancer cells form spheroids on the surface, allowing immune cells and larger molecules, such as monoclonal antibodies, to penetrate the cancerous structures, and (3) the possible reactivation of immune cells by immune checkpoint inhibitors may be observed via killing/destroying effects on cancer structures.

Key words 3D cell culture, Immuno-oncology, Immune checkpoint inhibitors, Viability assay

1 Introduction

Therapies with immune checkpoint inhibitors (ICIs) have become a breakthrough in cancer treatment. In recent years, drugs targeting PD-1 and CTLA-4, such as nivolumab and ipilimumab, have demonstrated remarkable clinical efficacy in many patient subsets. Moreover, numerous clinical trials are ongoing to develop new immune checkpoint blockade inhibitors [1, 2]. Many in vitro studies dedicated to studying their biological activity utilize either two-dimensional (2D) cell cultures or mouse models, each of which presents strengths but on the other hand, also has a set on own limitations [3–5].

2D models used for drug efficacy testing are easy and relatively quick to set up and obtain results. Moreover, 2D cultures are widely used, described, and accessible to a wide range of researchers. 2D

Sweta Rani and Lukasz Skalniak (eds.), *IMMUNO-model in Cancer: Methods and Protocols*, Methods in Molecular Biology, vol. 2959, https://doi.org/10.1007/978-1-0716-4734-9_11, © The Author(s) 2026

co-culture models of breast cancer cells with PBMCs in immune checkpoint examination have been presented so far [6, 7]. However, an increasing number of studies demonstrate that 2D culture systems do not fully recapitulate tumor microenvironment, cancer phenotypes, and physiology [8, 9].

Mouse models allow for in vivo drug testing and investigation of absorption, distribution, metabolism, and excretion (*ADME*) [10]. However, it is evidenced that the murine tumor microenvironment does not fully reflect the human tumor niche [11]. It has been also demonstrated that there is a different affinity between mouse and human PD-L1 protein for the designed PD-1/PD-L1 inhibitors [12]. Immunodeficient mice act as an advanced model to study human immune cell-cancer mechanisms, but they are expensive and present numerous challenges in their generation, which may limit their use in preclinical research [13, 14].

Compared to 2D models, 3D models are considered more physiologically relevant and better at replicating the complexities of tumor biology. Furthermore, in contrast to murine models, 3D models are cheaper, faster, and can study human immune system interactions. So far, Saraiva et al. described the 3D co-culture model with MDA-MB-231 breast cancer cells and PBMCs underlying the potency of the method for immunotherapies. However, no immune checkpoint inhibitors have been tested using this model so far [15].

Several 3D models based on the co-culture of organoids derived from patients with PBMCs have already been described in the literature [16, 17]. Organoids that can be derived from the patient's cells retain the heterogeneity of tumor cells and preserve the characteristics of tumor tissues. This allows for personalized medicine development [18, 19]. However, their use in high-throughput screening is challenging due to high costs, time required for development, and limited lifespan [20, 21].

A major advantage of the 3D co-culture model that we propose is that cancer cells (RL95-2 cell line, endometrium carcinoma) are grown in the scaffold-based 3D culture system (hydrogel LifeGel®) that mimics extracellular matrix (ECM) [22]. What is more, cancer spheroids are generated on the top of the hydrogel so they can be easily penetrated by immune cells represented by PBMCs and also immune checkpoint inhibitors. The general experimental workflow is presented in Fig. 1.

2   Materials

2.1   Cell Culture

1. RL95-2—human endometrial carcinoma cells were delivered from our collaborator Recepton Sp. z o.o.

RL95-2 cells were cultured and seeded in the medium: D-MEM:F12 medium, 0.005 mg/mL insulin, 10% (v/v) FBS (*see* **Note 1**).

2. In our assays, we used cryopreserved PBMCs obtained from Recepton Sp. z o.o. (*see* **Note 2**). Prior to cryopreservation, PBMCs were isolated from whole blood of healthy donors and isolated from buffy coats using gradient centrifugation.

 PBMCs were cultured in medium: RPMI 1640, 10% (v/v) FBS, 2 mM L-glutamine.

3. Co-culture of RL95-2 cells and PBMCs was provided in RPMI 1640, 10% (v/v) FBS, 2 mM L-glutamine.

4. LifeGel® 96-well plates (cat. no. L912141912).

5. Phosphate-buffered saline (PBS) without calcium and magnesium.

6. L-Trypsin-EDTA 0.02% (v/v).

7. CO_2 cell-culture incubator.

2.2 Viability Assay

1. CellTiter-Blue® Cell Viability Assay (Promega).

2.3 Laboratory Equipment

1. CO_2 incubator.

2. Optical microscope.

3. Microplate reader.

2.4 Other

1. Immune checkpoint inhibitors.

3 Methods

3.1 Seeding Cells (DAY 0)

1. Seed RL95-2 cells at 96-well LifeGel® plate at the density of 8000 cells/well in total volume 150 µL/well.

3.2 Change of the Culture Medium (DAY 4 and 6)

1. Warm culture medium [DMEM:F12 medium, 0.005 mg/mL insulin, 10% (v/v) FBS].

2. Remove the plate from the incubator.

3. Remove 120 µL of medium per well (*see* **Note 3**).

4. Add 120 µL of prewarmed culture medium per well.

5. Place the plate back into the incubator.

3.3 Thawing PBMCs and Starting a Co-culture (DAY 7)

3.3.1 Thawing PBMCs

1. Warm RPMI 1640 medium supplemented with 10% FBS (v/v) to 37 °C.

2. Prepare a 50 mL Falcon tube and transfer 8 mL of warmed RPMI 1640 medium per every five million of thawed PBMCs. If desired, several cryovials from the same PBMCs donor can be combined into one 50 mL Falcon tube.

3. Transfer the cryovials to a 37 °C water bath.

   Keep the cryogenic tubes s in the bath until the cells are thawed, gently flick them occasionally during thawing (*see* **Note 4**).

4. Disinfect the cryovial from the outside to avoid contamination.

5. Transfer thawed PBMCs into a culture medium in 50 mL Falcon tube (*see* point 2) (*see* **Note 5**).

   Add the cells to the medium very slowly, drop by drop, while gently swirling the Falcon tube.

6. Leave the cells in the Falcon tube in the CO_2 incubator at 37 °C for about 20–30 min.

7. Centrifuge the cells at $500 \times g$ for 7 min.

8. Remove the supernatant and add complete RPMI 1640. At this step, we always add 2 mL of medium for every five million of PBMCs.

9. Incubate PBMCS at 37 °C, 5% CO_2 for about 2 h to provide them with a "resting time" after thawing (*see* **Note 6**).

10. Centrifuge PBMCs: $500 \times g$, 7 min.

11. Remove the supernatant, and resuspend the pellet in the desired volume of warm complete RPMI medium.

12. Count the cells using Trypan Blue or equivalent method.

13. Dilute PBMCs to a final working concentration: 1.35×10^6 live cells/mL (*see* **Note 7**).

*3.3.2 Setting Up a Co-culture (See **Note 8**)*

1. Prepare dilutions of the immune checkpoint inhibitors that will be tested. Use the RPMI-1640 culture medium (*see* **Note 9**). Remember to ensure that your working concentrations are 2× higher than the final concentrations.

2. Remember about conditions: only culture medium and only the inhibitors' solvent conditions.

3. Remove the medium from the LifeGel® plate with growing RL95-2 cells (*see* **Note 3**).

4. Add 75 µL/well of prepared inhibitors dilutions (*see* point 1).

5. Seed PBMCs by adding 75 µL/well of prepared PBMCs solution. The total number of cells will be 100,000 PBMCs per well (*see* point 14).

3.4 Verification of Cancer Cell Viability in Co-culture in the Presence of Immune Checkpoint Inhibitors (DAY 12) (See **Note 10)**

1. Take microscope images of the 3D cultures for each condition (control, checkpoint inhibitors, etc.) (*see* **Note 11**).

2. Equilibrate CellTiter-Blue® to room temperature. Protect from light.

3. Remove experimental plates from the incubator and add 25 µL/well of CellTiter-Blue®.

A

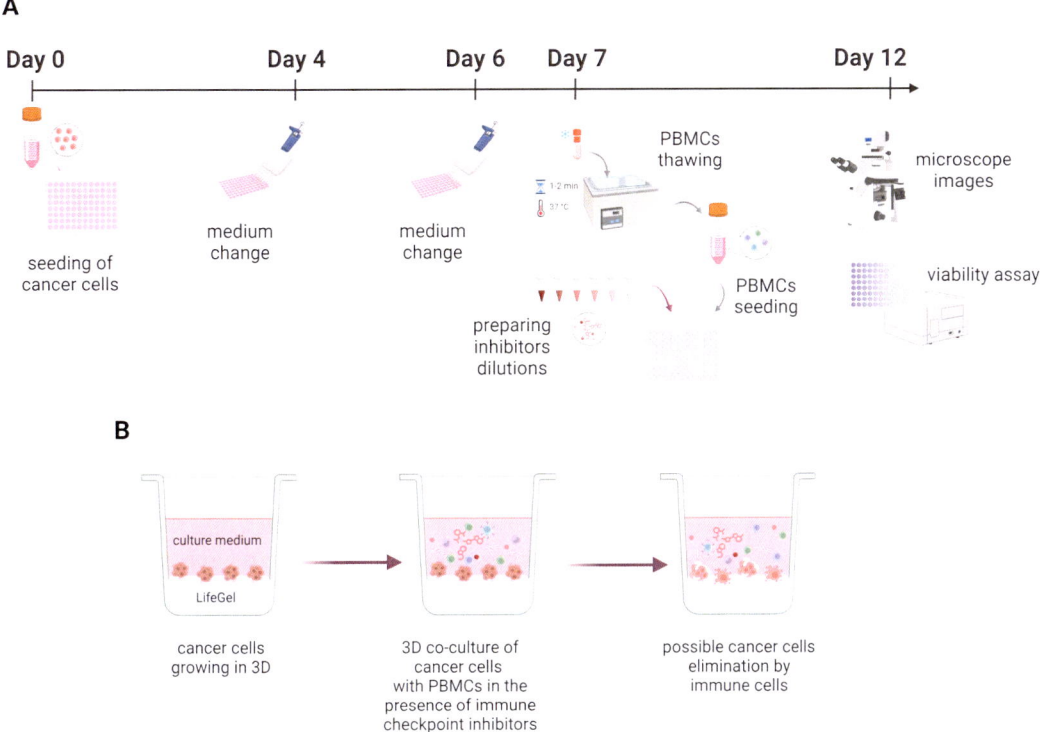

B

Fig. 1 Summary of the experimental design. (**a**) Schematic representation of the procedures conducted on the indicated days of the experiment. (**b**) Close-up view of the culture well at successive stages throughout the experiment. (This figure was created with BioRender.com)

4. Incubate in the cell culture incubator for 6 h.

5. Shake the experimental plate for 10 s and read the fluorescence at 570/615 nm.

6. Calculate the results: Subtract the average fluorescence values of the culture medium background from all experimental well fluorescence readings. Create a plot of fluorescence that indicates cell viability versus tested immune checkpoint inhibitors in several concentrations (*see* **Note 12**). We presented our example results in Fig. 2.

4   Notes

1. In the assay, other cancer cell lines can be used depending on the expression of immune checkpoints.

Using LifeGel® technology, the 3D cell culture of various types of immortalized cancer cell lines, as well as patient-derived xenograft (PDX) cells and patient-derived cells, can be provided.

2. In our experiments, we use cryopreserved PBMCs; however, freshly isolated cells from donors can also be utilized.

3. When removing the medium, place the pipette tip at a 45° angle and gently aspirate from one place of the well, without touching the LifeGel®.

   See the Instructional video "How to perform 3D Cell Culture with LifeGel?" https://real-research.com/movies/

4. Typically, cell thawing takes about 2 min. It is very important to transfer the cells to a fresh medium immediately after thawing. Do not keep the cells in the cryovial once they are thawed.

5. We recommend using a 1 mL-single-channel pipette when transferring PBMCs. Pipette the cells to the medium very slowly, drop by drop, while gently swirling the Falcon tube.

6. Resting time (1–24 h) after thawing PBMCs is described in the literature as desirable to recapitulate the surface marker expression of fresh cells [23, 24].

7. In our assay, we used PBMCs without previous stimulation that provide the activation signal via the TCR/CD3 complex. The cytotoxic activity of PBMCs against cancer cells in our example experiment (Fig. 2) was observed for 3 per 6 preselected PBMCs donors (preselection based on 2D direct co-culture of PBMCs with cancer cells). Several studies have been conducted comparing non-stimulated and stimulated conditions [15, 25].

8. When setting up a co-culture remember also that the "only cancer cells" condition, "only PBMCs" condition, and "only cancer cells + immune checkpoint inhibitors" conditions need to be included.

9. Co-culture is conducted in RPMI 1640 medium supplemented with 10% FBS, adjusted for PBMCs. In our previous experiments, we confirmed the viability of RL95-2 cells under 3D culture conditions in the RPMI 1640 medium.

10. We provide the CellTiterBlue® Cell Viability Assay protocol optimized for 3D culture on LifeGel® plates.

11. Based on the microscope images, an analysis of parameters such as the cancer cell size and sphericity of cancer cells in 3D culture can be performed using image analysis software.

12. The metabolic activity of PBMCs in this essay is at the background level. Therefore, the obtained measurement results reflect the metabolic activity and, consequently, the viability of cancer cells.

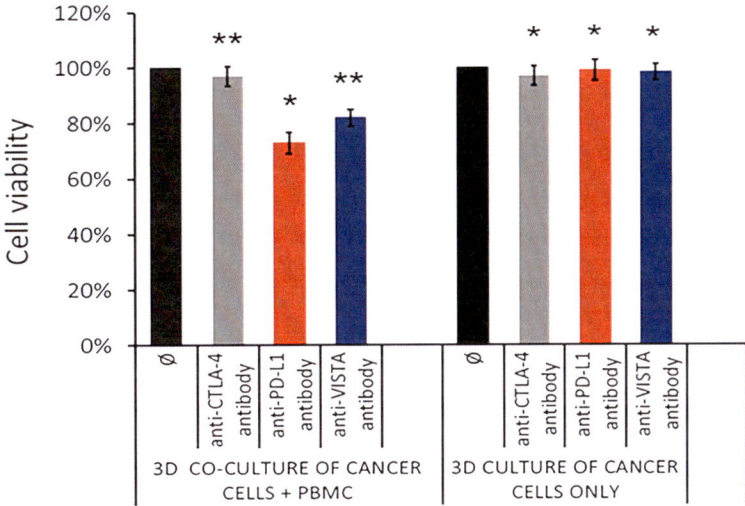

Fig. 2 Cancer cell viability measured using CellTiter-Blue®. In the assay, monoclonal antibodies targeting immune checkpoints were tested, each at a final concentration of 100 nM: anti-CTLA-4 (ipilimumab), anti-PD-L1 (atezolizumab), anti-VISTA (onvatilimab). The data are presented as the mean of three PBMC donor samples $\pm$ SD, * indicates statistical significance $p < 0.05$ for comparison with "culture medium only" (black bars on the graph) condition

Acknowledgments

This publication is based upon work from COST Action IMMUNO-model, CA21135, supported by COST (European Cooperation in Science and Technology).

References

1. Maritaz C, Broutin S, Chaput N et al (2022) Immune checkpoint-targeted antibodies: a room for dose and schedule optimization? J Hematol Oncol 15:1–16

2. Shiravand Y, Khodadadi F, Kashani SMA et al (2022) Immune checkpoint inhibitors in cancer therapy. Curr Oncol 29:3044–3060

3. Zhang C, Sui Y, Liu S et al (2024) In vitro and in vivo experimental models for cancer immunotherapy study. Curr Res Biotechnol 7: 100210

4. Bosenberg M, Liu ET, Yu CI et al (2023) Mouse models for immuno-oncology. Trends Cancer 9:578–590

5. Chulpanova DS, Kitaeva KV, Rutland CS et al (2020) Mouse tumor models for advanced cancer immunotherapy. Int J Mol Sci 21:1–15

6. Grubczak K, Kretowska-Grunwald A, Groth D et al (2021) Differential response of mda-mb-231 and mcf-7 breast cancer cells to in vitro inhibition with ctla-4 and pd-1 through cancer-immune cells modified interactions. Cells 10:1–19

7. Saleh R, Toor SM, Khalaf S et al (2019) Breast cancer cells and PD-1/PD-L1 blockade upregulate the expression of PD-1, CTLA-4, TIM-3 and LAG-3 immune checkpoints in CD4+ T cells. Vaccines 7:1–13

8. Fitzgerald AA, Li E, Weiner LM (2021) 3D culture systems for exploring cancer immunology. Cancers (Basel) 13:1–19

9. Ostendorf BN (2024) Recapitulating the tumor microenvironment in a dish, one cell type at a time. Cell Rep Methods 4:100800

10. Zhang D, Luo G, Ding X et al (2012) Preclinical experimental models of drug metabolism and disposition in drug discovery and development. Acta Pharm Sin B 2:549–561

11. Mestas J, Hughes CCW (2004) Of mice and not men: differences between mouse and human immunology. J Immunol 172:2731–2738

12. Magiera-Mularz K, Kocik J, Musielak B et al (2021) Human and mouse PD-L1: similar molecular structure, but different druggability profiles. iScience 24:101960

13. Chen J, Liao S, Xiao Z et al (2022) The development and improvement of immunodeficient mice and humanized immune system mouse models. Front Immunol 13:1–13

14. Chen B, Liu H, Liu Z et al (2023) Benefits and limitations of humanized mouse models for human red blood cell-related disease research. Front Hematol 1:1–12

15. Saraiva DP, Matias AT, Braga S et al (2020) Establishment of a 3D co-culture with MDA-MB-231 breast cancer cell line and patient-derived immune cells for application in the development of immunotherapies. Front Oncol 10:1–13

16. Zhou G, Lieshout R, Tienderen GS van, et al (2022) Modelling immune cytotoxicity for cholangiocarcinoma with tumour-derived organoids and effector T cells. Br J Cancer 127:649–660

17. Jeong S-R, Kang M (2023) Exploring tumor-immune interactions in co-culture models of T cells and tumor organoids derived from patients. Int J Mol Sci 24:14609

18. Wang Z (2024) Unveiling the potential: patient-derived organoids in cancer research and treatment. Oral Oncol Rep 9:100240

19. Wensink GE, Elias SG, Mullenders J et al (2021) Patient-derived organoids as a predictive biomarker for treatment response in cancer patients. NPJ Precis Oncol 5:30

20. Foo MA, You M, Chan SL et al (2022) Clinical translation of patient-derived tumour organoids- bottlenecks and strategies. Biomark Res 10:10

21. Bae J, Choi YS, Cho G et al (2022) The patient-derived cancer organoids: promises and challenges as platforms for cancer discovery. Cancers (Basel) 14:1–24

22. Abuwatfa WH, Pitt WG, Husseini GA (2024) Scaffold-based 3D cell culture models in cancer research. J Biomed Sci 31:7

23. Browne DJ, Miller CM, Doolan DL (2024) Technical pitfalls when collecting, cryopreserving, thawing, and stimulating human T-cells. Front Immunol 15:1–10

24. Wang L, Hückelhoven A, Hong J et al (2016) Standardization of cryopreserved peripheral blood mononuclear cells through a resting process for clinical immunomonitoring—development of an algorithm. Cytometry A 89:246–258

25. Palermo B, Panetta M, Campo G et al (2020) A cytofluorimetric assay to evaluate T cell polyfunctionality. Methods Enzymol 631:61–76

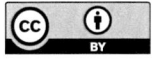

Chapter 12

Immunocompetent Preclinical Mouse Models of Brain Cancer

Ángel F. Álvarez-Prado

Abstract

Brain cancer represents a critical public health issue with thousands of newly diagnosed patients per year in Europe and the United States facing a dismal prognosis. The tumor immune microenvironment (TIME) has recently emerged as a key player promoting brain tumor growth and shaping responses to therapy. Consequently, new strategies have been developed to target the immune component of brain cancers and foster ant-tumoral immune responses, although they have only proven effective in a subset of patients. Therefore, it is of utmost importance to understand the dynamic biology of the TIME upon therapeutic intervention. Here, I describe different immunocompetent preclinical mouse models of primary and metastatic brain cancer, which allow a comprehensive exploration of the role of the immune system in tumor progression and response to therapy.

Key words Brain cancer, Preclinical models, Immunocompetent, Tumor microenvironment, Glioblastoma, Brain metastasis

1 Introduction

Primary glioblastoma and brain metastatic (BrM) tumors are respectively the most aggressive and frequent forms of brain cancer in adults [1–10]. Approximately 15,000 new glioblastoma patients are diagnosed per year in Europe [3] and the United States [4], and it is estimated that between 20% and 40% of all cancer patients will develop metastasis to the brain [9, 10], most frequently arising from lung (40–50%), breast (15–25%), and melanoma (5–10%) primary tumors [9, 10]. Patients with glioblastoma or BrM tumors face a dismal prognosis, with a median overall survival post-diagnosis between 6 and 15 months [1–10]. Therefore, there is an urgent clinical need to develop new therapies against these fatal cancers.

The tumor immune microenvironment (TIME), that is, all immune cells surrounding cancer cells in the tumor, has recently emerged as a fundamental regulator of cancer progression and

Sweta Rani and Lukasz Skalniak (eds.), *IMMUNO-model in Cancer: Methods and Protocols*, Methods in Molecular Biology, vol. 2959, https://doi.org/10.1007/978-1-0716-4734-9_12, © The Author(s) 2026

responses to therapy in primary and metastatic brain malignancies [11–13]. Indeed, recent therapeutic advances have focused on targeting the immune component of brain tumors, with promising but limited success to date [5, 6, 14–22]. A better understanding of the intricate and evolving microenvironmental landscape of brain tumors is thus critical to expand the therapeutic repertoire to effectively target these dismal diseases.

In this chapter, I will describe different immunocompetent preclinical mouse models of primary and metastatic brain cancer, including genetic mouse models of glioblastoma (based on the RCAS/NTV-a system [23]); and transplantable glioblastoma (GL261 [24]) and brain metastatic breast (PyMT-BrM3 [25]), lung (Sv2T3-BrM1 [26]), and melanoma (YUMM1.1-BrM4 [27]) cell lines.

The RCAS/NTv-a system is based on the somatic cell-specific transfer of DNA into neural progenitors, the cells of origin of glioblastoma tumors [23]. The system has two main components: (i) DF-1 chicken fibroblasts transduced with Replication-Competent ALV-Splice acceptor (RCAS) retroviral vectors and (ii) NTv-a transgenic mice. RCAS vectors allow the introduction of specific genetic alterations, such as overexpression of oncogenes or downregulation of tumor suppressor genes, in a cell-specific manner. NTv-a transgenic mice express the Tv-a viral receptor, which is essential for RCAS virus entry to the cell, under the control of the nestin promoter. This restricts the gene transfer to nestin-expressing neural progenitors, the cells of origin of glioblastomas. By intracranially injecting DF1 cells containing RCAS vectors, oncogenes (such as *hPDGF-B*) can be selectively overexpressed; and tumour suppressors (such as *Trp53*) silenced to generate glioblastoma tumors.

The BrM models described here are based on intracardiac transplant of cell lines with tropism for the brain. In brief, the PyMT-BrM3 cell line was established by intracardiac injection and three rounds of in vivo selection of a metastatic cell line that was originally derived from the MMTV-Polyoma Middle T-antigen (PyMT) breast cancer model [25] (C57BL/6 background). When injected intracardially into immunocompetent isogenic hosts, PyMT-BrM3 cells circulate in the blood, extravasate, seed, and give rise to multiple metastatic lesions throughout the brain parenchyma. SV2T3-BrM1 [26] cells originate from a metastatic cell line derived from a $Kras^{G12D}$; $Tp53^{flox/flox}$ lung cancer model and YUMM1.1-BrM4 [27] from Yale University Mouse Melanoma 1.1 (YUMM1.1) cells, which underwent the same procedure for one and four rounds, respectively. SV2T3-BrM1 and YUMM1.1-BrM4 cells spontaneously metastasize to the brain when intracardially injected into immunocompetent C57BL/6 hosts.

All these models recapitulate the components and complexity of the TIME of glioblastomas and brain metastatic tumors, therefore serving as valuable preclinical platforms to test novel therapies and understand mechanisms of response and resistance.

2   Materials

2.1   Immuno-competent Preclinical Mouse Models of Glioblastoma

2.1.1   Genetically Engineered Mouse Models (GEMMs): RCAS/NTv-a System

Experimental models: mouse strains

- Nestin-Tv-a (Tg(NES-TVA)J12Ech) mice: 4.5 to 7 weeks old.
- Nestin-Tv-a;*Ink4a/Arf*$^{-/-}$ (Tg(NES-TVA)J12Ech; Cdkn2a^{tm1Rdp}) mice: 4.5 to 7 weeks old.

Experimental models: cell lines

- DF-1 RCAS-hPDGF-B-HA cells (*see* **Notes 1** and **2**).
- DF-1 RCAS-sh*Tp53* cells (*see* **Notes 1** and **2**).

Reagents

- Dulbecco's Modified Eagle Medium (DMEM, Gibco), 10% fetal bovine serum (FBS, Gibco), 1% penicillin/streptomycin (Pen-Strep, Gibco) medium: prepare solution by mixing DMEM, FBS (1:10), and penicillin (10,000 units/mL)/streptomycin (10,000 μg/mL) (1:100) stock solutions (as an example, to prepare 500 mL, mix 445 mL DMEM, 50 mL FBS, and 5 mL Pen-Strep stocks). Warm medium at 37 °C for 30 min before use.
- Trypsin 0.25% EDTA (Gibco).
- 0.4% Trypan blue solution (Gibco).
- Bupivacaine/lidocaine solution: mix stock 0.5% bupivacaine (Carbonstesin, Aspen Pharma Schweiz) 5:9 with stock 2%, 20 mg/mL lidocaine (Streuli Pharma), and dilute the mix 1:2 in 1× PBS.
- Buprenorphine solution: dilute stock 0.3 mg/mL buprenorphine (Temgesic, Indivior Schweiz) 1:15 in 1× PBS.
- 70% ethanol.
- 70% ethanol wipes.
- Iodine wipes.
- ViscoTears liquid gel (Alcori/Novartis).
- Vetbond tissue adhesive (3 M).
- Bepanthene antiseptic cream (Bayer).
- Isoflurane liquid for inhalation (Attane, Minrad).
- Paracetamol.

Other materials

- Neubauer counting chamber hemocytometer.
- Brightfield microscope.
- Heating pad.
- Mouse stereotaxic device.
- Isoflurane vaporizer for small animals and rodents.
- Mouse anesthesia system for stereotaxic surgery (Stoelting).
- Cordless Micro Drill (Stoelting).
- Induction chamber for anesthesia.
- Clipper/Trimmer (Aesculap Exacta).
- 10 µL Hamilton 1800 gas tight syringe (Hamilton)
- 1 mL insulin syringe (BD Micro-Fine)
- 0.5 mL insulin syringe (BD Micro-Fine)
- Forceps (F.S.T.) (2 units).
- Cotton sticks.
- Disposable scalpel (Swann Morton).
- Bed mat (Molicare).

2.1.2 Orthotopic Transplant of Mouse Glioblastoma Cell Lines

Experimental models: mouse strains

- Wild-type C57BL/6 J mice (Charles River): 6–10 weeks old.

  Experimental models: cell lines

- GL261 cell line (see **Notes 1** and **2**).

  Reagents

- Same as indicated in Subheading 2.1.1.

  Other materials

- Same as indicated in Subheading 2.1.1.

2.2 Immuno-competent Preclinical Mouse Models of Brain Metastasis

Experimental models: mouse strains

- Wild-type C57BL/6 J mice (Charles River): 6–10 weeks old.

  Experimental models: cell lines

- PyMT-BrM3 (breast to brain metastasis, *see* **Notes 1** and **2**).
- Sv2T3-BrM1 (lung to brain metastasis, *see* **Notes 1** and **2**).
- YUMM1.1-BrM4 (melanoma to brain metastasis, *see* **Notes 1** and **2**).

Reagents

- DMEM/F-12 GlutaMAX (Gibco) 10% FBS (Gibco) 1% Pen-Strep (Gibco) medium: prepare solution by mixing DMEM/F-12 GlutaMAX, FBS (1:10) and Pen-Strep (1:100) stock solutions (as an example, to prepare 500 mL, mix 445 mL DMEM, 50 mL FBS, and 5 mL Pen-Strep stocks). Warm medium at 37 °C for 30 min before use.

- 1× HBSS (Gibco).

- 1× PBS.

- Depilatory cream (Veet).

- Isoflurane liquid for inhalation (Attane, Minrad).

Other materials

- Clipper/trimmer (Aesculap Exacta).

- Heating pad.

- Isoflurane vaporizer for small animals and rodents.

- Induction chamber for anesthesia.

- 25G, 80 mm Safety-multifly needle (Starstedt).

- 15 mL plastic syringe (BD Plastipak).

- 26G needle (Braun).

- 30G needle (Braun).

- 1 mL plastic syringe.

- 70 μm cell strainer.

- Gauze.

- Tape.

3 Methods

3.1 Immunocompetent Preclinical Mouse Models of Glioblastoma

3.1.1 Genetically Engineered Mouse Models

1. Calculate the number of DF1 cells required. NTv-a mice are injected with 1.5×10^5 DF1-hPDGF-B and 1.5×10^5 DF1-sh$Tp53$ cells per mouse; NTv-a; $Ink4a/Arf^{-/-}$ mice are injected with 2×10^5 DF1-hPDGF-B cells per mouse. Prepare at least double of the required number of DF1 cells.

2. Thaw DF-1 cells and expand them in DMEM 10% FBS Pen-Strep (*see* **Notes 1** and **2**) inside an incubator at 37 °C and 5% CO_2. Keep them in culture at least 1.5 weeks prior to intracranial injection.

3. Calculate required amount of bupivacaine/lidocaine (bupi/lido) and buprenorphine solutions: 50 μL bupi/lido and 100 μL buprenorphine per mouse. Prepare at least 15% excess to account for syringe dead volumes.

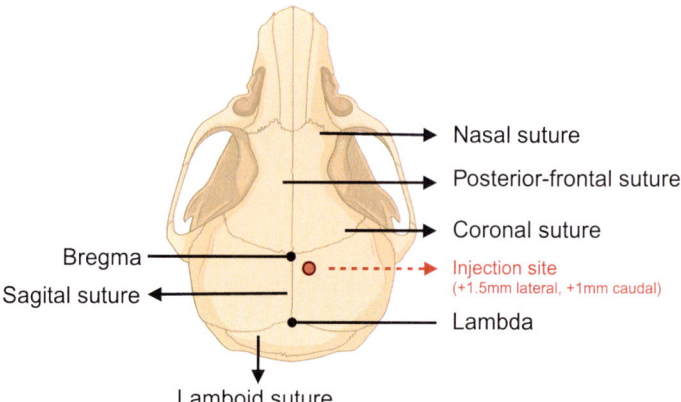

Nasal suture

Posterior-frontal suture

Coronal suture

Bregma

Injection site
(+1.5mm lateral, +1mm caudal)

Sagital suture

Lambda

Lamboid suture

Fig. 1 Anatomical representation of the mouse skull indicating injection site for DF-1 cells

4. Harvest and count DF-1 cells: slowly remove culture medium, rinse cells with $1\times$ PBS once and add trypsin solution. Incubate at 37 °C until cells start to detach, then neutralize trypsin by adding DMEM 10% FBS 2:1. Take an aliquot of the cell suspension and add trypan blue solution 1:1. Count alive cells on a Neubauer chamber.

5. Adjust DF-1 cells concentration. Spin cells at 4 °C 400 G for 5 min and resuspend the pellet in the appropriate volume of DMEM 1% FBS. Note that cells need to be resuspended in DMEM FBS 1% (not 10%) for injection. NTv-a mice, adjust DF1-hPDGF-B and DF1-sh*Tp53* to 1.5×10^5 cells/μL, and mix 1:1 (*see* **Note 3**); NTv-a; *Ink4a/Arf*$^{-/-}$ mice, adjust DF1-hPDGF-B to 2×10^5 cells/μL (*see* **Note 4**). Keep cells in ice until injection.

6. Set up the surgery environment: clean up surfaces with 70% ethanol, place a bed mat on the surface, assemble induction chamber, isoflurane vaporizer, and stereotaxic device.

7. Load a 1 mL insulin syringe with buprenorphine solution and a 0.5 mL insulin syringe with bupi/lido solution.

8. Turn on O_2 pump and keep pressure between 1.5 and 2 mmHg and isoflurane flux to 2%.

9. Restrain the mouse and add ViscoTears to the eyes to prevent corneal drying during surgery.

10. Introduce mouse in the induction chamber and wait until it is anesthetized.

11. Resuspend DF-1 cells by pipetting up and down and load Hamilton syringe with 10 μL cell suspension.

12. Restrain the mouse and shave the head from approximately 2 mm from the eyes to approximately 2 mm before the ears.

13. Clean the mouse skin with an ethanol wipe first and then an iodine wipe.

14. Inject 50 µL of bupi/lido solution subcutaneously under the scalp of the mouse for local analgesia.

15. Inject 100 µL of buprenorphine solution subcutaneously in the neck of the mouse for systemic long-term analgesia.

16. Place the mouse in the stereotaxic device, ensuring that the mouse front teeth are placed in the incisor bars and the head is immobilized by the lateral ear bars.

17. Clean skin with an iodine wipe and make a small incision (between 3 and 5 mm) to expose the skull for the craniotomy.

18. Localize the injection site. Coordinates for injection are 1.5 mm lateral, 1 mm caudal, and 2 mm deep from bregma (see Fig. 1).

19. Place a 0.8 mm carbide steel burr in the micro drill and drill a hole in the skull.

20. Place the Hamilton syringe at the injection site using the guides in the stereotaxic device, wait 10 s' for the syringe to stabilize, and slowly inject 2 µL of the DF-1 cell suspension (total of 3×10^5 cells for NTv-a mice; 2×10^5 cells for NTv-a; $Ink4a/Arf^{-/-}$ mice). Wait 10 s and slowly remove the syringe.

21. Remove mouse from the stereotaxic device.

22. Close the incision in the skin by bringing the two skin ends together (one under the other) and applying VetBond tissue adhesive. Avoid leaving rolled or folded skin, especially close to the eyes, where mice can scratch themselves and reopen the wound.

23. Wait until the adhesive is dry and apply Bepanthen (antiseptic) using a cotton stick.

24. Place the mouse on a warm pad until it recovers from anesthesia and return to its cage.

25. Add paracetamol (final concentration of 2 mg/mL) to the drinking water for pain relief. Keep the treatment for 1 week.

26. Mice must undergo close visual inspection daily for the first 48 h postsurgery (*see* **Note 5**).

27. Turn off O_2 and isoflurane vaporizers, disassemble equipment, and clean surfaces.

3.1.2   Orthotopic Inoculation of Glioblastoma Cell Lines

Follow the same steps described in Subheading 3.1.1, but adjust the GL261 cell concentration to 5×10^4 cells/µL in DMEM 1% FBS. A total of 10^5 cells in a final volume of 2 µL will be injected (*see* **Note 6**).

3.2 Immuno-competent Preclinical Mouse Models of Brain Metastasis

3.2.1 Breast to Brain Metastasis

1. Calculate number of PyMT-BrM3 cells required: 10^5 cells per mouse will be intracardially injected into C57BL/6 J hosts (*see* **Note** 7). Prepare cells in excess to control for pipetting errors/syringe dead volume: it is advised to prepare 2.5× the number of cells required.

2. Thaw PyMT-BrM3 cells and culture them in DMEM/F-12 GlutaMAX 10% FBS 1% Pen-Strep (*see* **Notes 1** and **2**) inside an incubator at 37 °C and 5% CO_2.

3. Change culture medium 24 h after thawing.

4. Harvest and count PyMT-BrM3 cells: slowly remove culture medium, rinse cells with 1x PBS once, and add trypsin solution. Incubate at 37 °C until cells start to detach, then neutralize trypsin by adding DMEM/F-12 GlutaMAX 10% FBS 2:1. Centrifuge cells at 4 °C 300 × *g* for 5 min, and resuspend in 1× HBSS. Filter cell suspension through a 70 μm cell strainer. Take an aliquot of the cell suspension and add trypan blue solution 1:1. Count alive cells on a Neubauer chamber.

5. Adjust PyMT-BrM3 cells concentration to 10^3 cells/μL. Spin cells at 4 °C 300 G for 5 min and resuspend the pellet in the appropriate volume of 1× HBSS. Place cells on ice until injection. Cells will be injected in a final volume of 100 μL.

6. Set up isoflurane vaporizer, induction chamber, and isoflurane mask. Turn on O_2 pump and keep pressure between 1.5 and 2 mmHg and isoflurane flux to 2%.

7. Shave mice. Anesthetize mice into an induction chamber with 2% isoflurane. Restrain mice and shave the skin covering the thoracic cage using a clipper, be careful to avoid clipper burn. Apply a thin layer of depilatory cream using a glove or cotton swab. Allow a contact time of 30–60 s and immediately wipe off the depilatory cream using warm water and gauze. Do not leave depilatory cream in contact with the mouse skin for longer periods, since it can cause chemical burns. If hair remains, dry the area and repeat the process once.

8. Fit the isoflurane mask to keep mouse anesthetized under 2% isoflurane and place it in a supine position. Use tape to fix the mouse to the surgery table surface and prevent unwanted movements during cell injections.

9. Resuspend PyMT-BrM3 cells by pipetting up and down and load a 1 mL syringe with a 26G needle with 100 μL of cell suspension. Aspirate a bit of air before loading the syringe with the cells, so that there is space for blood to flow in (*see* **step 11**).

10. Insert syringe in the second left intercostal space of the mouse, approximately 1 mm away from the sternum to get into the left ventricle apex of the heart. Blood backflush from the heart into the syringe needle should be observed.

11. Slowly inject 100 μL of cell suspension into the left ventricle of the heart.

12. Place the mouse on a warm pad until it recovers from anesthesia and return to its cage.

3.2.2 Lung to Brain Metastasis

Follow the same steps described in Subheading 3.2.1 with the following changes:

- **Steps 2–4**: SV2T3-BrM1 cells (*see* **Notes 1, 2** and **8**) are resuspended in DMEM/F-12 GlutaMAX, 10% FBS, 1% Pen-Strep at a concentration of 6.7×10^4 cells/mL and seeded in 30 μL drops in the lid of a petri dish. The lid is inverted, PBS is added to the bottom of the dish to prevent evaporation and cells are incubated for 12 h inside a cell incubator at 37 °C and 5% CO_2. Four hanging drops (approximately 120 μL volume) per mouse will be inoculated in the left ventricle apex.

- **Steps 10–12**: to minimize the outgrowth of SV2T3-BrM1 cells in the injection site and pericardium, a dual syringe system is employed. A multifly needle (25G, 80 mm) attached to a syringe filled with 1× PBS is inserted into the left ventricular apex of the mouse. Blood backflush from the heart into the needle should be observed. Four hanging drops (approximately 120 μL volume) are loaded into a second syringe with a 30G needle. The cell suspension is then slowly injected into the catheter of the multifly needle and immediately flushed with PBS from the syringe attached to the multifly needle until the cell suspension is completely transferred to the mouse heart. See Fig. 2 for a schematic representation of the dual syringe setup.

3.2.3 Melanoma to Brain Metastasis

Follow the same steps described in Subheading 3.2.1 with the following changes:

- **Steps 2–4**: 5×10^4 YUMM1.1-BrM4 cells (*see* **Notes 1, 2, 9, 10,** and **11**) per mouse will be intracardially injected. Adjust cell concentration to 5×10^2 cells/μL in an appropriate volume of 1× HBSS. Cells will be injected in a final volume of 100 μL.

- **Steps 10–12**: to minimize the outgrowth of YUMM1.1-BrM4 cells in the injection site and pericardium, the same dual injection system described in Subheading 3.2.2 is employed (*see* Fig. 2).

4   Notes

1. All cell lines described in this chapter must routinely undergo morphology and growth dynamics analyses and be tested for mycoplasma contamination.

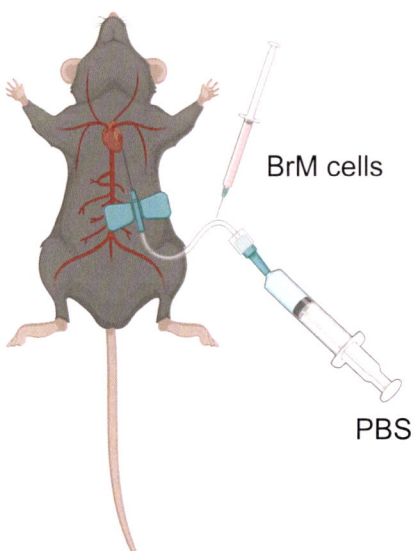

BrM cells

PBS

Fig. 2 Schematic representation of the dual syringe system for intracardial injection of lung- and melanoma-BrM cell lines

2. Cell lines doubling times: DF1, 22 h; GL261, 80–100 h; PyMT-BrM3, 24 h; SV2T3-BrM1, 24 h; YUMM1.1-BrM4, 48–72 h.

3. NTv-a mice intracranially injected with DF1 cells containing RCAS-hPDGFB and RCAS-sh*Tp53* vectors develop glioblastoma tumors with a penetrance of approximately 80%. Tumor onset is between 4 and 5 weeks postinjection and median survival approximately 2–3 weeks post-tumor detection. Please note that the TIME in these mice is wild type.

4. NTv-a;*Ink4a/Arf*$^{-/-}$ mice intracranially injected with DF1 cells containing the RCAS-hPDGFB vector develop glioblastoma tumors with a penetrance of approximately 95%. Tumor onset occurs at 4 weeks, and median survival is approximately 2 weeks post-tumor detection. Please note that the TIME in these mice is knocked out for *Ink4a/Arf*.

5. Success rate of the intracranial surgery is 100% when performed appropriately. Mice recover from anesthesia and have a normal exploratory behavior in 2–5 min. If animals appear distressed or show any symptoms, please follow humane endpoint evaluation criteria guidelines according to local regulations.

6. C57BL/6J mice intracranially injected with 10^5 GL261 cells develop glioblastoma tumors with a penetrance of 95–100%. Tumor onset is 3 weeks, and survival is approximately 1–2 weeks post-tumor detection. Please note that the TIME in these mice is wild type.

7. C57BL/6J mice intracardially injected with 10^5 PyMT-BrM3 cells (breast-BrM) develop BrM tumors with a penetrance of 90%. Tumor onset is approximately 40 days post-injection, and survival is between 50 and 60 days postinjection. Mice may develop metastasis to other sites, mainly in the ovaries and adrenal gland. Please note that the TIME in these mice is wild-type.

8. C57BL/6J mice intracardially injected with SV2T3-BrM1 (lung-BrM) cells develop BrM tumors with a penetrance of 70–80%. Tumor onset is approximately 21 days postinjection, and survival is around 28 days postinjection. Mice may develop pericardial tumors and metastasis to other sites, including meningeal and extracranial tumors mainly in the eyes. Please note that the TIME in these mice is wild type.

9. C57BL/6J mice intracardially injected with 5×10^4 YUMM1.1-BrM4 (melanoma-BrM) cells develop BrM tumors with a penetrance of 40%. Tumor onset is approximately 20 days postinjection, and survival is between 40 and 50 days postinjection. Mice develop pericardial tumors and metastasis to other sites, mainly intrathoracic and in the adrenal gland. YUMM1.1-BrM4 cells can only be used to model the initial stages of brain metastasis (micrometastasis), due to the outgrowth of cancer cells in the pericardium. Please note that the TIME in these mice is wild type.

10. Additional mouse and human cell lines with tropism to the brain and the ability to form BrM tumors are available through the Brain Metastasis Cell Lines Panel. All details are available in the original publication [28].

11. Magnetic resonance imaging (MRI) can be employed to monitor tumor growth in all the models presented in this chapter in a longitudinal and noninvasive manner.

Acknowledgments

This work was supported by The Brain Tumor Charity Future Leaders Program (FL_2021_/1_10602) and FNR ATTRACT Grant (A24/BM/18696400) to A.A-P. The author would like to express his gratitude to Prof. Johanna Joyce and all lab members who were involved in the development of the breast-, lung-, and melanoma-BrM models presented in this chapter; all scientists from the nineteen laboratories that contributed to the Brain Metastasis Cell Lines Panel; Prof. Eric Holland and all lab members who developed the RCAS/NTv-a system; and Prof. David P Rall and all lab members who developed the GL261 glioblastoma cell line. This publication is based upon work from COST Action

IMMUNO-model, CA21135, supported by COST (European Cooperation in Science and Technology).

References

1. Louis DN, Perry A, Reifenberger G, von Deimling A, Figarella-Branger D, Cavenee WK et al (2016) The 2016 World Health Organization classification of tumors of the central nervous system: a summary. Acta Neuropathol (Berl) 131:803–820

2. Wen PY, Kesari S (2008) Malignant gliomas in adults. N Engl J Med 359:492–507

3. Crocetti E, Trama A, Stiller C, Caldarella A, Soffietti R, Jaal J et al (2012) Epidemiology of glial and non-glial brain tumours in Europe. Eur J Cancer 48:1532–1542

4. Ostrom QT, Gittleman H, Liao P, Vecchione-Koval T, Wolinsky Y, Kruchko C et al (2017) CBTRUS statistical report: primary brain and other central nervous system tumors diagnosed in the United States in 2010–2014. Neuro-Oncol 19:1–88

5. Stupp R, Mason WP, van den Bent MJ, Weller M, Fisher B, Taphoorn MJB, et al (2009) Radiotherapy plus concomitant and adjuvant temozolomide for glioblastoma [Internet]. https://doi.org/10.1056/NEJMoa043330. Accessed 11 Jan 2019

6. Ostrom QT, Gittleman H, Stetson L, Virk SM, Barnholtz-Sloan JS (2015) Epidemiology of gliomas. In: Raizer J, Parsa A (eds) Current understanding and treatment of gliomas. Springer International, Cham, pp 1–14. https://doi.org/10.1007/978-3-319-12048-5_1

7. Lambert AW, Pattabiraman DR, Weinberg RA (2017) Emerging biological principles of metastasis. Cell 168:670–691

8. Massagué J, Obenauf AC (2016) Metastatic colonization by circulating tumour cells. Nature 529:298–306

9. Valiente M, Ahluwalia MS, Boire A, Brastianos PK, Goldberg SB, Lee EQ et al (2018) The evolving landscape of brain metastasis. Trends Cancer 4:176–196

10. Boire A, Brastianos PK, Garzia L, Valiente M (2020) Brain metastasis. Nat Rev Cancer 20:4–11

11. Quail DF, Joyce JA (2017) The microenvironmental landscape of brain tumors. Cancer Cell 31:326–341

12. Bejarano L, Jordão MJC, Joyce JA (2021) Therapeutic targeting of the tumor microenvironment. Cancer Discov 11:933–959

13. de Visser KE, Joyce JA (2023) The evolving tumor microenvironment: from cancer initiation to metastatic outgrowth. Cancer Cell 41: 374–403

14. Steindl A, Brunner TJ, Heimbach K, Schweighart K, Moser GM, Niziolek HM et al (2022) Changing characteristics, treatment approaches and survival of patients with brain metastasis: data from six thousand and thirty-one individuals over an observation period of 30 years. Eur J Cancer 162:170–181

15. Suh JH, Kotecha R, Chao ST, Ahluwalia MS, Sahgal A, Chang EL (2020) Current approaches to the management of brain metastases. Nat Rev Clin Oncol 17:279–299

16. Sperduto PW, Yang TJ, Beal K, Pan H, Brown PD, Bangdiwala A et al (2017) Estimating survival in patients with lung cancer and brain metastases: an update of the graded prognostic assessment for lung cancer using molecular markers (lung-molGPA). JAMA Oncol 3: 827–831

17. Sperduto PW, Jiang W, Brown PD, Braunstein S, Sneed P, Wattson DA et al (2017) Estimating survival in melanoma patients with brain metastases: an update of the graded prognostic assessment for melanoma using molecular markers (melanoma-molGPA). Int J Radiat Oncol 99:812–816

18. Goldberg SB, Gettinger SN, Mahajan A, Chiang AC, Herbst RS, Sznol M et al (2016) Pembrolizumab for patients with melanoma or non-small-cell lung cancer and untreated brain metastases: early analysis of a non-randomised, open-label, phase 2 trial. Lancet Oncol 17: 976–983

19. Goldberg SB, Schalper KA, Gettinger SN, Mahajan A, Herbst RS, Chiang AC et al (2020) Pembrolizumab for management of patients with NSCLC and brain metastases: long-term results and biomarker analysis from a non-randomised, open-label, phase 2 trial. Lancet Oncol 21:655–663

20. Tawbi HA, Forsyth PA, Algazi A, Hamid O, Hodi FS, Moschos SJ et al (2018) Combined Nivolumab and Ipilimumab in melanoma metastatic to the brain. N Engl J Med 379:722–730

21. Tawbi HA-H, Forsyth PAJ, Hodi FS, Lao CD, Moschos SJ, Hamid O et al (2019) Efficacy and safety of the combination of nivolumab

(NIVO) plus ipilimumab (IPI) in patients with symptomatic melanoma brain metastases (CheckMate 204). J Clin Oncol 37:9501–9501

22. Long GV, Atkinson V, Menzies AM, Lo S, Guminski AD, Brown MP et al (2017) A randomized phase II study of nivolumab or nivolumab combined with ipilimumab in patients (pts) with melanoma brain metastases (mets): the anti-PD1 brain collaboration (ABC). J Clin Oncol 35:9508–9508

23. Hambardzumyan D, Amankulor NM, Helmy KY, Becher OJ, Holland EC (2009) Modeling adult gliomas using RCAS/t-va technology. Transl Oncol 2:89–95

24. Ausman JI, Shapiro WR, Rall DP (1970) Studies on the chemotherapy of experimental brain tumors: development of an experimental model. Cancer Res 30:2394–2400

25. Croci D, Santalla Méndez R, Temme S, Soukup K, Fournier N, Zomer A et al (2022) Multispectral fluorine-19 MRI enables longitudinal and noninvasive monitoring of tumor-associated macrophages. Sci Transl Med 14: eabo2952

26. Bejarano L, Kauzlaric A, Lamprou E, Lourenco J, Fournier N, Ballabio M et al (2024) Interrogation of endothelial and mural cells in brain metastasis reveals key immune-regulatory mechanisms. Cancer Cell 42:378–395.e10

27. Saltarin F, Wegmüller A, Bejarano L, Ildiz ES, Zwicky P, Vianin A et al (2023) Compromised blood-brain barrier junctions enhance melanoma cell intercalation and extravasation. Cancer 15:5071

28. Valiente M, Van Swearingen AED, Anders CK, Bairoch A, Boire A, Bos PD et al (2020) Brain metastasis cell lines panel: a public resource of organotropic cell lines. Cancer Res 80:4314–4323

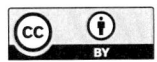

Chapter 13

Cancer Patient-Derived Scaffolds as In Vitro Preclinical Models for Immunotherapy Screening

Diogo Estêvão, Maria J. Oliveira, and Tânia B. Cruz

Abstract

The extracellular matrix (ECM) is a complex network of macromolecules that provides physical structure support for tissues and acts as a reservoir for multiple growth factors and signaling mediators modulating the behavior of both cancer and stromal cells within the tumor microenvironment (TME). This key element of the tumor milieu significantly influences various cancer features such as cell differentiation, proliferation, angiogenesis, immune escape, invasion, and metastasis. Therefore, to accurately mimic tumors, it is essential that in vitro models include ECM components. Therefore, to develop 3D biomimetic models for studying cancer, researchers have explored various approaches, including scaffolds made from natural or synthetic polymers and ceramics. However, decellularized ECM derived from patient tumors presents a distinctive model since it preserves the native ECM architecture, biomechanical properties, and molecular composition. Here, we spotlight innovative and advanced protocols to obtain 3D models based on patient-derived decellularized ECM as high-throughput strategies for cancer research, particularly to immunotherapy screening.

Key words Patient-derived scaffolds, Extracellular matrix, Decellularization, Biomimetic models, Therapy screenings

1 Introduction

The extracellular matrix (ECM) is a complex network of macromolecules that provides a physical structure to support tissues constituting a reservoir of signaling molecules. Over the last years, in the oncology field, attention has been given to the influence of this noncellular component on both cancer and non malignant stromal cells, fibroblasts, adipocytes, endothelial, and immune cells. The ECM is an extremely dynamic element of the tumour microenvironment (TME) [1] known to modulate the behavior of cells through its biochemical and biomechanical properties [2, 3]. These are significantly changed during tumor development and often enable cellular transformation, angiogenesis, inflammation, immune escape, invasion, and metastasis [4, 5]. Furthermore,

Sweta Rani and Lukasz Skalniak (eds.), *IMMUNO-model in Cancer: Methods and Protocols*, Methods in Molecular Biology, vol. 2959, https://doi.org/10.1007/978-1-0716-4734-9_13, © The Author(s) 2026

the tumor ECM properties are also described to influence therapy response and to impact therapy resistance [6–8]. Considering the relevant role of the ECM and the lack of effective protocols that mimic native tissues conditions failing to recapitulate the complexity of the TME, it is essential to employ biomimetic 3D models in drug discovery and development [9, 10]. Currently, there are several 3D tumor models available, from bio-fabricated tissues to organotypic 3D-bioactive models [11–13]. The use of decellularized ECM derived from cancer patients' native tissues as a scaffold for cellular components allows the maintenance of tissue architecture and physiology, representing an interesting model, for example, to reduce drug attrition rates and to uncover therapy resistant mechanisms [8, 14, 15]. Decellularization protocols are diverse and mainly rely on the combination of physical, chemical, and enzymatic methodologies to eliminate cellular components, while maintaining ECM architecture and biochemical features [16, 17]. In this chapter, we describe one protocol for efficient removal of cells from native tumor tissues with subsequent repopulation with specific populations as cancer and/or immune cells, to dissect molecular mechanisms or perform different screening assays.

2   Materials and Solutions

All solutions should be prepared with ultrapure water (prepared by purifying deionized water, to attain a sensitivity of 18 MΩ-cm at 25 °C) and analytical grade reagents. Unless indicated otherwise, prepare and store all reagents at room temperature (RT). Follow all waste disposal regulations when disposing of waste materials.

2.1 Sample Collection and Storage

1. Prepare 50 mL sterile plastic tubes with 10–20 mL Hanks' balanced salt solution (HBSS) to collect each tissue sample. Maintain at 4 °C until sample collection.

2. Reserve optimal cutting temperature compound (OCT) to embed tissue samples before freezing steps (see **Note 1**).

3. Label Peel-A-Way® Disposable Histology Molds and aluminum foil squares, one per tissue sample.

4. Prepare an isopentane bath (−55 °C) by prechilling the solution with liquid nitrogen (see **Note 2**). For that, pour liquid nitrogen into a square-base container, fill a 100 mL glass beaker with 4 cm of isopentane, and place the beaker onto the liquid nitrogen to chill the solution. Always work under the flow hood for safety.

2.2 Tissue Decellularization

1. Prepare one petri dish for washing steps and a scalpel or a biopsy punch (Cat. no. BPP-40F) for preparation of sample fragments (*see* **Note 6**).

2. For the decellularization procedure, according to the number of required samples, prepare sterile 24-well plates.

3. Phosphate-buffered saline (PBS) 1×: weigh 200 g of NaCl, 15.25 g of Na$_2$HPO$_4$, 5 g of KCl, 5 g of KH$_2$PO$_4$, and transfer to a 1 L graduated cylinder. Add water to a volume of 800 mL and mix. Adjust pH to 7.4 with HCl. Complete volume to 1 L with distilled water, autoclave to sterilize, and store at room temperature (RT).

4. Hypotonic buffer A: weigh 1.21 g of Trizma base (10 mM) and 1 g EDTA (0.1%), transfer to a 1 L graduated cylinder. Add water to a volume of 800 mL and mix. Adjust pH to 7.8 with HCl. Complete volume to 1 L with distilled water, autoclave to sterilize, and store at RT. Before using the solution, add 10 µg/mL gentamicin to the required volume to minimize bacterial growth.

5. Hypotonic buffer B: weigh 1.21 g of Trizma base (10 mM) and transfer to a 1 L graduated cylinder. Add water to a volume of 800 mL and mix. Adjust pH to 7.8 with HCl. Complete volume to 1 L with distilled water, autoclave to sterilize, and store at RT.

6. 0.2% SDS solution: weigh 0.5 g sodium dodecyl sulfate (0.2% SDS) (*see* **Note 3**) and transfer to a 500 mL glass flask. Add 250 mL of hypotonic buffer B (10 mM Tris) and mix. Adjust pH to 7.8 with HCl, autoclave to sterilize, and store at RT. Before using the solution, add 10 µg/mL gentamicin to the required volume.

7. DNAse solution: weigh 2.42 g of Trizma base (20 mM) and 0.19 g of MgCl$_2$ (2 mM), and transfer to a 1 L graduated cylinder. Autoclave to sterilize and store at RT. Before using the solution, add 50 U/mL DNAse (*see* **Note 4**) and 10 µg/mL gentamicin to the required volume. For longer time storage, aliquot the solution and store at −20 °C.

2.3 Extracellular Matrix Repopulation

1. Prepare U-bottom 96-well plates for repopulation steps according to experimental needs and a sterile needle.

2. RPMI 1640 complete medium: 500 mL of medium supplemented with 10% (50 mL) inactivated foetal bovine serum and 1% (5 mL) Pen/Strep (100 U/mL penicillin and 100 ng/mL streptomycin).

3. Phosphate-buffered saline (PBS) 1×: weigh 200 g of NaCl, 15.25 g of Na$_2$HPO$_4$, 5 g of KCl, 5 g of KH$_2$PO$_4$, and transfer to a 1 L graduated cylinder. Add distillled water to a volume of

800 mL and mix. Adjust pH to 7.4 with HCl. Complete volume to 1 L with water, autoclave to sterilize, and store at RT.

2.4 Screening Assays

1. For histology procedures, standard formalin and paraffin solutions will be required.

2. For scanning electron microscopy, standard solutions of 0.1 M cacodylate buffer and 2.5% glutaraldehyde (in 0.1 M sodium cacodylate) will be required.

3. For cell retrieval from the repopulated scaffolds, a solution of accutase (GRISP, Cat. no. GTC01) will be needed and flow cytometry buffer should be prepared (PBS 1x supplemented with 0.01% of sodium azide and 2% bovine serum albumin).

3   Methods

3.1 Sample Collection and Storage

1. To collect the tissue sample, place each specimen to the corresponding labeled 50 mL tube containing HBSS with tweezer assistance. If possible, proceed immediately to storage or, alternatively, keep it at 4 °C for a maximum of 2 h.

2. For storage, take one labeled Peel-A-Way® Disposable Histology Mold and fill the bottom with OCT medium. Place the tissue sample at the center of the mold and cover it with OCT compound completely, as demonstrated in Fig. 1.

3. Hold the mold with a tweezer and place it in the prechilled isopentane. Keep it under the isopentane bath until the OCT has solidified and turned white.

4. Retrieve the mold from the isopentane and decant the excess solution.

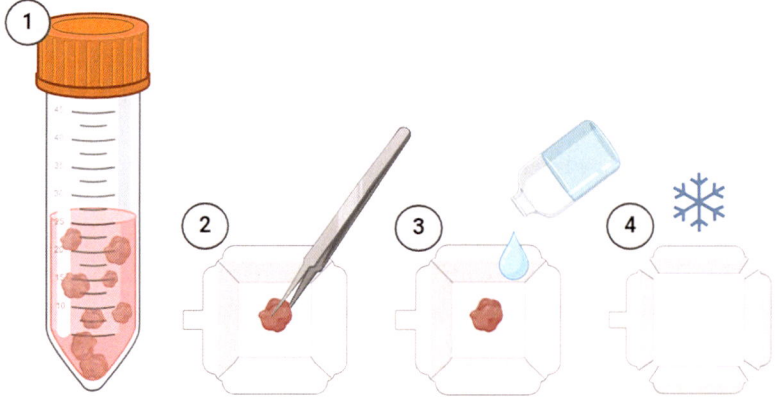

Fig. 1 Schematic view of tissue sample collection and storage (1). Tube containing specimens in HBSS, (2) sample transfer into the cryomold, (3) embedding in OCT, (4) isopentane chilling bath to freeze specimen

5. Wrap the mold in the labeled aluminum foil square and immediately place the cryomold on dry ice.

6. Store frozen embedded tissue samples in a container at $-80\ °C$ until further use.

3.2 Tissue Decellularization

1. Take the frozen sample from $-80\ °C$ (*see* **Note 5**) and leave it on ice to thaw gently.

2. Transfer the tissue to a petri dish and wash it twice with PBS 1x to remove all the OCT.

3. Slice the sample to 3 mm^2 pieces using a scalpel or a biopsy punch (*see* **Note 6**) and transfer each tissue piece into a well of a 24-well plate (Fig. 2).

4. Add 1 mL of hypotonic buffer A per well with sample and incubate the fragments for 18 h at RT with 160 rpm agitation (use a horizontal shaker with light agitation to attain solution embedding into the sample).

5. Remove the solution from each well and carefully add 1 mL PBS 1×. Incubate for 1 h at RT with 160 rpm agitation.

6. Repeat **step 5** twice to wash the fragments.

7. Prewarm the 0.2% SDS solution at 37 °C in a water bath to assure that the detergent is completely dissolved and add 1 mL per well to cover each fragment.

8. Incubate for 24 h at RT with 160 rpm agitation.

9. Remove the solution from each well and carefully add 1 mL hypotonic buffer B. Incubate for 20 min at RT with 160 rpm agitation (use a horizontal shaker with light agitation to attain solution embedding into the sample).

10. Repeat **step 9** twice to wash the fragments.

11. Add 1 mL DNase solution to each well and incubate for 3 h at 37 °C with 160 rpm agitation (*see* **Note 7**).

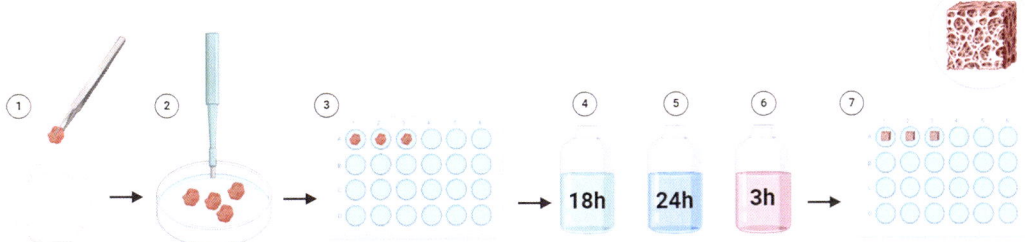

Fig. 2 Schematic view of tissue sample decellularization protocol (1). Unfreeze specimens in OCT, (2) transfer the sample into a petri dish and divide it into 3 mm^2 fragments, (3) transfer each fragment into one well of a 24-well plate, (4) hypotonic buffer incubation for cell rupture, (5) SDS action for membrane dissociation, (6) DNase treatment for DNA digestion, (7) scaffold wash with PBS 1× and storage until further use

12. Remove the solution, add very carefully 1 mL PBS 1× to each well, and incubate for 20 min at RT with 160 rpm agitation (use a horizontal shaker with light agitation to attain solution embedding into the sample).

13. Repeat **step 12** twice to wash the fragments.

14. Leave the sample in PBS 1× with gentamicin, to minimize bacterial growth, and store at 4 °C, after sealing the plate with aluminum foil (*see* **Note 8**).

3.3 Extracellular Matrix Repopulation

1. Take the decellularized fragments from 4 °C and, in the flow hood (*see* **Note 9**), transfer the required scaffolds into wells of a U-bottom 96-well plate (one matrix per well).

2. Wash it twice with PBS 1× to remove all storage solution, including gentamicin.

3. Add 200 μL of RPMI 1640 complete medium to each well and incubate 30 min at 37 °C with 5% CO_2.

4. Proceed with the preparation of the cell suspension to repopulate the matrix (choose cell type according to experimental requirements, namely cancer cell lines or primary monocytes).

5. Wash the cells with PBS 1× and count them to obtain the desired number of cells per mL.

6. To a new 15 mL sterile tube, transfer the number of cells required to repopulate each scaffold (*see* **Note 10**).

7. Centrifuge cell suspension at 1200 rpm ($300 \times g$) for 5 min at 4 °C.

8. Remove all the supernatant carefully and resuspend the pellet in a final volume of 20 μL of RPMI 1640 complete medium.

9. Remove all the medium from each well containing decellularized specimens.

10. Carefully move the scaffold into the center of the well.

11. Add the 20 μL of the previously prepared cell suspension, containing the desired number/population of cells, on top of each matrix.

12. Carefully add the cell suspension to the decellularized matrix, gently pipetting up and down (always avoid air bubbles).

13. Incubate the repopulated scaffold at 37 °C with 5% CO_2 for 18 h.

14. Gently transfer the repopulated matrix to a new well by using a sterile needle.

15. Carefully add 200 μL of RPMI 1640 complete medium to each matrix-containing well.

16. Incubate repopulated decellularized matrix at 37 °C with 5% CO_2 for the required days (*see* **Note 11**). At this point, treatment with different compounds can be applied.

17. Change the medium every 2 days.

3.4 Screening Assays

3.4.1 Preparation of Repopulated Scaffolds for Histology

1. After treatment exposure, remove culture medium from each repopulated matrix.

2. Add 200 µL of PBS to wash the sample gently.

3. Remove PBS and add 200 µL of formalin.

4. Incubate samples in formalin during 24 h to fix repopulated scaffolds.

5. Proceed with standard paraffin-embedding and histology studies.

3.4.2 Preparation of Repopulated Scaffolds for Scanning Electron Microscopy

1. After treatment exposure, remove culture medium from each repopulated matrix.

2. Add 200 µL of PBS to wash the sample gently.

3. Remove washing buffer and add 500 µL of fixation buffer containing 2.5% glutaraldehyde (in 0.1 M sodium cacodylate), for 30 min at RT (fixation step).

4. Remove fixation buffer and wash in 500 µL standard 0.1 M cacodylate buffer.

5. Store sample in fresh 0.1 M cacodylate buffer at 4 °C until further use in the standard protocol of scanning electron microscopy.

3.4.3 Recovery of Cells from Repopulated Matrices to Perform Flow Cytometry

1. After repopulation and treatment exposure, collect the medium from each repopulated scaffold into a 1.5 mL tube and store at −80 °C (*see* **Note 12**).

2. Next, add 200 µL of accutase to each repopulated sample to dissociate cell aggregates.

3. Incubate 30 min at 37 °C in a humidified atmosphere with 5% CO_2.

4. Afterward, add 600 µL of RPMI 1640 with 10% FBS to inactivate accutase action.

5. Mix gently to recover the cells from each decellularized matrix and transfer the cell-containing medium into a clean 1.5 mL tube (*see* **Note 13**).

6. Add fresh 200 µL of RPMI 1640 with 10% FBS to each matrix-containing well and gently wash the sample to recover the maximum of cell numbers from the scaffold.

7. Collect the medium and add into the tube used in **step 5**.

8. Count cells in a haemocytometer and dilute into the desired concentration.

9. Transfer the desired number of cells to each well of a 96-well plate (U-bottom).

10. Add 150 μL of ice-cold flow-cytometry buffer to each cell-containing well and proceed with standard flow-cytometry protocols for staining or live/dead assessment.

4 Notes

1. The optimal cutting temperature (OCT) compound is a cryo-preservation medium suitable for tissue sample storage. The OCT method results in excellent morphological preservation being ideal for small specimens, retrieved from cancer patient surgeries, to be archived at −80 °C. The OCT can be easily removed by simply thawing the specimen on ice or by rinsing the sample in a cold PBS solution.

2. Isopentane bath may be achieved with liquid nitrogen or dry ice. If using dry ice, prepare a polystyrene box with 5–10 cm of dry ice and place a glass beaker on top. Fill the beaker with 4 cm of isopentane and leave it to chill until −55 °C.

3. Always wear a mask when weighing SDS. This ionic detergent is harmful and toxic in contact with skin or the eyes. To avoid exposing your co-workers to SDS, use the fume hood to weigh and dissolve this detergent. A low concentration of SDS is used to avoid extracellular matrix degradation.

4. To prepare the DNase solution, add 50 U/mL of the enzyme to the solution by calculating the volume from the U/mL provided in the stock solution.

5. Tissue decellularization may be achieved by either using OCT-embedded samples kept at −80 °C or using freshly col-lected specimens.

6. To obtain fragments sized for decellularization process, it is highly important to slice the tissue sample into 3 mm^2 either with a grid and a scalpel or a biopsy punch. Make sure every replicate has the same exact size to guarantee reproducibility of the decellularization protocol.

7. During the decellularization protocol, it is expected that each tissue fragment reduces in size, turns white-like, and gains a degree of viscosity. In every step, one should be careful when removing or adding each solution to avoid sample damage, particularly upon DNase treatment.

8. After decellularization, the scaffolds may be stored at 4 °C, in PBS 1× supplemented with gentamicin and fungizone

(optional), for 1–2 months without losing their integrity. Before using long-term stored decellularized samples, one should make sure there is no microbial contamination.

9. Perform all the repopulation procedure in the flow hood to guarantee a sterile environment.

10. When performing the repopulating of decellularized matrices, the number of cells per scaffold should be first assessed in a pilot experiment, considering the model of study and the cancer cell replication time. However, for cancer cell lines we recommend using 5×10^4 cells and for monocytes or macrophages 25×10^4 cells.

11. When performing the repopulation of decellularized matrices with cancer cell lines, we recommend culturing for 3 days. If using monocytes or macrophages, we recommend culturing repopulated scaffolds for 10–13 days.

12. The conditioned medium used in the repopulated matrices maintenance can be recovered and stored at −80 °C until further use. It may be applied in zymography, ELISA, metabolomics, or other assays.

13. **Steps 5** and **6** should be performed carefully once the decellularized scaffolds are viscous samples and may cause difficulties in pipetting. Nevertheless, it is important to wash well each matrix to recover most cells essential to proceed to flow cytometry.

Acknowledgments

This publication is based upon work from COST Action IMMUNO-model, CA21135, supported by COST (European Cooperation in Science and Technology). Diogo Estêvão was supported by the a PhD scholarship by FCT- Portuguese Science Foundation (UI/BD/151551/2021). MJ Oliveira acknowledges the support of Ipatimup- Institute of Pathology and Immunology of the University of Porto through the KRASMet project.

References

1. Hynes RO (2009) The extracellular matrix: not just pretty fibrils. Science 326:1216–1219

2. Pickup MW, Mouw JK, Weaver VM (2014) The extracellular matrix modulates the hallmarks of cancer. EMBO Rep 15:1243–1253

3. Marques-Magalhães Â, Cruz T, Costa ÂM et al (2022) Decellularized colorectal cancer matrices as bioactive scaffolds for studying tumorstroma interactions. Cancer 14(2):359

4. Hanahan D (2022) Hallmarks of cancer: new dimensions. Cancer Discov 12(1):31–46

5. Winkler J, Abisoye-Ogunniyan A, Metcalf KJ, Werb Z (2020) Concepts of extracellular matrix remodelling in tumour progression and metastasis. Nat Commun 11:5120

6. Denys H, Braems G, Lambein K et al (2009) The extracellular matrix regulates cancer progression and therapy response: implications for

prognosis and treatment. Curr Pharm Des 15(12):1373–1384

7. Chen L, Zhang D, Zheng S, Li X, Gao P (2022) Stemness analysis in hepatocellular carcinoma identifies an extracellular matrix gene-related signature associated with prognosis and therapy response. Front Genet 30(13):959834

8. Pinto ML, Rios E, Silva AC et al (2017) Decellularized human colorectal cancer matrices polarize macrophages towards an anti-inflammatory phenotype promoting cancer cell invasion via CCL18. Biomaterials 124:211–224

9. Nunes AS, Barros AS, Costa EC et al (2019) 3D tumor spheroids as in vitro models to mimic in vivo human solid tumors resistance to therapeutic drugs. Biotechnol Bioeng 116:206

10. Horvath P et al (2016) Screening out irrelevant cell-based models of disease. Nat Rev Drug Discov 15:751–769

11. Devarasetty M, Dominijanni A, Herberg S et al (2020) Simulating the human colorectal cancer microenvironment in 3D tumor-stroma co-cultures in vitro and in vivo. Sci Rep 10:9832

12. Piccoli M, D'Angelo E, Crotti et al (2018) Decellularized colorectal cancer matrix as bioactive microenvironment for in vitro 3D cancer research. J Cell Physiol 233:5937–5948

13. Kondo J, Ekawa T, Endo H et al (2019) High-throughput screening in colorectal cancer tissue-originated spheroids. Cancer Sci 110:345–355

14. Hoshiba T (2019) Decellularized extracellular matrix for cancer research. Materials 12:1311

15. Ferreira LP, Gaspar VM, Mano JF (2020) Decellularized extracellular matrix for bioengineering physiomimetic 3D in vitro tumor models. Trends Biotechnol 38:1397–1414

16. Taylor DA, Sampaio LC, Ferdous Z et al (2018) Decellularized matrices in regenerative medicine. Acta Biomater 74:74–89

17. Cruz TB, Carvalho FA, Matafome PN et al (2021) Mice with type 2 diabetes present significant alterations in their tissue biomechanical properties and histological features. Biomedicine 10(1):57

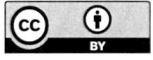

Chapter 14

An Indigenous Workflow for Generating CD19 CAR-T Cells

Muthuganesh Muthuvel and Sunil Martin

Abstract

FDA-approved CD19 CAR T cell therapy for treating B-cell lineage malignancies gave impetus to the adoptive immune/cell and gene therapy field. Although tested to a considerable extent, side effects such as immune effector cell-associated neurotoxicity syndrome (ICANS), immune effector cell-associated hematotoxicity (ICAHTs), the high cost of the therapy, and often complicated logistics make the accessibility of this CAR therapy far from the reach of many eligible patients. Therefore, the development of a safe, cost-effective, streamlined indigenous workflow for T-cell expansion, transduction, and CAR T-cell characterization is essential in a preclinical as well as clinical setting. We have optimized a method to develop CD19 CAR T cells from peripheral blood T cells from healthy donors. In this chapter, we describe an indigenous protocol for the generation and characterization of CD19 CAR T cells via lentiviral transduction to understand the immunology or possible downstream applications.

Key words CD19 CAR T cells, Lentiviral production, Antitumor functions, Flow cytometry

1 Introduction

B-lineage malignancies that are refractory/relapsed after standard care therapy remain an unmet medical need across the globe [1]. Chimeric antigen receptor (CAR) T cells are modular in vitro-modified receptors that are engineered to target tumor cells against a specific antigen. They are T cells derived from the patient and genetically modified to express CAR on the T-cell surface that can, when reintroduced into the patient's body, target and kill cancer cells [2]. CAR T-cell immunotherapy is an important and effective means of treating blood cancers with high mortality [3]. The widely employed second generation CD19 CAR structure ideally consists of a single chain variable fragment derived from variable regions of light and heavy chain (V_L and V_H) of a monoclonal antibody connected to a transmembrane domain through a hinge region and intracellular signaling domain consisting of CD3ζ with an additional co-stimulatory domain typically derived from CD28 or 4-1BB [4, 5].

Sweta Rani and Lukasz Skalniak (eds.), *IMMUNO-model in Cancer: Methods and Protocols*, Methods in Molecular Biology, vol. 2959, https://doi.org/10.1007/978-1-0716-4734-9_14, © The Author(s) 2026

Over the years, the CAR configurations have been progressively modified toward achieving a higher degree of safety and efficacy [6]. Although CAR therapy demonstrated outstanding clinical response, toxicity, off-tumor effect, and cost remain a challenge in the clinic [3, 7]. Cytokine release syndrome (CRS) and immune effector cell-associated neurotoxicity syndrome (ICANs) pose a major risk in CAR T cell-based immunotherapy coupled with the problem of an untenable price tag of product and process flow [8–10]. Ongoing research aims to optimize the production workflow to reduce the cost of CAR T cells product without compromising safety and efficacy. CAR T-cell therapy developed and produced in the United States is priced around $500,000, making the therapy extremely expensive [11, 12]. A recent protocol to develop indigenous CAR T cells from India significantly reduced the cost of production. With the introduction of India-based NexCAR19, the cost of CAR therapy has decreased to approximately $50,000 [13]. Due to the sheer demand for CAR T products and reduced supplies, more indigenous protocols need to be developed to cater to patients who relapsed after stem cell transplantation [14].

Here, we describe a protocol for generating CD19 CAR T cells by isolating peripheral blood T cells, which are subsequently activated with CD3 + CD28+ beads in the presence of IL-15 and IL-7. The activated T cells are lentivirally transduced with a titer-optimized and safe pseudoviral SIN vector, which is then used to engineer T cells at a low multiplicity of infection (MOI) of 10 for enhanced safety. The generated CAR T cells are characterized on day 7 by phenotyping, proliferation, CAR expression, viability, and antitumor function.

2   Materials

2.1   Equipment

1. Biosafety cabinet—BSL-2.
2. Swinging bucket centrifuge.
3. Ultracentrifuge (Beckman Coulter Life Sciences).
4. 70 Ti fixed-angle titanium rotor.
5. 26.3 mL polycarbonate bottle.
6. Cell counter (Corning®).
7. Counting chamber.
8. FACS analyzer.
9. 5 mL round bottom tubes.
10. 50-, 15-, and 1.5-mL centrifuge tubes.
11. Cryovials.
12. Serological pipettes.

13. CO_2 incubator.

14. 24- and 48-well plates.

15. 100 mm and 50 mm culture dishes.

16. 0.45 μm PVDF syringe filter.

17. 20 mL syringe.

18. EasySep™ Magnet (STEMCELL Technologies).

19. 10 mL ethylenediaminetetraacetic acid (EDTA)-coated tubes.

20. FACS tubes.

21. Parafilm.

22. 96-well U-bottom plate.

2.2 Reagents

1. Dulbecco's Modified Eagle Medium (DMEM).

2. Roswell Park Memorial Institute Medium (RPMI).

3. Heat-inactivated fetal bovine serum (FBS).

4. CTS™ OpTmizer™ T-cell expansion basal medium.

5. 1× Dulbecco's phosphate-buffered saline (DPBS) without calcium and magnesium.

6. Phosphate-buffered saline (PBS).

7. 0.1% bovine serum albumin (BSA).

8. Trypan blue.

9. 2.5 M calcium chloride.

10. 2× hepes-buffered saline (HBS) buffer (pH 7) (*see* **Note 2**).

11. CAR transfer plasmid (the construct was a generous gift from Dr. Trent Spencer, Emory University, and further modified in the lab).

12. Packaging plasmids (pMDLg/pRRE and pRSV-Rev, Addgene) (*see* **Note 1**).

13. Envelope plasmid (pMD2.G, Addgene).

14. Human recombinant IL-15 (*see* **Note 1**).

15. Human recombinant IL-7 (*see* **Note 1**).

16. Complete DMEM: DMEM with 10% FBS and 1% Pen-Strep.

17. Complete RPMI: RPMI with 10% FBS and 1% Pen-Strep.

18. FACS buffer: 2% FBS in 1× PBS.

19. Human embryonic kidney (HEK) 293T cell line.

20. NALM-6 cell line.

21. Trypsin-EDTA (0.05%).

22. EasySep™ human T-cell isolation kit (STEMCEL™ Technologies).

23. Polybrene.

24. 4% paraformaldehyde (PFA).

25. Peripheral blood.

26. Dynabeads™ Human T-Activator CD3/CD28 for T-cell expansion and activation.

27. GolgiPlug (protein transport inhibitor).

28. LIVE/DEAD™ Fixable Aqua Dead Cell Stain Kit.

29. Permwash buffer.

30. Bleach solution.

2.3 Antibodies and Stains

The reagents mentioned below are used for CAR T cell phenotyping. *See* also **Note 3**.

1. Antihuman CD3 PE/Cyanine7 (BioLegend, cat. no. 344816).

2. Antihuman CD8 Pacific Blue (BioLegend, cat. no. 300928).

3. Antihuman CD4 Brilliant Violet 785 (BioLegend, cat. no. 317442).

4. Antihuman CD45RA Brilliant Violet 650 (BioLegend, cat. no. 304136).

5. Antihuman CD27 Brilliant Violet 605 (BioLegend, cat. no. 302830).

6. 7-AAD (dead-cell staining reagent, BioLegend, cat. no. 420404).

7. Antihuman CD107a (LAMP-1) APC/Cyanine7 (BioLegend, cat. no. 328630).

8. Antihuman IFN-γ PE (BioLegend, cat. no. 506507).

3 Methods

All the cell-culture experiments should be carried out in a BSL-2 biosafety cabinet. Media should be prewarmed in a 37 °C water bath before the experiments or when specified otherwise. The CO_2 incubator is maintained at 37 °C and 5% CO_2 unless specified otherwise.

3.1 Lentiviral Production

The following protocol is for making a third-generation lentiviral vector by using HEK 293T as a producer cell line (*see* **Note 4**).

3.1.1 HEK293T Cells for Transfection

1. Seed 4×10^6 HEK 293T cells in 10 mL of complete DMEM (10% FBS) in a 100 mm dish. Incubate the cells in the incubator.

2. Cells are ready for transfection when the confluency reaches about 70%.

3. On attaining the desired confluency, remove the media, add 10 mL of fresh, prewarmed complete DMEM, and prepare transfection complex using the calcium phosphate method.

4. Preparation of transfection complex: Add 10 μg of transfer vector, 5 μg of pMDLg/pRRE, 2.5 μg of pRSV-Rev, 2.5 μg of pMD.2G to 25 μL of 2.5 M calcium phosphate, followed by addition of 250 μL of 2× HBS buffer (*see* **Note 2**). The total volume is made up to 500 μL using sterile water.

5. Incubate the transfection complex at room temperature for 30 min.

6. Add the transfection mixture to the dish containing HEK 293T cells and mix the media by tilting it slowly. Return the dish to the incubator.

7. After 24 h, discard the media from the plate carefully into a bottle containing bleach solution (*see* **Note 6**).

8. Add fresh, prewarmed 10 mL of complete DMEM without disturbing the cells.

9. Keep the dish back in the incubator.

3.1.2 Harvesting of Lentiviral Particles

1. After 48 h, harvest the culture media from the dish in the 50 mL tube and add prewarmed fresh media to the cells. Store the 48 h collection in a 4 °C refrigerator (*see* **Note 7**).

2. After 72 h, collect the media from the dish and combine it with the 48 h collection.

3. Filter the collected supernatants with a 0.45 μm PVDF syringe filter.

4. Transfer the filtered supernatant to the ultracentrifuge tubes (26.3 mL polycarbonate bottle).

5. Keep another tube with another virus or water to balance the ultracentrifuge. Make sure the balance is equal by measuring it in weighing balance (*see* **Note 8**).

6. Put the bottle carefully into the 70 Ti rotor and centrifuge it at $80,000 \times g$ for 2 h at 4 °C.

7. After centrifugation, carefully discard the supernatant, suspend the pellet in 200 μL of OpTmizer™ (1/100th of the original sample volume), and store at −80 °C.

3.1.3 Determination of Lentiviral Titre

The CAR construct is linked to GFP as a receptor protein. GFP can be used for titration by flow cytometry (Fig. 1a).

1. Seed HEK 293T cells at 0.7×10^6 cells/well in a 6-well plate and 2 mL of complete DMEM per well.

2. After 24 h of seeding, trypsinize one well and perform cell count to measure the cell number. Take 5 μL of virus and

a.

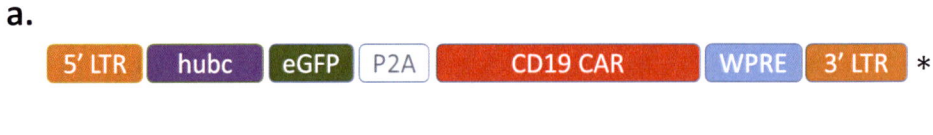

b.

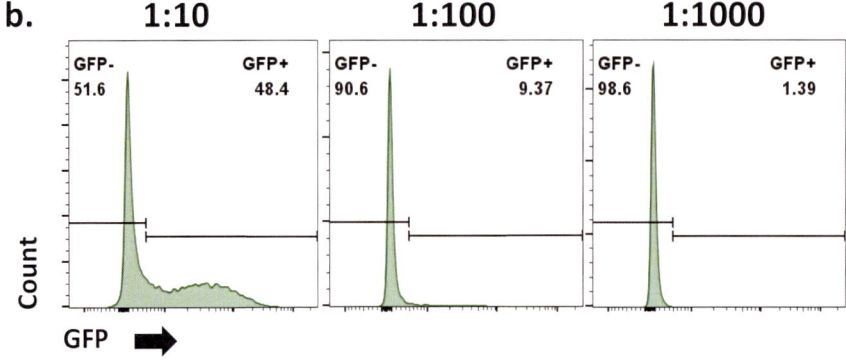

c. Transducing Units (TU/mL) = <u>No. of cells x (% of expression/100) x Dilution Factor</u>
Virus volume (mL)

From dilution 1:100 = <u>1,000,000x (0.093) x100</u>
0.05
= 1.8x10^7 TU/mL

Fig. 1 Generation and titration of lentiviral vectors. (**a**) Schematic representation of CAR lentiviral vector. The CAR transgene is driven by hubc promoter with eGFP as a surrogate marker. (**b**) Titration of lentivirus by FACS. (**c**) Formula for calculating titration and multiplicity of infection (MOI). The titre was calculated from 1:100 dilutions. * *LTR* long terminal repeat, *hubc* human ubiquitin c, *eGFP* enhanced green fluroscent protein, *WPRE* Woodchuck hepatitis virus posttranscriptional regulatory element

serially dilute it with media (1:10, 1:100, and 1:1000) (Fig. 1b).

3. Add the serially diluted virus to the cells along with polybrene (8 μg/mL).

4. After 48 h of incubation, collect the cells and fix them with 4% PFA solution.

5. Measure the GFP expression by flow cytometry and calculate the titer following the formula (Fig. 1c).

$$\text{Transducing units (TU/mL)} = \frac{\text{No. of cells} \times (\% \text{ of expression}/100) \times \text{dilution factor}}{\text{Virus volume (mL)}}$$

6. Calculate the MOI using the following formula and use an MOI of 10 for primary T-cell transduction.

$$\text{Multiplicity of Infection (MOI)} = \frac{\text{Virus volume (mL)} \times \text{titre (TU/mL)}}{\text{No. of cells}}$$

3.2 Generation of CAR T Cells

3.2.1 Isolation of T Cells

1. Collect 2–5 mL peripheral blood from the volunteers in EDTA-coated tubes with informed consent (*see* **Note 5**).

2. Take 1.5 mL of whole blood in a 5 mL round bottom tube and add 75 μL of human T-cell isolation cocktail (*see* **Note 9**).

3. Vortex the RapidSpheres™ and add 75 μL to the tube, mix it well, and incubate it for 5 min at room temperature.

4. Mix the sample with 2 mL of 1× DPBS and place the tube without the lid into the purification magnet for 5 min at room temperature.

5. Grasping the magnet, invert the magnet with the tube in a continuous motion, pouring the enriched cell suspension into a new 5 mL tube.

6. Mix the above-obtained cell suspension with 75 μL of Rapid-Spheres™ and incubate it for 5 min at room temperature.

7. Keep the tube in the magnet for 5 min.

8. Repeat **step 5**.

9. Centrifuge the cell suspension at $300 \times g$ for 5 min and wash the cells with 2 mL of 1× DPBS.

10. Post-wash, add 1 mL of media, and perform cell counting with trypan blue using cell counter.

3.2.2 Baseline Phenotyping of T Cells

1. Take 1×10^5 cells in six different FACS tubes for phenotyping by flow cytometry and label the tubes as follows:
   - Unstained.
   - CD3.
   - CD4.
   - CD8.
   - CD27.
   - CD45RA.
   - 7-AAD
   - Mixed (all antibodies).

2. Add 2 μL of hCD3 antibody to the tube labeled as CD3 and mix well.

3. Add 2 μL of hCD4 antibody to CD4 and mixed tubes.

4. Add 2 μL of hCD8 antibody to CD8 and mixed tubes.

5. Add 2 μL of hCD27 antibody to CD27 and mixed tubes.

6. Add 2 μL of hCD45RA antibody to CD45RA and mixed tubes.

7. Keep all tubes at 4 °C or on ice, wrapped with aluminum foil for 30 min keep them in the dark.

8. Wash the cells twice with FACS buffer.

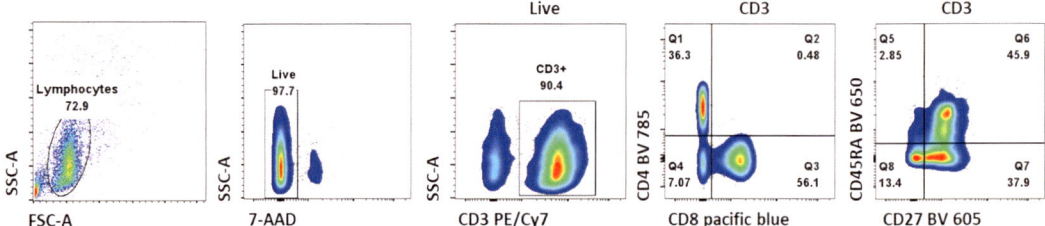

Fig. 2 Baseline phenotype of T cells. The lymphocyte population on FSC/SSC is gated followed by the exclusion of dead cells by gating on 7-AAD negative population. From the CD3 (PE/Cyanine7) positive population, CD4 (BV 785), CD8 (pacific blue), CD27 (BV 605), and CD45RA (BV 650) are gated

Table 1
Antibody combination to phenotype the CAR T cells

SI. no	Antibodies	Phenotype
1	CD3 (+)	Total T cells
2	CD3 (+) CD4 (+)	Helper T cells
3	CD3 (+) CD8 (+)	Cytotoxic T cells
4	CD27 (+) CD45RA (−)	Central memory T cells
5	CD27 (+) CD45RA (+)	Naïve T cells
6	CD27 (−) CD45RA (+)	Effector memory RA positive T cells (EMRA)
7	CD27 (−) CD45RA (−)	Effector memory T cells

9. Add 5 µL of 7-AAD to tubes labeled as 7-AAD and mix.

10. Analyze the samples using a flow cytometer (Fig. 2, Table 1). Perform compensation with a single antibody-stained tube (*see* **Note 10**).

3.2.3 Expansion of T Cells: Day 0

1. Seed $0.5 \times 10^6/0.5$ mL isolated T cells in a 24-well plate using OpTmizer™ media and add 10 ng/mL of IL-15 and IL-7 (*see* **Note 11**).

2. Add 12.5 µL of CD3/CD28 Dynabeads into a 1.5 mL centrifuge tube and mix it with 1 mL of 0.1% BSA in PBS (*see* **Note 12**).

3. Place the tube in a magnetic stand for 3 min and remove the supernatant.

4. Resuspend the beads in 50 µL of media. Mix well and add the suspension to the cells.

5. Place the cells in the incubator.

3.2.4 Transduction of T Cells: Day 2

1. After 48 h (Day 2), add lentiviral particles at an MOI of 10 with 8 µg/mL of polybrene.

2. Seal the plate with parafilm and centrifuge at 300 g for 30 min at 37 °C (acceleration and break at 1).

3. After centrifugation, remove the parafilm and return the plate to the incubator.

3.2.5 De-Beading of T Cells and Revival of Tumor Cells

1. After 24 h of transduction, collect the plated cells in a 1.5 mL tube and place it on the magnetic stand for 5 min. Collect the supernatant and centrifuge at $300 \times g$ for 5 min.

2. Remove the supernatant and resuspend the cells with 1 mL of fresh media containing IL-15 and IL-7.

3. Count the cells and seed 1×10^6 cells per mL of media. Also, count every 2 days and add media according to the cell number. Maintain the media volume at 1×10^6 cells/mL (*see* **Note 13**).

4. Concurrently, revive a vial of NALM-6 cell line in T25 flask in complete RPMI media (*see* **Note 14**).

3.2.6 Phenotyping of CAR T Cells on Day 7

1. On day 7, measure the CD3, CD4, CD8, CD45RA, CD27, and GFP markers by flow cytometry.

2. The CAR construct has GFP as a surrogate protein, therefore, CAR transduction can be measured by measuring GFP (Fig. 3).

3.2.7 Assessing the Antitumor Function of CAR T Cells on Day 8

After 8 days of expansion, the cells are ready to be validated by measuring their antitumor functions. The antitumor function of CAR T cells can be measured using a flow cytometer-based degranulation and interferon gamma production assay (*see* **Notes 15** and **17**).

1. Collect both effector cells (CAR T cells) and target cells (NALM-6) in two different 15 mL tubes and count the cells.

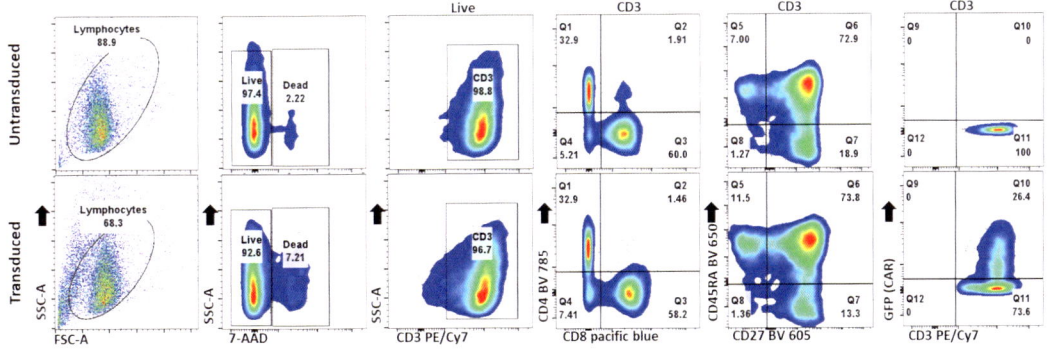

Fig. 3 The phenotype of CAR-T cells. Phenotyping of CAR T cells on day 8. Transduction efficiency is monitored by measuring GFP expression

Table 2
Plate design for degranulation and cytokine release assay (96-well plate)

UT cells	UT cells + NALM-6	CAR T cells	CAR T cells + NALM-6
UT cells	UT cells + NALM-6	CAR T cells	CAR T cells + NALM-6
UT cells	UT cells + NALM-6	CAR T cells	CAR T cells + NALM-6

2. Seed the cells in a 96-well U-bottom plate at a 1:1 ratio of effector and target (1×10^5 each of the effector and target) in fresh 100 µL of OpTmizer media (Table 2).

3. Add 5 µL of hCD107a antibody to each well and incubate the plate in the incubator for an hour (*see* **Note 16**).

4. After an hour, add 0.5 µL GolgiPlug, mix well by pipetting, and place the plate in the incubator for 5 h.

5. After incubation, collect the cells in 5 mL FACS tubes.

6. Wash the cells by adding 1 mL of FACS buffer and centrifuge at $300 \times g$ for 5 min. Discard the supernatant and repeat the washing step.

7. Resuspend the cells in 50 µL of FACS buffer containing 0.5 µL fixable live/dead aqua dye and incubate the tubes at 4 °C or on ice for 30 min.

8. Postincubation, wash the cells twice with FACS buffer and resuspend them in a total volume of 50 µL containing 2 µL of CD3 antibody. Incubate at 4 °C or on ice for another 30 min and wash twice with FACS buffer.

9. Add 200 µL of 4% PFA to the pellet and mix it by overtaxing for 2–5 s.

10. Incubate the cells for 15 min at 4 °C and wash twice with FACS buffer.

11. Add 500 µL of 1× permwash buffer to the cells and incubate it for 15 min on ice. Wash twice with FACS buffer.

12. Add 50 µL of 1× permwash buffer containing 5 µL of IFN-γ antibody. Incubate in the dark for 30 min at 4 °C or on ice.

13. Wash twice with FACS buffer and resuspend the pellet in 200–300 µL of FACS buffer. Perform the analysis using FACS.

14. Gating is performed on CD3+ and GFP+ to measure the CD107a and IFNγ from CAR T cells (Fig. 4).

4   Notes

1. Once the plasmids are isolated, validation should be carried out via restriction digestion and sanger sequencing. Store the

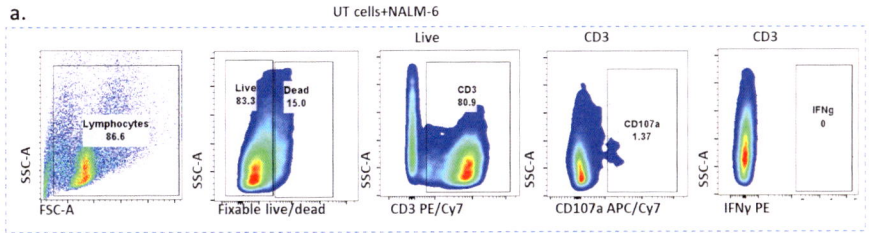

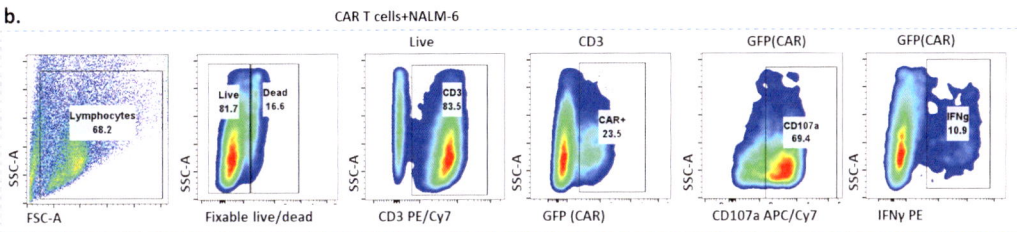

Fig. 4 Degranulation and cytokine assay. The expression of CD107a (APC/Cyanine7) and IFNγ (PE) as measured from 7-AAD-, CD3+, and CAR+ cells in **a**, CAR-untransduced T cells cocultured with NALM-6 cells and **b**, CAR-transduced T cells cocultured with NALM-6 cells

plasmids at −20 °C, while IL-15 and IL-7 are stored at −80 C in multiple aliquots to keep the freeze-thaw cycles at a minimum.

2. Ensure that the pH of 2× HBS buffer is maintained at 7. Any minor changes in the pH can reduce the transfection efficiency.

3. Store the FACS antibodies at 4 °C in dark or cover them with an aluminum foil. All the staining must be carried out in 4 °C or on ice in the dark as antibodies are sensitive to light and temperature.

4. The HEK 293T cells should be passaged less than four times. Higher passage numbers can affect lentiviral production and quality.

5. Special care must be taken during the handling of human blood. Consent must be obtained prior to collection of blood from healthy donors.

6. Bleach solution should be used to disinfect blood sample tubes, virus production apparatuses, and the workspaces.

7. Do not store the media containing the virus for more than 3 days as it can affect the virus yield.

8. Ultracentrifuge tubes and rotor must be prechilled by keeping them inside at 4 °C. Switch on the ultracentrifuge machine 30 min prior and set the temperature to 4 °C.

9. Use 50 μL of human T-cell isolation cocktail and Rapid-Spheres™ for 1 mL blood (50 μL/mL).

10. If performing multicolour FACS, always keep single stained cells to compensate for the fluorescence bleed-through.

11. Reconstitute IL-15 and IL-7 in a way that 10 μL volume contains 10 ng of the protein. Therefore, for 1 mL of culture, 10 μL of IL-15/IL-7 can be added.

12. The concentration of the Dynabeads is one million per 25 μL. For one million of cells, add 25 μL of Dynabeads to achieve a 1:1 ratio.

13. Replacement with fresh media should be performed only during de-beading/replacing viral media. Any addition to the media after that should be additional media containing cytokines, calculated based on the cell number.

14. NALM-6 is a cell line of B-cell acute lymphoblastic leukemia (B-ALL), expressing CD19 antigen. The antitumor function of generated CAR T cells can be measured against it.

15. Currently, our protocol is optimized for expanding the CAR T cells only up to 8 days, thus minimizing exhaustion. However, expansion can be increased up to 14 days.

16. CD107a is a marker of degranulation. When a CAR T cell engages with an antigen, CD107a will be expressed on its cell surface. The percentage of degranulation can be measured by flow cytometry using specific antibodies.

17. Apart from degranulation and cytokine release, the antitumor function of CAR T cells can be assessed by cytotoxicity, antigen-specific proliferation, and by using xenograft mice models.

Acknowledgments

This work was funded by the Department of Biotechnology, Ministry of Science and Technology, Government of India, through the grant number BT/PR40655/MED/31/443/2020.

This publication is based upon work from COST Action IMMUNO-model, CA21135, supported by COST (European Cooperation in Science and Technology). We thank Maithreyi Prakash for helping to draft the manuscript.

References

1. Cappell KM, Sherry RM, Yang JC, Goff SL, Vanasse DA, McIntyre L, Rosenberg SA, Kochenderfer JN (2020) Long-term follow-up of anti-CD19 chimeric antigen receptor T-cell therapy. J Clin Oncol 38:3805–3815. https://doi.org/10.1200/JCO.20.01467

2. Guedan S, Calderon H, Posey AD, Maus MV (2019) Engineering and design of chimeric antigen receptors. Mol Ther Methods Clin Dev 12:145–156

3. Sterner RC, Sterner RM (2021) CAR T cell therapy: current limitations and potential

strategies. Blood Cancer J 114(11):1–11. https://doi.org/10.1038/s41408-021-00459-7

4. Heyman B, Yang Y (2018) New developments in immunotherapy for lymphoma. Cancer Biol Med 15:189. https://doi.org/10.20892/J.ISSN.2095-3941.2018.0037

5. Brudno JN, Lam N, Vanasse D, Shen Y, Rose JJ, Rossi J, Xue A, Bot A, Scholler N, Mikkilineni L, Roschewski M, Dean R, Cachau R, Youkharibache P, Patel R, Hansen B, Stroncek DF, Rosenberg SA, Gress RE, Kochenderfer JN (2020) Safety and feasibility of anti-CD19 CAR T cells with fully human binding domains in patients with B-cell lymphoma. Nat Med 26:270–280. https://doi.org/10.1038/S41591-019-0737-3

6. Muthuvel M, Srinivasan H, Louis L, Martin S (2022) Engineering off-the-shelf universal CAR T cells: a silver lining in the cloud. Cytokine 156:155920. https://doi.org/10.1016/J.CYTO.2022.155920

7. Flugel CL, Majzner RG, Krenciute G, Dotti G, Riddell SR, Wagner DL, Abou-el-Enein M (2022) Overcoming on-target, off-tumour toxicity of CAR T cell therapy for solid tumours. Nat Rev Clin Oncol 201(20):49–62. https://doi.org/10.1038/s41571-022-00704-3

8. Rejeski K, Greco R, Onida F, Sánchez-Ortega I, Bonini C, Sureda A, Gribben JG, Yakoub-Agha I, Subklewe M (2023) An international survey on grading, diagnosis, and management of immune effector cell-associated hematotoxicity (ICAHT) following CAR T-cell therapy on behalf of the EBMT and EHA. HemaSphere 7:e889. https://doi.org/10.1097/HS9.0000000000000889

9. Velasco R, Mussetti A, Villagrán-García M, Sureda A (2023) CAR T-cell-associated neurotoxicity in central nervous system hematologic disease: is it still a concern? Front Neurol 14:1144414. https://doi.org/10.3389/FNEUR.2023.1144414/BIBTEX

10. Zhao Y, Niu C, Cui J (2018) Gamma-delta (γδ) T cells: friend or foe in cancer development? J Transl Med 16:3. https://doi.org/10.1186/S12967-017-1378-2

11. Roddie C, O'Reilly M, Dias Alves Pinto J, Vispute K, Lowdell M (2019) Manufacturing chimeric antigen receptor T cells: issues and challenges. Cytotherapy 21:327–340. https://doi.org/10.1016/J.JCYT.2018.11.009

12. Fiorenza S, Ritchie DS, Ramsey SD, Turtle CJ, Roth JA (2020) Value and affordability of CAR T-cell therapy in the United States. Bone Marrow Transplant 55:1706–1715

13. Mallapaty S (2024) Cutting-edge CAR-T cancer therapy is now made in India—at one-tenth the cost. Nature 627:709–710. https://doi.org/10.1038/D41586-024-00809-Y

14. Kochenderfer JN, Dudley ME, Kassim SH, Somerville RPT, Carpenter RO, Stetler-Stevenson M, Yang JC, Phan GQ, Hughes MS, Sherry RM, Raffeld M, Feldman S, Lu L, Li YF, Ngo LT, Goy A, Feldman T, Spaner DE, Wang ML, Chen CC, Kranick SM, Nath A, Nathan D-AN, Morton KE, Toomey MA, Rosenberg SA (2014) Chemotherapy-refractory diffuse large B-cell lymphoma and indolent B-cell malignancies can be effectively treated with autologous T cells expressing an anti-CD19 chimeric antigen receptor. J Clin Oncol 33:540–549. https://doi.org/10.1200/JCO.2014.56.2025

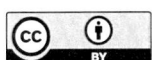

Chapter 15

Using Epigenetic Data to Deconvolute Immune Cells in Cancer from Blood Samples

Hatim Boughanem, Sotiris Ouzounis, Maurizio Callari, Rebeca Sanz-Pamplona, Manuel Macias-Gonzalez, and Theodora Katsila

Abstract

DNA methylation plays a crucial role in regulating gene expression and is a hallmark of epigenetic dysregulation in human tumors. High-throughput DNA methylation profiling can unravel intricate patterns in cancer. Moreover, understanding immune cell dynamics is essential for comprehending cancer progression and treatment response. Using DNA methylation data in immune cells, we can apply deconvolution algorithms estimate proportions of major immune cell types, providing insights into immune status and its implications in cancer. Functional analysis can identify specific overrepresented or underrepresented immune cell subsets, potentially uncovering novel biomarkers or therapeutic targets. This pipeline presents a detailed workflow in RStudio for DNA methylation studies and immune cell deconvolution, enhancing reproducibility and efficiency. The workflow integrates preprocessing, analysis, and visualization steps, facilitating robust inference of cell-type proportions from DNA methylation data.

Key words Immune cells, Blood, Cancer, Epigenetic, 450K, EPIC

1 Introduction

DNA methylation plays a crucial role in the regulation of gene expression. Epigenetic dysregulation is considered the hallmark of human tumors, offering valuable insights into disease mechanisms and potential therapeutic targets [1]. Utilizing high-throughput DNA methylation profiling platform holds promise for unraveling the intricacies of DNA methylation patterns in cancer studies. Moreover, understanding the composition and dynamics of immune cells within the tumor microenvironment and peripheral blood is essential for comprehending cancer progression and treatment response [2].

Characterizing immune cell proportions within blood samples is pivotal for understanding immune system dynamics in health and disease. Utilizing DNA methylation data, immune cell deconvolution algorithms enable estimation of major immune cell types,

Sweta Rani and Lukasz Skalniak (eds.), *IMMUNO-model in Cancer: Methods and Protocols*, Methods in Molecular Biology, vol. 2959, https://doi.org/10.1007/978-1-0716-4734-9_15, © The Author(s) 2026

including T cells, B cells, natural killer cells, and myeloid cells. Presentation of immune cell proportions provides valuable insights into immune status and its potential implications in cancer progression and treatment response. Furthermore, functional analysis offers a systematic approach to deciphering the biological significance of immune cell profiles. By comparing observed immune cell proportions with predefined immuno-profiling sets, enrichment analysis identifies overrepresented or underrepresented immune cell subsets within samples. Calculation of enrichment scores elucidates the functional relevance of immune cell composition in the context of cancer biology, potentially uncovering novel biomarkers or therapeutic targets [3].

Leveraging DNA methylation analysis and immune cell estimation in cancer studies holds immense potential for unraveling the complex interplay between epigenetic regulation and immune response. Through meticulous data preparation, utilization of relevant software packages, and integration of RStudio pipelines, comprehensive insights into DNA methylation patterns and immune cell dynamics can be attained. Here, we offer a detailed pipeline analysis workflow in Rstudio to enhance reproducibility and efficiency in the context of DNA methylation studies and immune cell deconvolution. This includes facilitate seamless integration of preprocessing, analysis, and visualization steps. This enhances robust inference of sample-specific cell-type proportions from DNA methylation data (Fig. 1).

Therefore, the objectives of this chapter are:

– Understanding the considerations when designing DNA methylation experiments.

– Discussing the steps involved in taking *idat.* files.

– Computing and assessing QC metrics at every step in the workflow.

– Identifying differentially methylated positions and regions.

– Analyzing immune cells within your blood sample.

2   Materials and Methods

2.1 EPIC and 450K Dataset

Our analysis will utilize the *idat.* files, and its related data sheet. This pipeline requires input data in the form of *idat.* files, which represent two distinct color channels before normalization. *idat.* files offer the most comprehensive dataset as they encompass measurements on control probes. While Genome Studio files can be utilized alongside this package, their functionality is limited due to the absence of control probe information. Moreover, Genome Studio output is typically normalized using methods within Genome Studio itself, which are often deemed less effective.

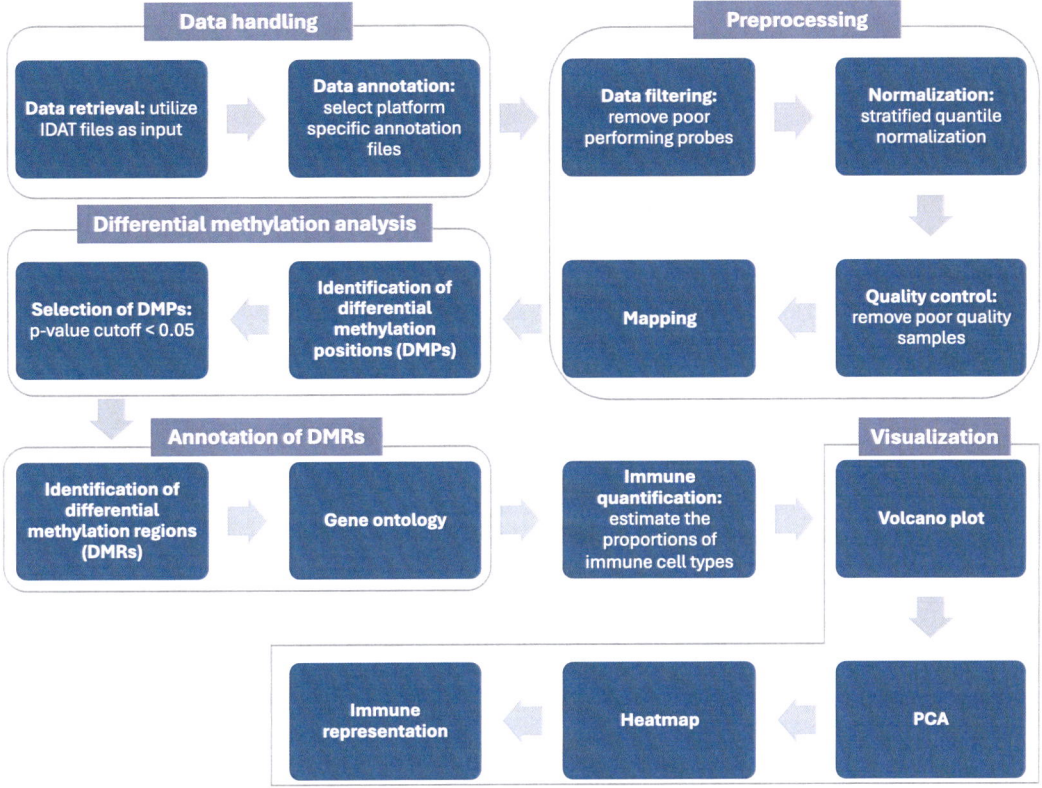

Fig. 1 Workflow of the pipeline. Visualization of a generalized pipeline for the deconvolution of methylation data to quantify immune cell proportions in cancer from blood samples. The pipeline consists of six major steps: (1) Data handling, (2) preprocessing, (3) differential methylation analysis, (4) annotation of differential methylation regions, (5) immune quantification, (6) visualization

For this purpose, we will use a public dataset containing as an example of genome-wide DNA methylation profiling of peripheral blood mononuclear cells (PBMCs) in both normal and breast cancer samples, provided by Wang T. et al. (2023) [4]. Of course, you can use your own dataset to run this example, with some adjustment that are clearly indicated along the pipeline. The Illumina Infinium 850k Human DNA Methylation BeadChip was utilized to obtain DNA methylation profiles across approximately 820,000 CpGs in PBMC samples. The samples included five newly diagnosed breast cancer (GSM7593324, GSM7593325, GSM7593326, GSM7593327, GSM7593328) patients and five normal controls (GSM7593399, GSM7593400, GSM7593401, GSM7593402, GSM7593403) to simplify the model. The users can access to this data by the following link: https://www.ncbi.nlm.nih.gov/geo/query/acc.cgi?acc=GSE237036

Additionally, this chapter also covers the 450K platform in detail. It is designed to facilitate switching between platforms, ensuring the use of both platforms depending on the samples available for analysis.

2.2 Computational Resources

RStudio can be installed from the RStudio website: http://www.rstudio.com/, or can be downloaded for all platforms using the link: https://rstudio.com/products/rstudio/download/. The whole analysis is conducted within the R/Bioconductor environment. R (version 4.0.0) should be downloaded and installed from the CRAN website (https://cran.r-project.org/). Bioconductor (version 3.11) can be installed from within the R console using the following commands:

```
if (!requireNamespace("BiocManager", quietly = TRUE)) {
install.packages("BiocManager")
}
BiocManager::install(version = "3.14")
```

2.3 Main Packages Needed

You can install all necessary packages for the analysis from CRAN and Bioconductor. To process *idat.* files, you need to install specific packages: "minfi" for raw data and metadata retrieval, and "IlluminaHumanMethylationEPICmanifest" for genomic annotation on the EPIC platform. For the 450 K platform, use the "IlluminaHumanMethylation450kmanifest" package [5].

```
# You can use each package, you need depending on the platform
you have
BiocManager::install(c('minfi', 'limma' 'IlluminaHumanMethy-
lationEPICmanifest', 'IlluminaHumanMethylation450kmanifest'))
BiocManager::install("IlluminaHumanMethylationEPICanno.
ilm10b4.hg19")

BiocManager::install("DMRcate")
BiocManager::install("FlowSorted.Blood.EPIC")
install.packages("ggfortify")
BiocManager::install("ComplexHeatmap")
BiocManager::install("clusterProfiler")
```

For the visualization of graphs and manipulation of data, it is required to install the packages "ggplot2" and "dplyr," among others.

```
BiocManager::install(c('ggplot2', 'dplyr', 'tibble', 'ggre-
pel'))
```

For regulatory factors enrichment analysis, the package "org.Hs.eg.db" is required for the conversion of the gene names from Entrez ID to Gene Symbols.

```
BiocManager::install('org.Hs.eg.db')
```

For extracting the data that we will use in this example, please install GEOquery and Biobase packages following the next script:

```
BiocManager::install(c('GEOquery', 'Biobase'))
```

For identifying and analyzing differentially methylated regions (DMRs) from Whole Genome Bisulfite Sequencing (WGBS) and Illumina Infinium Array (450K and EPIC) data, we utilize the DMRcate package:

```
BiocManager::install("DMRcate")
```

For deconvoluting the cell type composition in whole blood samples analyzed with the Illumina HumanMethylationEPIC, we will install the package FlowSorted.Blood.EPIC [6]:

```
BiocManager::install("FlowSorted.Blood.EPIC")
```

Finally, please check that all the packages were installed successfully by loading them one at a time using the library() function.

2.4 Creating Annotation File and Data Environment

Depending on the platform we are using, the following script is specially designed for EPIC. In case you are using the 450 K platform, you can replace "IlluminaHumanMethylationEPICanno.ilm10b4.hg19" with "annEPIC" and using "IlluminaHumanMethylation450kanno.ilmn12.hg19," with "ann450K." This modification ensures that the appropriate annotation files are used for the different platforms, allowing the script to accurately process the data. It is crucial to use the correct manifest and annotation files to avoid any discrepancies in the genomic analysis and ensure that the data interpretation is accurate and reliable for your specific platform.

```
# load package
library(minfi)
annEPIC <- getAnnotation("IlluminaHumanMethylationEPICanno.
ilm10b4.hg19")
```

2.5 Creating Data Information Sheet

We will use data from the paper published by Wang T. et al. (2023) https://www.ncbi.nlm.nih.gov/geo/query/acc.cgi?acc=GSE23 7036. Specifically, we will use DNA methylation data from peripheral blood mononuclear cells, including samples from five patients with breast cancer and five normal controls. The samples included five newly diagnosed breast cancer patients (GSM7593324, GSM7593325, GSM7593326, GSM7593327, GSM7593328) and five normal controls (GSM7593399, GSM7593400, GSM7593401, GSM7593402, GSM7593403). To download these samples, you can manually access the dataset using the following link: https://www.ncbi.nlm.nih.gov/geo/query/acc.cgi?acc=GSE237036. Alternatively, you can use the GEOquery package to access and download the data using the following script. We will also download the supplementary data from GSE47915, which contains all the raw data we need. This process may take some time.

```r
# Load packages
library(GEOquery)
library(Biobase)
library(minfi)


# We will create a file in the desktop named GSE237036, in
which we will download the idat files. We create a function
checking if the directory exist or if it should be created
check_dir<-function(dir_path){
# Check if the directory exists
if (!dir.exists(dir_path)) {
# If the directory does not exist, create it
dir.create(dir_path)
cat("Directory created:", dir_path, "\n")
  } else {
cat("Directory already exists:", dir_path, "\n")
  }


}


# We initailize the working directory of our project
work_dir <- getwd()


# Utilizing the function created above to create the following
directories if they do not exist
dir_path1 <- paste0(work_dir,"/GSE237036") # Directory regard-
ing the data required
dir_path2 <- paste0(work_dir,"/GSE237036/Data") # for the idat
files
dir_path3 <- paste0(work_dir,"/GSE237036/Info") # for the
dataset's information


# Define the URL of the raw data file to be downloaded
raw_dat_url <- "https://ftp.ncbi.nlm.nih.gov/geo/series/
GSE237nnn/GSE237036/suppl//GSE237036_RAW.tar"
# Define the destination file path where the raw data file will
be saved
destfile <- paste0(work_dir,"/GSE237036/GSE237036_RAW.tar")
```

```
# Download the raw data file from the specified URL to the
destination file path
download.file(raw_dat_url, destfile, "curl", quiet = FALSE,
mode = "w",
 cacheOK = TRUE)
# Directory where the tar file will be extracted
out_dir <- paste0(work_dir,"/GSE237036/Data/")
# Extract the contents of the tar file into the specified
directory
untar(destfile, files = NULL, list = FALSE, exdir = out_dir)


# We download the sample sheet with information about the
samples. getGEO function retrieves GEO data corresponding to
the specified GEO accession number (GSE237036). The sample
sheet will be saved in the specified directory
targets <- getGEO(GEO = 'GSE237036', destdir =paste0(-
work_dir,"/GSE237036"))


# Define the URL of the processed matrix data file to be
downloaded
matrix_url <- "https://ftp.ncbi.nlm.nih.gov/geo/series/
GSE237nnn/GSE237036/suppl/GSE237036_matrix_processed.txt.gz"
# Destination file path where the processed matrix data file
will be saved
destfile <- paste0(work_dir,"/GSE237036/GSE237036_matrix_pro-
cessed.txt.gz")
# Download the processed matrix data file from the specified
URL to the destination file path
download.file(matrix_url, destfile, "curl", quiet = FALSE,
mode = "w",
 cacheOK = TRUE)
# File path where the uncompressed matrix data will be saved
out_dir2 <- paste0(work_dir,"/GSE237036/GSE237036_matrix_pro-
cessed.txt")
# Uncompress the downloaded gzipped matrix data file to the
specified destination file path
gunzip(destfile, destname = out_dir2)
```

The getGEOSuppFiles function creates a folder named GSE237036 in your working directory, containing the GSE47915_RAW.tar file, which we will extract in the next step. The getGEO function imports the metadata. We can extract the metadata from the GSE237036 object using the following command. Additionally, we will select the 10 samples that we will use for the analysis, using the package dplyr. if you do not want to preselect the files, just go to the next step.

```
# Select the object
targets <- pData(phenoData(targets[[1]]))

# We select the files that we will use
library(dplyr)
targets <- targets %>%
filter(geo_accession %in% c("GSM7593324", "GSM7593325",
"GSM7593326", "GSM7593327", "GSM7593328",
  "GSM7593399", "GSM7593400", "GSM7593401", "GSM7593402",
"GSM7593403"))
```

(Optional) If you have your own data stored on your computer or if you manually downloaded the data, please follow the next script to import and process your data accordingly.

```
# Load idat files and sample sheet, previously stores in a file
named GSE237036, located in your favorite file. Just place the
url of the file into the read.metharray.sheet
baseDir <- system.file("Your location", package = "minfiData")
targets <- read.metharray.sheet("Your location") # if your
file named EPIC containing idat. and sample sheet is located
in the Desktop, put "~/Desktop/EPIC"
# Preselect the samples we will use for the analysis
targets <- targets %>%
filter(geo_accession %in% c("GSM7593324", "GSM7593325",
"GSM7593326", "GSM7593327", "GSM7593328",
  "GSM7593399", "GSM7593400", "GSM7593401", "GSM7593402",
"GSM7593403"))
```

In the case that you have your own data, just replace location of your file by a directory or file that contain both *idat*. files and sample sheet. Now it is turn to load *idat*. From the file GSE237036 and match with the sample sheet. The initial step in minfi involves reading the *idat*. files using the built-in function read.450 k.exp. for 450K and read.metharray.exp. for EPIC (850 K). Users have various options available: you can specify the sample file names along with the directory path to read them, or you can specify the directory containing the files. In the latter scenario, all files with the *idat*. Extension within the directory will be imported into R. Additionally, users can import a sample sheet and utilize it to load the data into a RGChannelSet object. For more detailed guidance, please refer to the minfi vignette.

```
# Extract the supplementary file URLs from the targets object
tmp_targets <- targets$supplementary_file
# Extract the relevant part of the file names from the URLs,
starting from the 68th character to the end of the string
my_targets <- substr(tmp_targets,68,nchar(tmp_targets))
```

```
# Create a data frame with a single column named "Basename"
containing the extracted file names
my_targets2 <- data.frame("Basename"=my_targets)
# Read the methylation array data using the specified base
directory and targets data frame
RGset <- read.metharray.exp(
 base = out_dir, # Base directory where the raw data files are
located. If your file names EPIC contains another file namer
idat, in which contains idat. files, put: "~/Desktop/EPIC/
idat"
 targets = my_targets2, # Data frame containing the basenames
of the files to be read. Put only targets in you upload your
own data
 extended = TRUE, # Read extended format of the array data
 recursive = FALSE, # Do not search directories recursively
 verbose = FALSE, # Suppress verbose output
 force = TRUE # Force reading of the data even if some files
are missing
 )


head(RGset)
```

2.6 Quality Control, Normalization, and Mapping

Poor-performing probes can obscure biological signals in the data and are typically filtered out before conducting differential methylation analysis. Since the signals from these probes are unreliable, removing them reduces the number of statistical tests performed, thereby lowering the multiple testing penalty. We filter out probes that have failed in one or more samples based on their detection p value. This ensures that only high-quality, reliable probes are used in the analysis, improving the accuracy and robustness of the results. After filtering, it is important to normalize the data to correct for technical variations and ensure comparability across samples. Various normalization methods, such as quantile normalization or functional normalization, can be applied depending on the specific characteristics of the dataset. Proper normalization is crucial for minimizing batch effects and other technical artifacts that could confound the biological interpretation of the data. Finally, quality control checks should be performed to assess the effectiveness of the filtering and normalization steps. Visualizations such as density plots, boxplots, and multidimensional scaling (MDS) plots can help to identify any remaining issues with the data and ensure that it is ready for downstream analysis. By rigorously preparing the data in this way, we can maximize the reliability and interpretability of the differential methylation analysis results.

```
detP <- detectionP(RGset)
failed <- detP > 0.01
```

```
keep <- colMeans(detP) < 0.05
RGset <- RGset[,keep]
targets <- targets[keep,]

rm(detP, failed, keep)
```

This function performs stratified quantile normalization pre-processing. The normalization procedure is applied separately to the methylated (Meth) and unmethylated (Unmeth) intensities. The type I and type II probe signals are aligned by first quantile normalizing the type II probes across samples, and then interpolating a reference distribution to normalize the type I probes. Because probe types and regions are confounded and DNA methylation (DNAm) distributions vary across regions, the probes are stratified by region before applying this interpolation. It is important to note that this algorithm relies on the assumptions necessary for quantile normalization and is not recommended for cases where global changes are expected, such as in cancer vs. normal comparisons. This normalization procedure is similar to one previously presented by Nizar Touleimat and Jörg Tost (2012). The different options for this function include:

- If fixMethOutlier is TRUE, the function corrects outliers in both the methylated and unmethylated channels when small intensities are close to zero.
- If removeBadSamples is TRUE, it removes poor quality samples using the previously discussed QC criteria.
- It performs stratified subset quantile normalization if quantileNormalize = TRUE and stratified = TRUE.
- It predicts the sex (if not provided in the sex argument) using the getSex function and normalizes males and females separately for the probes on the X and Y chromosomes.

```
GRset.quantile <- preprocessQuantile(RGset, fixOutliers =
TRUE,
 removeBadSamples = TRUE, badSampleCutoff = 10.5,
 quantileNormalize = TRUE, stratified = TRUE,
 mergeManifest = FALSE, sex = NULL)
```

In addition to filtering based on detection p values, it is also common to remove probes that map to multiple locations in the genome or overlap with known single nucleotide polymorphisms (SNPs) and sex chromosomes. These probes can introduce noise and potential biases into the analysis. By applying these additional filtering steps, we can further enhance the quality of the methylation data and increase the confidence in our findings.

```
keep <- !(featureNames(GRset.quantile) %in% annEPIC$Name[an-
nEPIC$chr %in%c("chrX","chrY")])
mSetSqFlt <- GRset.quantile[keep,]
mSetSqFlt <- dropLociWithSnps(mSetSqFlt)
rm(keep, GRset.quantile)
```

Another common metric for describing methylation levels is the M value, which is the log2 ratio of the intensities of the methylated probe to the unmethylated probe. An M value close to 0 indicates similar intensities between the methylated and unmethylated probes, suggesting the CpG site is approximately half-methylated, assuming the intensity data has been properly normalized. Positive M values indicate that more molecules are methylated than unmethylated, while negative M values indicate the opposite. While Beta- and M values are related, beta values are generally preferred for graphically representing methylation levels because percentage methylation has a more intuitive biological interpretation. However, due to their distributional properties, M values are more statistically valid for differential methylation analysis. A thorough comparison of both metrics can be found here.

```
mVals <- getM(mSetSqFlt)
bVals <- getBeta(mSetSqFlt)
```

3   Results

3.1   Differential Methylation Positions

After all this preprocessing and filtering, we can finally address the main biological question: which CpG sites are differentially methylated between the different cell types? To answer this, we will design a linear model using *limma*. We are interested in pairwise comparisons between the four cell types, accounting for variation between individuals. This analysis is conducted on the matrix of M values using limma, which provides t-statistics and associated p values for each CpG site. A convenient way to manage multiple comparisons is to use a contrasts matrix alongside the design matrix. The contrasts matrix allows for linear combinations of the design matrix columns corresponding to the comparisons of interest, effectively focusing the analysis on these comparisons. Next, these contrasts are fitted to the model, and the function eBayes is used to calculate the statistics and p values for differential expression. This function ranks genes based on the evidence for differential methylation. We would not go into detail about this statistical framework here, but more information can be found in the *limma* documentation. Using the topTable function in *limma*, you can extract differentially methylated genes for each comparison/contrast. To order these by p value, set sort.by = "p." The results for the first comparison can be saved as a data.frame by setting coef = 1. The coef parameter explicitly refers to the column in the contrasts matrix that corresponds to the comparison of interest. Additionally, you can enhance the list of CpGs by including a genelist parameter in the topTable function. This helps retrieve the location of the CpG, the nearest gene or CpG island, and other relevant information.

```
library(limma)
# Create a new variable with groups if needed
targets$Sample_group <- ifelse(targets$source_name_ch1 ==
"normal PBMCs sample", "0", ifelse(targets$source_name_ch1
== "BC PBMCs sample", "1", NA))
table(targets$Sample_group)


# Here, you can add to the model such variables you consider to
adjust for
design <- model.matrix(~ targets$Sample_group, data=targets)


# Fit
fit <- lmFit(mVals, design)


# contrast.matrix <- makeContrasts(1-0,levels=design)
# fit2 <- contrasts.fit(fit, contrast.matrix)
fit2 <- eBayes(fit)


# Use a specific column for genome annotation
annEPICsub <- annEPIC[match(rownames(mVals),annEPIC$Name),
c(1:4,12:19,22:31,35:39:ncol(annEPIC))]


# Obtain Differentially methylated positions (DMP)
DMP <- topTable(fit2, num=Inf, coef=2, confint = TRUE,
genelist=annEPICsub)
DMP$UCSC_RefGene_Name <- sub(";.*", "", DMP$UCSC_RefGene_Name)


# Select the significant DMP
DMP <- subset(DMP, adj.P.Val < 0.05)


# Check the DMPs
sum(DMP$adj.P.Val < 0.05, na.rm=TRUE)
summary(decideTests(fit2))


# Write an Excel file with DMPs if needed
# install.packages("writexl")
# library(writexl)
# write_xlsx(DMP, "DMP.xlsx")
```

3.2 Differential Methylation Regions

Often, differential methylation at a single CpG site is not highly informative or can be difficult to detect. Therefore, identifying whether multiple nearby CpGs (or regions) are concordantly differentially methylated is often more insightful. Several Bioconductor packages provide functions for identifying differentially methylated regions (DMRs) from 450 k data. Some of the most popular options include the dmrFind function in the charm package, which has been somewhat replaced for 450 k arrays by the bumphunter function in minfi, and the dmrcate function in the DMRcate package. Each is based on different statistical methods, but we will use dmrcate here because it is based on limma, allowing us to use the design and contrast matrix we defined earlier. We will start again with our matrix of *M* values. For this type of analysis, the matrix must be annotated with the chromosomal positions of the CpGs and their gene annotations. Since the initial step involves running the limma differential methylation analysis for single CpGs, we need to specify the design matrix, contrast matrix, and the contrast of interest.

```
library(DMRcate)
myannotation <- DMRcate::cpg.annotate(object = mVals,
 datatype = "array",
 what = "M",
 analysis.type = "differential",
 design = design,
 coef = 2,
 arraytype = "EPIC")
str(myannotation)

# Extract info
DMR <- dmrcate(myannotation, lambda=1000, C=2)
results.ranges <- extractRanges(DMR, genome = "hg19")
head(results.ranges)
results.ranges <- data.frame(results.ranges)

# Write an Excel file with DMPs if needed
# write_xlsx(x = results.ranges1, path = "DMR1.xlsx", col_-
names = TRUE)
```

3.3 Gene Ontology

An alternative method to detect DMRs involves predefining the regions to be tested. Unlike the previous approach, which defines regions based on heuristic distance rules, this method defines regions based on shared functions. We will use the mCSEA package, which includes three types of regions for 450K and EPIC arrays: promoter regions, gene bodies, and CpG Islands. mCSEA is based on gene set enrichment analysis (GSEA), a popular methodology for functional analysis designed to address certain limitations in the field of gene expression. In brief, CpG sites are ranked according to a metric (such as logFC or t-statistic), and an enrichment score (ES) is calculated for each region. This is done by traversing the entire ranked list of CpG sites, increasing the score when a CpG in the region is encountered and decreasing it when a CpG outside the region is encountered. A high ES indicates that the probes are found near the top of the ranked list, suggesting that the CpG sites in this region, on average, exhibit a higher methylation level. This approach is particularly effective for detecting smaller but consistent methylation differences.

In this case, we will apply this method to the output of the "naive-rTreg" comparison, ranking the CpGs by logFC differences. We will specify "promoters" as the type of region to be considered, although other options like CpG Islands or gene bodies can also be used. After obtaining a potentially extensive list of significantly differentially methylated CpG sites, one might question whether specific biological pathways are overrepresented in this list. In some cases, it is straightforward to link the top differentially methylated CpGs to genes that are biologically relevant to the cell types or samples being studied. However, with potentially thousands of significantly differentially methylated CpGs, gene set analysis (GSA) can be used to uncover meaningful biological patterns from these high-throughput data. The objective is typically to identify commonalities among the genes, using annotations from sources such as the Gene Ontology (GO) or Kyoto Encyclopedia of Genes and Genomes (KEGG).

This type of analysis can be performed using the gometh function in the missMethyl package. This function requires a character vector of the names (e.g., cg20832020) of the significant CpG sites and optionally, a character vector of all CpGs tested. Including all tested CpGs is recommended, especially if extensive filtering was done before the analysis, as it serves as the "background" from which any significant CpG could be chosen. For gene ontology testing, the user can set collection = "GO" (the default option). For testing KEGG pathways, collection = "KEGG" should be specified. In this tutorial, we will proceed with the results from the single-probe "naive vs rTreg" comparison and select all CpG sites with an adjusted p value of less than 0.05.

```
library(missMethyl)
# Get the significant CpG sites at less than 5% FDR
sigCpGs <- DMP$Name[DMP$P.Value<0.05]


# Get all the CpG sites used in the analysis to form the
background
all <- DMP$Name


# Run Gene Ontology Analysis, this may take a while
```

```r
GO <- gometh(sig.cpg=sigCpGs,
 all.cpg=all,
 collection = c("GO"),
 array.type = c("EPIC"),
 plot.bias = FALSE,
 equiv.cpg = TRUE,
 anno = annEPIC,
 sig.genes = TRUE)

# Run Gene Set Enrichment Analysis
# Add ENTREZID reference
library(org.Hs.eg.db)
library(clusterProfiler)

DMP$entrez <- mapIds(org.Hs.eg.db,
 keys=DMP$UCSC_RefGene_Name,
 column="ENTREZID",
 keytype="SYMBOL",
 multiVals="first")

# Select genes
original_gene_list <- DMP$logFC
names(original_gene_list) <- DMP$entrez
gene_list <- na.omit(original_gene_list)
gene_list <-sort(gene_list, decreasing = TRUE)
table(duplicated(gene_list))

# Run
organism = "org.Hs.eg.db"
gse <- gseGO(geneList=gene_list,
 ont ="ALL",
 keyType = "ENTREZID",
 nPerm = 10000,
 minGSSize = 3,
 maxGSSize = 800,
 pvalueCutoff = 0.05,
 verbose = TRUE,
 OrgDb = organism,
 pAdjustMethod = "none")

# Run KEGG Analysis
KEGG <- gometh(sig.cpg=sigCpGs,
 all.cpg=all,
 collection = c("KEGG"),
 array.type = c("EPIC"),
 plot.bias = FALSE,
 equiv.cpg = TRUE,
 anno = annEPIC,
 sig.genes = TRUE)
```

3.4 Immune Quantification

Peripheral blood is commonly used for DNA methylation analyses due to its easy accessibility through minimally invasive procedures. Emerging evidence suggests that specific DNA methylation changes in blood may reflect pathological states in target organs that are not easily accessible by biopsy. Blood DNA methylation profiles can also capture information on systemic exposures or diseases where single organ assessment is not feasible. Epigenome-wide association studies (EWAS) have shown that some DNA methylation changes reflect induced epigenetic alterations within blood cells, while others indicate changes in leukocyte subtype proportions related to pathophysiology. To address cell heterogeneity and potential confounding, both reference-based and non-reference-based techniques are employed, with applications detailed in previous studies. Deconvolution techniques, such as constrained projection/quadratic programming (CP/QP), estimate the relative proportions of blood cell types using DNA methylation signatures.

Initially pipelines for estimating leukocyte subtypes in adult blood were based on six adult male samples purified by flow cytometry and profiled using the Illumina HumanMethylation450K array (450K array). With the advent of the Illumina HumanMethylationEPIC array (EPIC array), which interrogates over 860,000 CpG sites, there is a need to assess the accuracy of cell deconvolution using existing 450 K reference signatures. The EPIC array includes additional genomic content in enhancer regions and DNase hypersensitive sites (DHS), crucial for hematopoietic development and differentiation.

The FlowSorted.Blood.EPIC package extends the reference library for blood cell proportion deconvolution using the EPIC array, aiming to improve the accuracy of cell composition estimates and address potential platform differences. DNA methylation was measured using the EPIC array on neutrophils, B cells, monocytes, NK cells, CD4+ T cells, and CD8+ T cells sorted with antibody beads. An iterative algorithm for Identifying Optimal Libraries (IDOL) from leukocyte differentially methylated regions (L-DMR) was applied to enhance the accuracy and efficiency of cell composition estimates obtained through cell mixture deconvolution. The package contains Illumina HumanMethylationEPIC (EPIC) DNA methylation microarray data from immunomagnetic sorted adult blood cell populations. This dataset, includes 37 magnetically sorted blood cell references and 12 additional samples. The data is formatted as an RGChannelSet object, which allows for seamless integration and normalization using most existing Bioconductor packages.

The code provided below is designed to estimate the proportions of various immune cell types in a given methylation dataset. This process involves several steps. First, the reference data is loaded, including the FlowSorted.Blood.EPIC dataset, which provides reference data for different blood cell types, and the IDOLOptimizedCpGs dataset, which contains optimized CpG probes for accurate cell type estimation. The target object, which includes sample sheet information, is utilized to extract relevant file names of the raw data files. A data frame named my_targets2 is created to hold these file names. The read.metharray.exp. function then reads the methylation data files specified in the my_targets2 data frame and stores the data in an object called RGset.

For estimating cell counts, the estimateCellCounts2 function is used with RGset as the input. This function estimates the proportions of different immune cell types by utilizing parameters such as the Noob preprocessing method (preprocessNoob), the IDOL optimization method for probe selection, and specifying cell types including CD8+ T cells, CD4+ T cells, NK cells, B cells, monocytes, and neutrophils. The FlowSorted.Blood.EPIC dataset is used as the reference set, and IDOLOptimizedCpGs are used for probe selection. The cell proportions are converted to percentages, rounding them to one decimal place for better readability. This framework provides a robust method for estimating immune cell proportions in blood samples using DNA methylation data.

```
library(FlowSorted.Blood.EPIC)

# Define the function below to retrieve the reference data from
ExperimentHub
libraryDataGet <- function(title) {
assign(title, ExperimentHub()[[query(
ExperimentHub(),
 title
 )$ah_id]])
}


# Load the FlowSorted.Blood.EPIC dataset, which provides
reference data for blood cell types
FlowSorted.Blood.EPIC <- libraryDataGet('FlowSorted.Blood.
EPIC')
# Load the IDOLOptimizedCpGs data, which contains optimized
CpG probes for cell type estimation
data("IDOLOptimizedCpGs")

# Estimate cell proportions in the given RGset using the
specified parameters
percEPIC <- estimateCellCounts2(
 RGset, # The methylation data set to be analyzed
  compositeCellType = "Blood", # Specify the composite cell
type as blood
  processMethod = "preprocessNoob", # Use the Noob preproces-
sing method
```

```
    probeSelect = "IDOL", # Select probes based on the IDOL
optimization method
  cellTypes = c("CD8T", "CD4T", "NK", "Bcell", "Mono", "Neu"),
  referencePlatform = "IlluminaHumanMethylationEPIC",
  referenceset = "FlowSorted.Blood.EPIC", # Use as reference
the FlowSorted.Blood.EPIC
  IDOLOptimizedCpGs = IDOLOptimizedCpGs # Provide the IDOL
optimized CpG probes
)

# Print the first few rows of the estimated cell proportions
print(head(percEPIC$counts))

# Convert the cell proportions to percentages and round to one
decimal place
percEPIC <- data.frame(round(percEPIC$prop * 100, 1))
```

4   Visualization

4.1 PCA

Principal Component Analysis (PCA) is a valuable tool for analyzing DNA methylation data from cancer and control patients, as it reduces the dimensionality of the dataset while retaining the most significant variation, thereby facilitating the identification of distinct methylation patterns that may differentiate cancerous tissues from normal tissues. In this case, we create a PCA from beta values, to use them as a valuable tool to separate two groups by DNA methylation (Fig. 2).

```
targets$Group <- ifelse(targets$source_name_ch1 == "normal
PBMCs sample", "Control",
ifelse(targets$source_name_ch1 == "BC PBMCs sample", "Can-
cer", NA))

# Create a data.frame for beta values to represent PCA
bVals_t <- t(bVals)
bVals_t <- data.frame(bVals_t)
pca_res <- prcomp(bVals_t, scale. = TRUE)

library(ggfortify)
autoplot(pca_res,
 data = targets,
 colour = 'Group',
 size = 5,
 addEllipses = TRUE,
 frame = TRUE, frame.type = 't')+
theme(title = element_text(size = 20))+
```

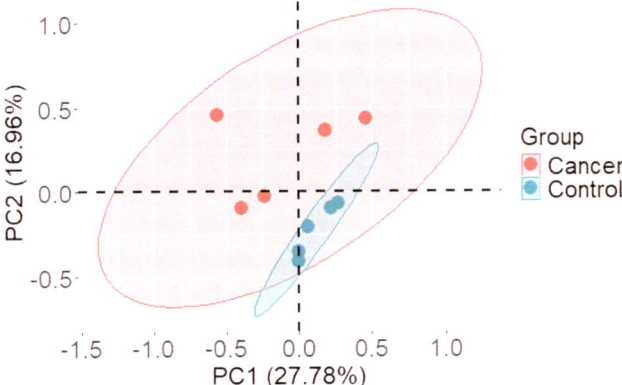

Fig. 2 PCA analysis using DNA methylation data. Tumor samples are in red circles and normal samples are in green circles

```
theme(axis.text = element_text(size = 20))+
theme(legend.text = element_text(size = 20))+
geom_hline(yintercept=0, linetype="dashed", color = "black",
size = 0.8) +
geom_vline(xintercept=0, linetype="dashed", colour= "black",
size = 0.8)
```

4.2 Volcano Plot

A volcano plot is a powerful visualization tool in the analysis of DNA methylation data from cancer and control patients. It allows researchers to quickly identify statistically significant differences in methylation levels between the two groups. By plotting the magnitude of change (e.g., fold change in methylation levels) on the X-axis and the statistical significance (e.g., p value) on the Y-axis, the volcano plot highlights individual CpG sites or regions that exhibit both large changes in methylation and strong statistical significance. This dual-axis approach helps in pinpointing potential epigenetic markers for cancer diagnosis or therapeutic targets, making the volcano plot an invaluable tool in cancer epigenetics research (Fig. 3).

```
library(tibble)
library(ggrepel)
DMP_adjusted <- subset(DMP, DMP$adj.P.Val <= 0.1)
DMP_adjusted <- DMP_adjusted %>%
mutate(
 Expression = case_when(logFC >= 0 & adj.P.Val <= 0.05 ~ "Up-
regulated",
 logFC <= 0 & adj.P.Val <= 0.05 ~ "Down-regulated",
 TRUE ~ "Unchanged")
 )
```

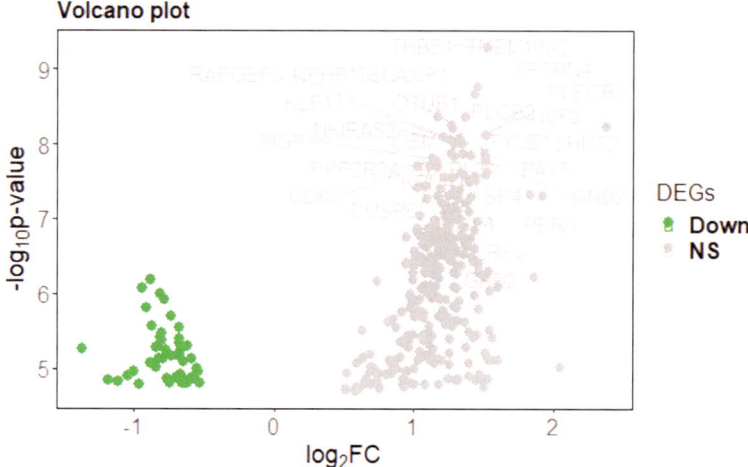

Fig. 3 Volcano plot for breast cancer vs normal, where the adjusted *p* value is less than 0.05

```
DMP_adjusted <- rownames_to_column(DMP_adjusted, var = "Head-
er")


# Add a column to the data frame to specify if they are UP- or
DOWN- regulated (log2fc respectively positive or negative)
DMP_adjusted$diffexpressed <- "NO"
# if log2Foldchange > 0.6 and pvalue < 0.05, set as "UP"
DMP_adjusted$diffexpressed[DMP_adjusted$logFC > 0 & DMP_ad-
justed$P.Value < 0.05] <- "UP"
# if log2Foldchange < -0.6 and pvalue < 0.05, set as "DOWN"
DMP_adjusted$diffexpressed[DMP_adjusted$logFC < 0 & DMP_ad-
justed$P.Value < 0.05] <- "DOWN"
# Explore a bit
head(DMP_adjusted[order(DMP_adjusted$P.Value) & DMP_adjusted
$diffexpressed == 'DOWN', ])


# Create a new column "delabel" to de, that will contain the
name of the top 30 differentially expressed genes (NA in case
they are not)
DMP_adjusted$delabel1 <- ifelse(DMP_adjusted$UCSC_RefGen-
e_Name %in% head(DMP_adjusted[order(DMP_adjusted$P.Value),
"UCSC_RefGene_Name"], 30), DMP_adjusted$UCSC_RefGene_Name,
NA)
DMP_adjusted$delabel2 <- ifelse(DMP_adjusted$Name %in% head(-
DMP_adjusted[order(DMP_adjusted$P.Value), "Name"], 30),
DMP_adjusted$Name, NA)


ggplot(data = DMP_adjusted, aes(x = logFC, y = -log10(P.
Value), col = Expression, label = delabel1)) +
```

```
theme_classic() +
# geom_vline(xintercept = c(-0.6, 0.6), col = "gray", linetype
= 'dashed') +
# geom_hline(yintercept = -log10(0.05), col = "gray", linetype
= 'dashed') +
geom_point(size = 3) +
scale_color_manual(values = c("green3", "grey", "red3"), # to
set the colours of our variable
 labels = c("Down", "NS", "Up")) +
labs(color = 'DEGs', #legend_title,
 x = expression("log"[2]*"FC"), y = expression("-log"[10]*"p-
value")) +
ggtitle('Volcano plot') +
geom_text_repel(max.overlaps = Inf, size = 5, face= "bold") +
theme(axis.text = element_text(size = 15)) +
theme(legend.text = element_text(size = 15, face= "bold")) +
theme(axis.title.x = element_text(size = 17, face = "bold")) +
theme(axis.title.y = element_text(size = 17, face = "bold")) +
theme(plot.title = element_text(size = 15, face = "bold")) +
theme(legend.title = element_text(size = 15)) +
theme(panel.border = element_rect(colour = "black", fill =
NA, size= 0.5),
 panel.grid.minor = element_blank(),
 panel.grid.major = element_blank())
```

4.3   Heatmap

Heatmaps are a crucial tool for visualizing DNA methylation data, as they provide an intuitive representation of methylation levels across numerous genomic regions and samples. This visualization technique can effectively highlight differences between cancer and control patients, making it easier to identify regions of the genome that are differentially methylated. By displaying complex data in a color-coded format, heatmaps facilitate the recognition of patterns and correlations that might be missed in traditional data tables. This ability to visually compare the methylation status across samples enables researchers to pinpoint specific genes or regions that could be involved in cancer development or progression, aiding in the discovery of potential biomarkers and therapeutic targets.

Moreover, heatmaps can be customized with annotations and clustering to further enhance data interpretation. For example, adding sample annotations for clinical variables or treatment groups can provide additional layers of insight, revealing how methylation patterns are associated with different clinical outcomes. The hierarchical clustering often applied in heatmap analyses groups similar samples and genomic regions together, which can uncover previously unrecognized subgroups within the data. This can lead to the identification of novel cancer subtypes or the

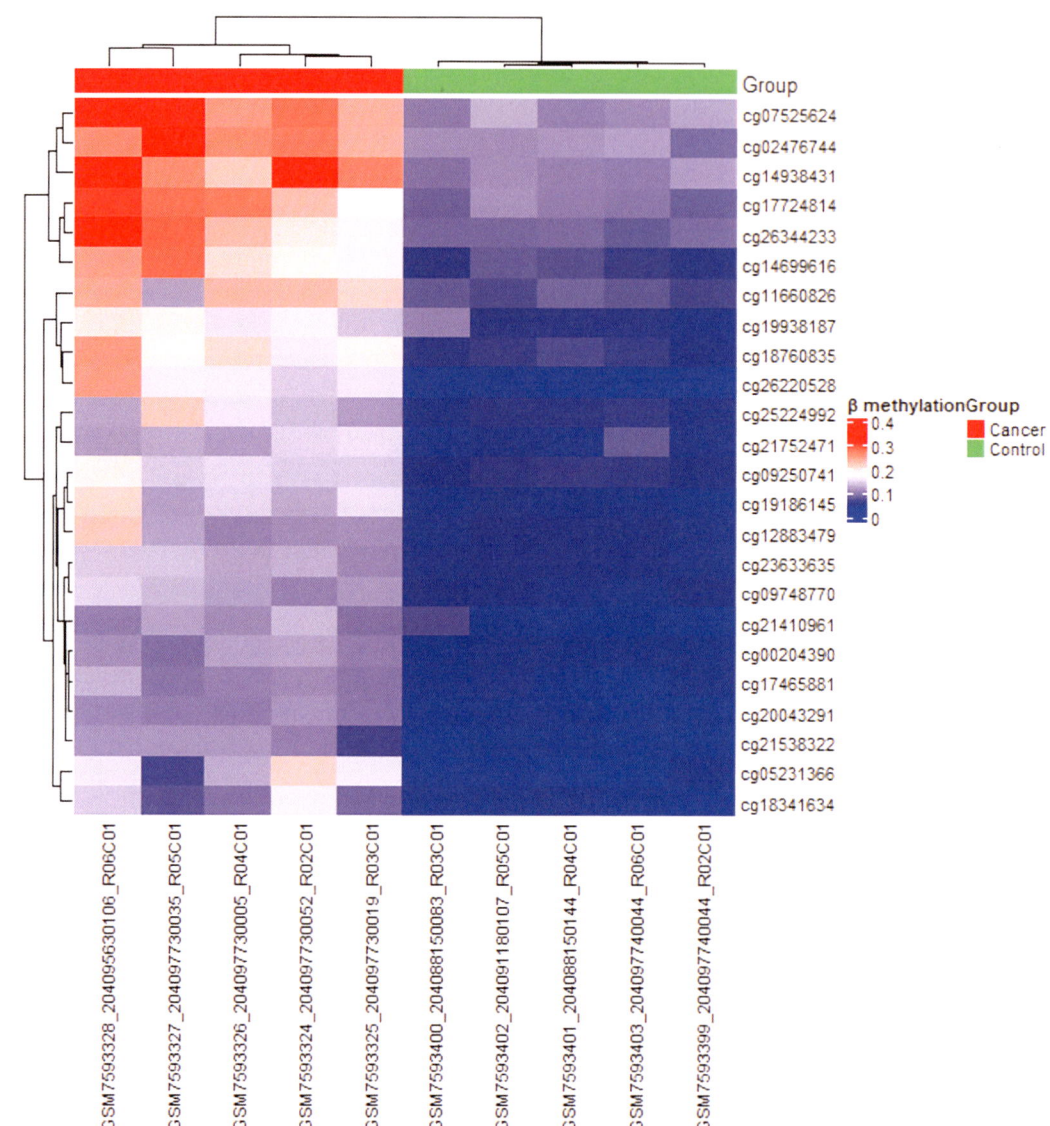

Fig. 4 Heatmap of DNA methylation positions, previously selected by adjusted *p* value less than 0.05 and an absolute log Fold Change greater than 1.5

elucidation of mechanisms underlying disease heterogeneity. In the context of integrative analyses, heatmaps can be used alongside other data types, such as gene expression or genetic mutations, to provide a comprehensive view of the epigenetic landscape and its interactions with other molecular alterations in cancer (Fig. 4).

```
library(ComplexHeatmap )
# Create data.frame for significant CpGs
DMP_subset <- subset(DMP, adj.P.Val<0.05 & abs(DMP$logFC) >
1.5)
```

```
idx = rownames(DMP_subset)

# Crear matrix of beta values from significant DMPs
bVals_significant <- data.frame(bVals[idx,])
bVals_significant <- as.matrix(bVals_significant)

# Create color of subsetting
col = list(Group = c("Control" = "green", "Cancer" = "red"))

# Create the heatmap annotation
ha <- HeatmapAnnotation(Group = as.factor(targets$Group), col
= col)

# Combine the heatmap and the annotation
library(ComplexHeatmap)
Heatmap(bVals_significant, name = "β methylation",
 top_annotation = ha,
 row_names_gp = gpar(fontsize = 10),
 column_names_gp = gpar(fontsize = 10))
```

4.4 GSEA and ORA

Gene Ontology (GO) and Kyoto Encyclopedia of Genes and Genomes (KEGG) analyses are indispensable tools in the realm of bioinformatics, providing valuable insights into the functional significance of genes and their involvement in various biological processes. These analyses offer a structured framework for annotating genes based on their molecular functions, biological processes, and cellular components, thereby unraveling the intricate interplay of genes within living organisms. The significance of results derived from GO and KEGG analyses lies in their ability to elucidate the underlying biological mechanisms driving complex biological phenomena. By associating genes with specific biological functions and pathways, these analyses facilitate the interpretation of high-throughput genomic data and enable researchers to discern meaningful patterns amidst vast datasets. This comprehension extends beyond individual genes, offering a holistic understanding of biological systems and their regulatory networks.

Furthermore, GO and KEGG analyses play a pivotal role in hypothesis generation and validation, guiding experimental studies aimed at deciphering the molecular basis of diseases, identifying therapeutic targets, and unraveling the intricacies of physiological processes. By pinpointing key pathways and biological functions enriched with relevant genes, these analyses provide valuable leads for further investigation, ultimately advancing our knowledge of disease mechanisms and therapeutic interventions. Moreover, the integration of GO and KEGG analyses with other omics data, such as transcriptomics, proteomics, and metabolomics, enables

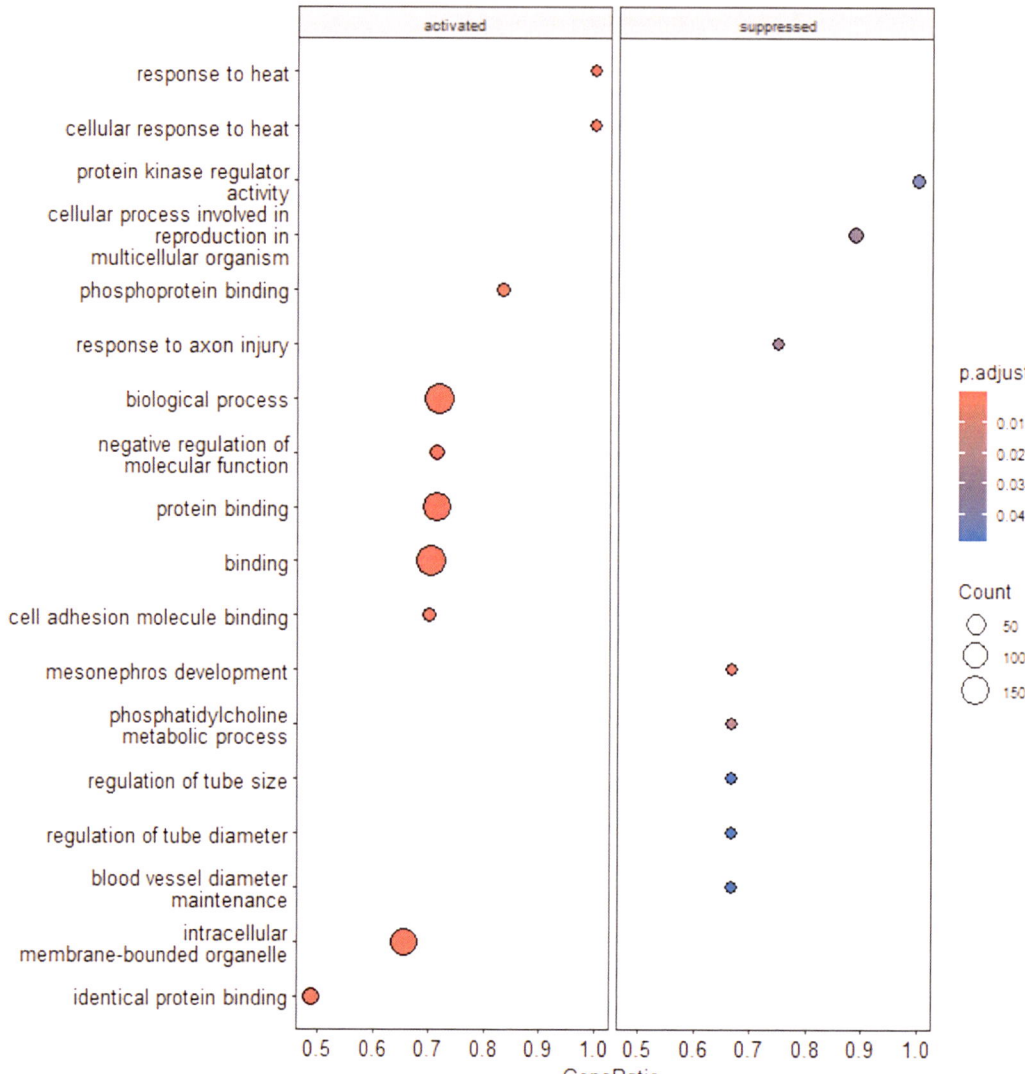

Fig. 5 Gene set enrichment analysis showing pathways activated and suppressed in cancer, by using DNA methylation analysis

comprehensive multi-omics investigations, facilitating a systems-level understanding of biological phenomena. This integrative approach fosters cross-disciplinary collaborations and accelerates discoveries in fields ranging from basic research to clinical applications. In conclusion, the results obtained from GO and KEGG analyses serve as a cornerstone in biological research, offering valuable insights into gene function, pathway regulation, and disease mechanisms. Their significance extends beyond mere data annotation, driving innovation and discovery in diverse areas of biomedical research.

```
library(multienrichjam)
library(enrichplot)

# GO
enr1 <- enrichDF2enrichResult(enrichDF = GO, keyColname =
"ONTOLOGY", geneColname = "SigGenesInSet", pvalueColname =
"P.DE", descriptionColname = "TERM", pvalueCutoff = 0.05)
 edox1 <- pairwise_termsim(enr1)
barplot(edox1, showCategory=30)

# KEGG
enr2 <- enrichDF2enrichResult(enrichDF = KEGG, keyColname =
"N", geneColname = "SigGenesInSet", pvalueColname = "P.DE",
descriptionColname = "Description", pvalueCutoff = 0.05)
edox2 <- pairwise_termsim(enr2)
barplot(edox2, showCategory=30)
```

The provided code utilizes the dotplot function from the enrichplot package to visualize the results of a gene enrichment analysis. Here's the detailed description of the code: dotplot(gse, showCategory = 10, split = ".sign"): This line generates a dot plot using the results of the gene enrichment analysis stored in the gse object. The showCategory parameter is set to 10, indicating that the top 10 categories will be displayed in the plot. The split parameter is set to ".sign", which splits the results into two panels based on the sign of the enrichment score. + facet_grid(. ~ .sign): This part of the code adds the facet to the plot, splitting the dots into two panels based on the sign of the enrichment score. In summary, this code generates a dot plot that displays the top categories of a gene enrichment analysis, with the results split into two panels based on the sign of the enrichment score. This provides a useful visualization of the gene enrichment analysis results, allowing for comparison of categories based on their enrichment sign (Fig. 5).

```
dotplot(gse, showCategory=10, split=".sign") + facet_grid(.~.
sign)
```

4.5 Immune Representation

For immune representation using estimateCellCounts function, you typically would not generate a dot plot directly from that function alone, as it returns estimated cell counts for various immune cell types. Instead, you might visualize the results in a bar plot or heatmap to represent the estimated counts of different immune cell types across samples. Customize the plot appearance, axis labels, titles, colors, and any other relevant aspects to make the visualization informative and visually appealing. Finally, interpret the generated plot to gain insights into the distribution of immune cell types across your samples, and how they may vary under different conditions or experimental groups (Fig. 6).

```
library(tidyr)
library(ggpubr)
# Create a barplot
data_long <- percEPIC %>%
pivot_longer(cols = c(CD8T, CD4T, NK, Bcell, Mono, Neu),
names_to = "variable", values_to = "valor")

dodge <- position_dodge(width = 0.9)
limits <- aes(ymax = mean + SD, ymin = mean)

ggplot(data_long) +
geom_boxplot(aes(x = as.factor(Group), y = valor, fill = as.
factor(Group))) +
facet_wrap(~ variable, scales = "free_y") +
```

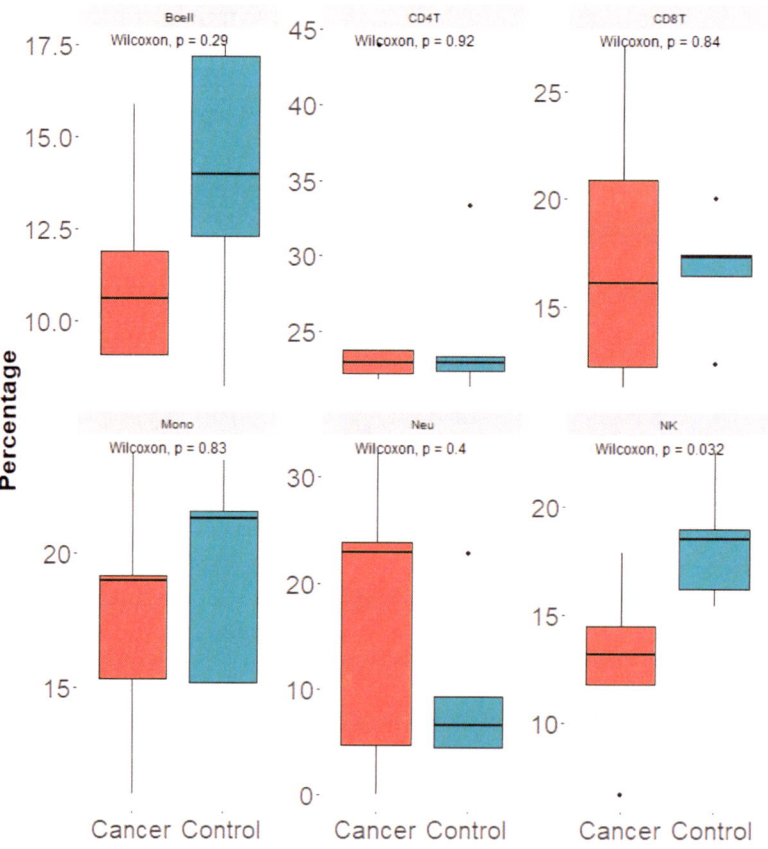

Fig. 6 Boxplot of DNA methylation deconvolution of immune cells located in the blood, including T cells, B cells, natural killers (NK), monocytes (mono), and neutrophils (neu). Wilcoxon test was used to calculate significant differences between groups

```
theme(legend.position = "none", text = element_text(size =
12)) +
labs(x = NULL, y = "Percentage") +
theme(axis.title = element_text(size = 20, face = "bold")) +
theme(axis.text = element_text(size = 20)) +
theme(legend.text = element_text(size = 20)) +
labs(color = "Participants") +
theme(legend.title = element_text(size = 20))+
scale_fill_manual(values = c("Cancer" = "#F8766D", "Control"
= "#00BFC4")) +
stat_compare_means(aes(x = as.factor(Group), y = valor, group
= as.factor(Group)))
```

5 Limitations

The RStudio workflow currently focuses on analyzing epigenetic data and estimating cell-type proportions specifically in blood samples. The current implementation of the pipeline has not been tested on tissue samples. However, as advancements in deconvolution methods continue and extended reference libraries are developed, the potential for its application broadens. Reference libraries containing purified cell subtypes, such as epithelial, mesenchymal, and progenitor cells, make deconvolution feasible also in solid tissue samples (PMID: 28977446). Thus, our pipeline could serve as a foundational framework, which with some fine-tuning, could be adapted to facilitate tissue deconvolution. Such efforts could integrate our workflow with tools like EpiSCORE (PMID: 32883324) to deconvolute bulk tissue samples of DNA methylomes. The working example of the workflow utilizes IDOL optimization algorithm (PMID: 26956433) and the FlowSorted. Blood.EPIC package which contains Illumina HumanMethylatio-nEPIC DNA methylation microarray data (PMID: 29843789). This dataset includes information for the following six cell populations: T lymphocytes (CD4+ and CD8+), B lymphocytes (CD19+), monocytes (CD14+), natural killer (NK) cells (CD56+) and Neutrophils (Neu). Consequently, our pipeline is limited by the available cell types. To extend the analysis to include additional cell populations, users can utilize the extended version of the Flow-Sorted.Blood.EPIC package (PMID: 35140201). The extended version supports a total of 12 different cell types: neutrophils (Neu), eosinophils (Eos), basophils (Bas), monocytes (Mono),B lymphocytes naive (Bnv), B lymphocytes memory (Bmem), T helper lymphocytes naive (CD4nv), T helper lymphocytes memory (CD4mem), T regulatory cells (Treg), T cytotoxic lymphocytes naive (CD8nv), T cytotoxic lymphocytes memory (CD8mem), and natural killer lymphocytes (NK). The usage of this package is restricted to research purposes and requires an academic license. Instructions for obtaining the license are provided in the readme file on their Github repository (https://github.com/immunomethylomics/FlowSorted.BloodExtended.EPIC).

The pipeline code has been tested for reproducibility on three major platforms: Windows, macOS, and Linux. An issue was found with the gene ontology analysis using KEGG, which produces an error on Linux. The entire pipeline relies on Bioconductor version 3.14 and has been tested with R versions 4.0.0 and 4.1.0. Users should be able to reproduce the pipeline using these versions. Additionally, it is expected that the pipeline can be reproduced with the latest version of R. Because the workflow depends on multiple packages, it is advised to set up an R project in an isolated environment using a package manager like "renv" to ensure reproducibility and minimize compatibility issues with package dependencies.

6 Notes

Code availability: https://github.com/SotirisOuzounis/ImmunoMethylation

Acknowledgments

This publication is based upon work from COST Action IMMUNO-model, CA21135, supported by COST (European Cooperation in Science and Technology). This study was supported by "Centro de Investigacion Biomédica en Red Fisiopatología de la Obesidad y Nutricion", which is an initiative of the "Instituto de Salud Carlos III" (ISCIII) of Spain, financed by the European Regional Development Fund, "A way to make Europe"/ "Investing in your future" (CB06/03), a grant from ISCIII (PI18/01399, PI21/00633) and a grant from Consejeria Universidad, Investigacion e Innovacion Junta de Andalucia (PY20-01270). HB is supported by a "Sara Borrell" postdoctoral contract (CD22/00053) from the Instituto de Salud Carlos III—Madrid (Spain), "Financiado por la Unión Europea—NextGenerationEU" y mediante el Plan de Recuperación, Transformación y Resiliencia. HB also received funding from the project 'PI24/00061', funded by the 'Instituto de Salud Carlos III (ISCIII)' and co-funded by the European Union. This work has been supported by Fondazione Michelangelo (Milan, Italy) and Breast Cancer Research Foundation (grant BCRF 21-181) from MC.

References

1. Esteller M (2008) Epigenetics in cancer. N Engl J Med 358(11):1148–1159. https://doi.org/10.1056/nejmra072067

2. Izquierdo AG, Boughanem H, Diaz-Lagares A, Arranz-Salas I, Esteller M, Tinahones FJ et al (2022) DNA methylome in visceral adipose tissue can discriminate patients with and without colorectal cancer. Epigenetics 17:665–676

3. Tien FM, Lu HH, Lin SY, Tsai HC (2023) Epigenetic remodeling of the immune landscape in cancer: therapeutic hurdles and opportunities. J Biomed Sci 30(1):1–23. https://doi.org/10.1186/s12929-022-00893-0

4. Wang T, Li P, Qi Q, Zhang S, Xie Y, Wang J et al (2023) A multiplex blood-based assay targeting DNA methylation in PBMCs enables early detection of breast cancer. Nat Commun 14(1):4724. https://pubmed.ncbi.nlm.nih.gov/37550304/

5. Aryee MJ, Jaffe AE, Corrada-Bravo H, Ladd-Acosta C, Feinberg AP, Hansen KD et al (2014) Minfi: a flexible and comprehensive Bioconductor package for the analysis of Infinium DNA methylation microarrays. Bioinformatics 30:1363

6. Salas LA, Koestler DC, Butler RA, Hansen HM, Wiencke JK, Kelsey KT et al (2018) An optimized library for reference-based deconvolution of whole-blood biospecimens assayed using the Illumina HumanMethylationEPIC BeadArray. Genome Biol 19(1):64. Available from: /pmc/articles/PMC5975716/

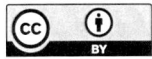

Chapter 16

Deciphering the Tumor Microenvironment Composition Using Bulk Transcriptomics: A Guide to Recent Advances and Open Challenges

Sotiris Ouzounis, Donya Zojaji, Sandra García-Mulero, Marco Barreca, Paolo Gandellini, Theodora Katsila, Rebeca Sanz-Pamplona, and Maurizio Callari

Abstract

Tumors are complex ecosystems comprising diverse cell types actively participating to carcinogenesis, tumor progression, and treatment response. Understanding the tumor microenvironment (TME) dynamics has become of primary importance, especially with the increasing clinical implementation of immunotherapy. Low and high-throughput single cell and spatial technologies are providing high-resolution strategies for the study of the tumor ecosystem. However, their cost and complexity limit widespread use. Bulk transcriptomics has become a widely used strategy to obtain the expression profile of large cohorts of tumors or preclinical models. Several methods implementing a deconvolution analysis have been developed to estimate from bulk transcriptomics the prevalence of multiple cell types to reconstruct the tumor ecosystem composition.

In this chapter, we introduce deconvolution analysis, the main steps, the recent advancements, and open challenges. Our emphasis lies on robust benchmarking methodologies, highlighting the importance of clear parameter definition and appropriate metric selection for reliable results across different software tools.

Using CIBERSORTx and BayesPrism, we conduct a practical analysis on triple-negative breast cancer (TNBC) datasets from The Cancer Genome Atlas (TCGA) dataset. We illustrate the impact of various factors such as preprocessing methods, reference datasets, and software choice on deconvolution outcomes.

Integrating insights from benchmarking analyses and real-world applications, we provide guidance to optimize and control for the quality of deconvolution analysis, weighting both its potential and limitations. Deconvolution analysis can contribute to unravelling the complexities of the tumor microenvironment, but further research is needed to enhance accuracy and reproducibility.

Key words Deconvolution, Cancer, Microenvironment, Bulk, Transcriptomics, TME, Immune, Cell type, Challenges

---

Sotiris Ouzounis, Donya Zojaji and Sandra García-Mulero are Co-First authors.

Rebeca Sanz-Pamplona and Maurizio Callari are Co-Last authors.

Sweta Rani and Lukasz Skalniak (eds.), *IMMUNO-model in Cancer: Methods and Protocols*, Methods in Molecular Biology, vol. 2959, https://doi.org/10.1007/978-1-0716-4734-9_16, © The Author(s) 2026

1   Introduction

Tumors are highly heterogeneous entities including cancer cells, but also non-tumoral cells embedded in the tumor microenvironment (TME) [1], a complex network of multiple molecules and cell types [2].

A major role has emerged for the immune system infiltrating neoplastic lesions. Active research is being carried on the role of immune cells in carcinogenesis, cancer progression and response to therapy. The immune system plays a key role in cancer prevention and elimination, in a process known as immune surveillance. For example, through the recognition of neoantigens, cancer cells could be attacked and eliminated by effector T cells [3]. However, the immune system has a dual role in cancer. Tumors can also recruit immune cells that provide an immunosuppressive tumor microenvironment. Moreover, the stromal cells resident in the tissue can also have effects on tumor growth, like cancer associated fibroblasts and endothelial cells. Understanding the cross talk between cancer, stromal and immune cells is a hot spot in cancer research [4]. Therefore, to study cancer, it is crucial to identify the immune and stromal composition of a tumor.

A number of old and new techniques allows the study of the TME. New sequencing approaches such as single cell RNA-seq and spatial transcriptomics have been developed allowing direct high-resolution measurements of distinct cell-type prevalence and phenotype [5]. However, these techniques are quite demanding in terms of costs, computational power, and expertise. In addition, sample preparation is quite cumbersome and time-consuming.

Deconvolution methods have emerged as indirect techniques to quantify immune and other TME cell infiltration. While these methods are not able to achieve the resolution of single-cell techniques, they can be applied to widely available bulk transcriptomics data estimating, for example, the TME composition in large cancer sample cohorts. This process of cell type quantification is widely used in immunogenomics, and many statistical methods have been developed for quantification of immune and stromal cell types from bulk expression data obtained by RNA-seq and microarrays [6] (Fig. 1).

Scientific literature in cancer research has plenty of examples demonstrating the utility of deconvolution methods applied to transcriptomics data. Applications include generation of new hypotheses and searching for new biomarkers, among others. For example, in a meta-analysis by Kamal et al., four independent transcriptomics datasets were interrogated using deconvolution methods. About 22 immune cell types were inferred, and the association between immune infiltration by each cell type and relapse-free survival was assessed in colorectal cancer. As a result,

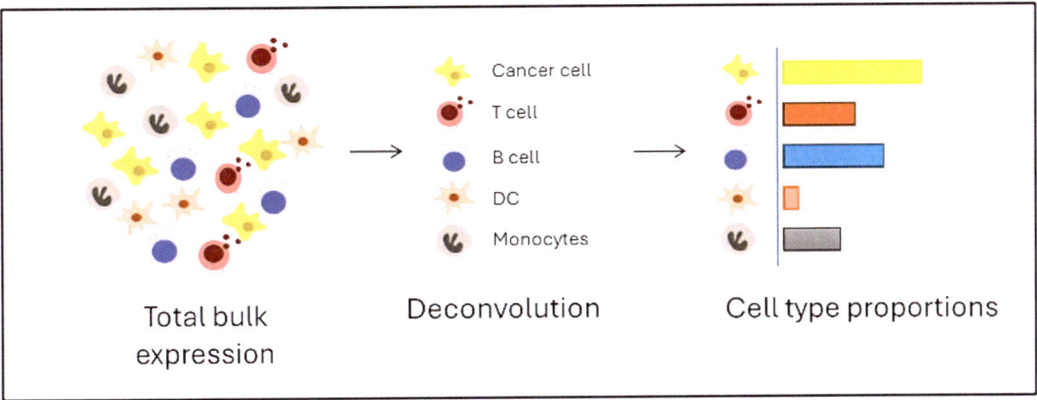

Fig. 1 Concept of immune cell infiltration estimation. From the total bulk RNA expression, it is possible to quantify the prevalence of distinct cell types infiltrating the tumor microenvironment

immune cell-type infiltration was found to be a better predictor of disease relapse than other expression-based biomarkers [7]. Specifically, CD4 and CD8 T cells and NK cells were found to be associated with better prognosis in this kind of tumor. Indeed, tumor infiltrating lymphocytes (TILs) have been associated with good prognosis in several cancer types [8]. On the contrary, infiltration of regulatory T cells (Tregs) has been described as a bad prognosis biomarker [9]. Immune cell infiltration could be also useful to generate new hypotheses. In a work by García-Mulero et al., metastatic samples from different cohorts were scored based on immune cell infiltration. Then, a cluster analysis was done, and three groups of samples emerged that were associated with immunotherapy response [10].

2   Available Methods and Key Steps of the Deconvolution Analysis

Systematic reviews summarising and benchmarking all the available tools have been reported elsewhere [11–13], but a summary of the most widely used open-source algorithms and their main features are listed in Table 1.

Deconvolution algorithms can be classified in various ways. Following the approach by Im and Kim [14], deconvolution algorithms can be categorized based on their methodology, prior knowledge of cell types, and methods of output. Based on the methodology used for inferring cell types, deconvolution tools can be divided into two categories: gene signature-based and fraction-based. Gene signature-based methods rely on the enrichment analysis of gene signatures. These methods are very useful for comparisons between phenotypes but cannot quantify inter-sample differences in cell-type abundance [15]. Fraction-based tools require a predefined reference matrix, which consists of expected

Table 1
Summary descriptive of methods for immune system infiltration estimation using transcriptomic profiles.

Tool	Approach	Cell fractions	Statistical method	Reference required	Cell-types	Applications	Reference
CIBERSORTx	Fraction-based	Relative/ Absolute	Support vector regression	Bulk and scRNA-seq	Custom	Immune profiling of tumors	[29]
EPIC	Gene signature	Relative/ Absolute	Constrained least squares regression	Bulk RNA-seq	Custom and predefined (six immune, two stromal, and unknown)	TME characterization	[36]
MCPcounter	Gene signature	Relative	Mean of marker gene expression	Bulk RNA-seq	Predefined (8 immune and 2 stromal)	TME characterization	[37]
TIMER	Fraction-based	Relative	ssGSEA	Bulk RNA-seq	Predefined (6 immune cells-types)	Immune profiling of tumors	[38]
quanTIseq	Fraction-based	Absolute	Constrained least squares regression	Bulk RNA-seq	Predefined (10 immune cell types)	Immune profiling of tumors	[39]
BayesPrism	Fraction-based	Relative	Bayesian framework	Bulk RNA-seq/ scRNA-seq	Custom	High resolution for high granularity	[30]
ConsensusTME	Gene signature	Relative	ssGSEA	Bulk RNA-seq	Custom and predefined from previous methods (18 cell types)	Combine multiple methods for comprehensive TME characterization	[40]

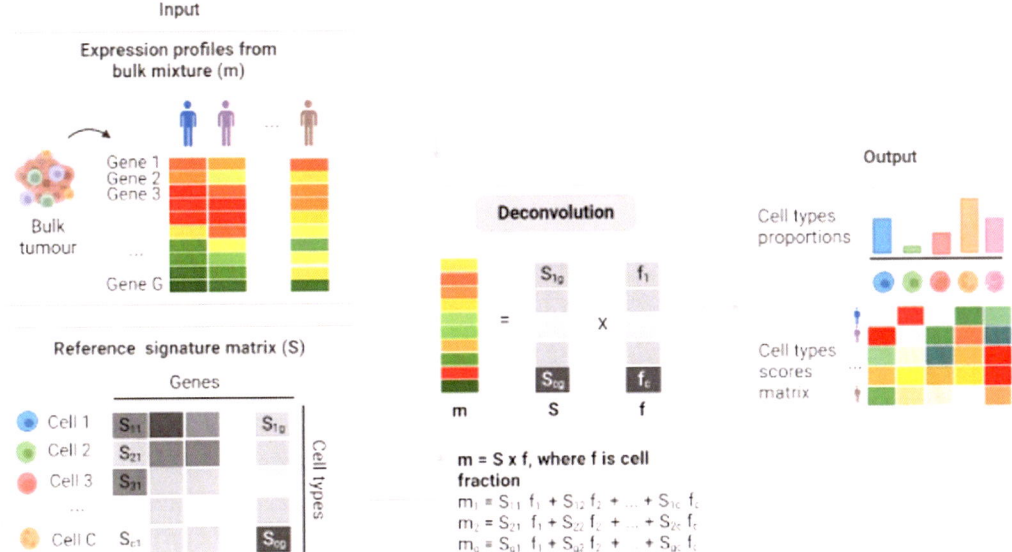

Fig. 2 Overview of deconvolution algorithms. Deconvolution from bulk transcriptomic data requires an expression matrix (m) from the bulk tissue and the cell-type specific reference signature matrix (S). The contribution of the different cell types can be inferred by regression models. The output of the deconvolution is a matrix of proportion scores per cell type and sample

values of gene expression for each cell type. This matrix is used to dissect the contribution of each signature profile to the aggregated bulk level of signal [16]. Furthermore, supervised or semi-supervised deconvolution methods can also be grouped based on the type of prior knowledge required. These include methods that rely on marker gene expression profiles, those that leverage single-cell RNA sequencing data to derive cell-type signatures, and those that account for gene expression variability within cell types.

Quantification methods can also be divided into two groups based on the abundance level: relative fraction or absolute fraction (Table 1). Relative methods estimate the relative abundance of each cell-type relative to each other, but do not provide information about the absolute quantification. The output of relative methods usually consists of enrichment scores and are useful for comparison across different samples or conditions (e.g., between different tumor types or disease states). Absolute scores, which account for the total proportions within a sample, provide more accurate and precise estimates of cell abundances, and allow both intra- and intercomparison of cell types [6].

Workflow in Fig. 2 explains fraction-based approaches that use an a priori defined reference matrix of expected values (S) and a gene expression matrix (m) from the interrogated sample. The bulk tissue representation (m) would result as the product of multiplying the reference signature (S) by the proportion contribution of each cell type (f). To dissect the contribution of each cell type to the bulk signal, different statistical approaches can be performed, from linear regression models to more sophisticated deep learning algorithms [16].

Below, we review the three main steps for performing comprehensive deconvolution pipelines.

2.1 Input Data Preparation: Normalization and Data Transformation

Optimal data preprocessing and normalization are key aspects for the correct performance of deconvolution analysis. In general, log transformation is widely used in RNA-seq data analysis. However, deconvolution algorithms can be affected by data transformations [17]; Cobos et al. performed a benchmark where they evaluated different transformation methods (linear, Log, Sqrt and VST) and found that all deconvolution methods performed at best when applied to linear data. Preprocessing steps like normalization are potentially crucial when handling gene expression data. For this reason, they tested 20 different normalization methods, and found that the choice of normalization strategy has a minor impact in certain deconvolution algorithms. Overall, linear TPM (transcripts per million) is a suitable RNA-seq input data in many deconvolution methods. However, some deconvolution methods expect the data to be normalized (or not) and with a specific strategy, thus it is recommended to carefully read the instructions and recommendations given by the authors [18].

2.2 Selection of the Most Appropriate Method and Reference

The choice of methodology depends on the research question and the goals of the analysis. It is a crucial step in the deconvolution process since different methods could show high disparities in their performance and in the obtained results (see section. 4). Many factors can contribute to this variability, such as the statistical algorithm and the quality of the reference signatures, as discussed below [18].

Often, the proposed algorithms come with one or multiple reference matrices or signatures, which can differ considerably from each other and represent the main source of variability. These reference signatures can vary in the gene markers selected, the number of cell types included (from six to dozens), the diversity of cells included (only immune cells or accounting also for stromal components and/or malignant cells), and the level of granularity (i.e., the specificity of cell-types; e.g., the different subtypes of T cells) [16]. Reference signatures can be generated from bulk RNA-seq (usually derived by flow cytometry sorted populations or in vitro cultured cells) or from single-cell RNA-seq. Moreover, cell-type-specific expression profiles could be generated starting from different tissues (PBMCs, healthy organs, tumor tissues, etc.), as well as different model organisms.

The choice of the most appropriate reference matrix or signatures has a major impact on the quality of the deconvolution results, as shown in the following sections. Ideally, the reference cell types should represent all cell types present in the bulk sample and their expression profile should be generated from tissues as similar as possible to the interrogated bulk sample. Deconvolution methods can overestimate (spillover effect) or even give positive results for absent cell types in the samples (background fraction prediction). This can happen when working with tumors with low immune infiltration and can lead to wrong conclusions. To deal with this problem, some methods like EPIC have added an "Unknown" category [13].

It is important to have the opportunity to use a custom reference matrix or signatures, possibly derived from the increasingly available single-cell RNA-seq data matching the bulk transcriptomics tissue. Moreover, it is common in the context of cancer research to use model organisms and derive nonhuman molecular data. The possibility of using custom references can consequently enable the opportunity to apply data deconvolution in this setting.

2.3 Output and Expected Results

The output of deconvolution algorithms consists of a matrix of proportion scores (Fig. 2), which can be further used for statistical comparisons among phenotypic groups, association studies and clustering analysis, among others. It is important to consider that the output can differ between different deconvolution methods due to the lack of standardized formats, normalization procedures, and scaling factors. Therefore, caution must be paid when attempting to integrate or compare outputs from different deconvolution methods, and careful consideration of methodological differences and validation against independent datasets may be necessary for robust interpretation. Often, additional metrics (e.g., root mean square error or RMSE and p values) providing some indication on the quality of the deconvolution process are provided.

3   Challenges in the Development and Benchmarking of Deconvolution Methods

Several challenges arise during the analysis of bulk transcriptomics from tumor samples using deconvolution methods. Over recent years, various approaches have been proposed and multiple tools have been developed to address these challenges [11, 19, 20]. Many tools aim to overcome known limitations of deconvolution, each offering unique features and benefits. However, despite the development of more robust and efficient tools, a major challenge has yet to be addressed. The challenge is to establish agreement among different tools, which is essentially affected by multiple different parameters of the deconvolution approaches. The agreement among computational tools can be generally defined as the consistency of results obtained from different software when applied to the same data. Therefore, the whole challenge is to design and perform valid benchmarking among existing methods. To achieve this, the parameters of the benchmarking must be clearly defined, and appropriate metrics should be established to measure the agreement among tools and to identify parameters that may introduce bias into the consistency of results. Benchmarking is also essential during the development of deconvolution tools and the strategy used could impact the final performance and comparability with other methods.

Benchmarking process typically involves evaluating the accuracy of tools and various other parameters, such as computational resources required, processing time, scalability, and ease of use [11]. Common methods for evaluating deconvolution algorithms make use of (1) simulated bulk (or pseudo-bulk) data from single-cell RNA-seq, (2) bulk expression profiles from both pure and mixed cell lines, (3) data from the same tissue samples analyzed with both bulk and single-cell RNA-seq, (4) bulk transcriptomics and flow-cytometry data, and (5) bulk transcriptomics paired with clinical data. In all five cases above, the input data are bulk transcriptomics data, yet the ground truth data used for the evaluation of each method differs [11].

In the first case, single-cell data is used as ground truth and a dataset of bulk samples is simulated according to the cell type composition of the ground truth. Deconvolution accuracy is then established by quantitatively comparing the cell-type proportions of each pseudo-bulk sample with the ground truth. This approach is rather biased since simulated data are produced based on several assumptions that are study specific. Currently, several computational tools exist for simulating scRNA-seq count matrices [21–23], enabling the creation of "gold-standard" datasets. Nevertheless, it is important to recognize that artificially generated scRNA-seq data for constructing bulk mixtures might not completely capture the complexity of real biological data, potentially resulting in biased and overestimated performance evaluation of deconvolution algorithms [12]. When an algorithm is designed using real data, it usually exhibits better accuracy, as in the second case where different cell lines are mixed in predefined rations, to generate bulk samples. In such instances, the deconvolution accuracy is measured by comparing the estimated cell-type proportions in bulk samples with the expression profiles of pure cell lines. Even though these methods offer a more realistic approach, in vitro datasets are low throughput (small sample size, few cell types), which can make them prone to lack of generalization. Consequently, this may limit agreement with other tools. Similar limitations arise when algorithms are designed based on both bulk and single-cell RNA-seq data produced from the same tissue. In such cases, single-cell data serve as the ground truth for cell proportions to evaluate the algorithm's accuracy. Simultaneously, a subset of the single-cell data is used to construct the signature matrix. Thorough data handling is required in this scenario since using the same single-cell data as both the ground truth and input for the signature matrix makes this approach susceptible to data leakage and, consequently, to over-fitting. Specifically, while bulk transcriptomics data are typically gathered from intact tissue, the cell-type proportions are often evaluated using cell suspensions and methods like single-cell RNA sequencing or fluorescence-activated cell sorting. However, these methods can alter cell proportions, not accurately reflecting the original tissue composition. Consequently, comparing inferred cell-type proportions from bulk data with those measured from single-cell assays can lead to misinterpretations during the evaluation of deconvolution methods. To address this issue one solution would be to create consistent ground truth data for transcriptomics by dissociating the tissue specimen into cell suspensions. Then, use a portion of the suspension for bulk RNA sequencing and another portion for single-cell-based assays. This approach ensures that both bulk and single-cell data are obtained from the same starting material. Additionally, other technical factors can influence the creation of gold standard dataset such as the variations in cryopre-served samples, stored under different conditions, may yield differ-ent proportions of "live" cells compared to fresh samples [24]. In the fourth approach, flow cytometry is used as the ground truth to determine the number of each cell type in bulk samples. While this provides a reliable reference for constructing the signature matrix in reference-based algorithms, it is important to note that flow cyto-metry is typically used for blood samples. Consequently, methods validated solely with flow cytometry may overfit to blood samples and perform poorly when applied to other tissue types. In the last case, there is no ground truth data available—only clinical informa-tion such as survival time, disease status, and treatment response. Hence, only an indirect association between the estimated cell-type proportions from bulk data deconvolution and those reported either in literature or previous cases can be inferred. This approach may not be considered as a valid method for evaluating an algo-rithm since it lacks direct quantitative validation. However, it can be employed when other quantitative data are lacking. Considering the above, it is important to note that the method used to design and evaluate a tool can significantly impact its reproducibility and generalization ability.

To define a reference dataset either from in silico or in vitro data, several quality control steps should be followed to ensure the quality of the (raw) experimental data. Especially for sequencing data, either bulk or single cell, a common quality control step is the removal of genes full of zeroes or with zero variance read counts across all samples within the dataset. Additionally, for single cell sequencing, to assure high quality of raw data, cells with low quality of sequences, low numbers of unique molecular identifiers (UMIs), and high fractions of ribosomal or mitochondrial content should be removed [25].

The generation of "gold-standard" datasets entails several challenges to be addressed, yet it is a crucial step for the quality control of the results. Toward the standardization of gold standard datasets and the benchmarking of the deconvolution algorithms, a recent study provides three "gold standard datasets" that were produced from imaging data with single-cell resolution [26]. This pipeline provides a high standard framework for benchmarking existing or new deconvolution algorithms while providing great reproducibility.

As mentioned above, a common factor that can influence the concordance of various tools analysing the same dataset is the preprocessing method employed. Sometimes, different tools require different preprocessing or normalization of the data and this could contribute to achieving discrepant estimations of cell type prevalences. Another parameter, often underestimated when comparing different algorithms, is the theoretical background according to which they are designed and the type of deconvolution algorithms used.

The evaluation of the agreement among different tools is also directly related to the metrics employed to quantitate the performance of the deconvolution method. The most common measure used to assess the accuracy of deconvolution algorithms is the correlation coefficient, which compares the computationally estimated cell-type proportions with the known proportions from the ground truth data. Pearson correlation is typically used, while Spearman correlation can also be employed. Pearson correlation indicates a linear relationship between estimated and ground truth data, while the Spearman coefficient reflects a monotonic relationship. Moreover, another proposed metric is correlation deviation [27]. This measure requires the sample size and the computation of the Pearson correlation between the estimated and the known counts per cell type. The formula of correlation deviation is provided below:

$$\text{Correlation deviation} = \sqrt{\frac{1}{n}\sum_{i=1}^{n}(1 - r_i)^2}$$

where n denotes the amount of different immune cell types found in the samples, r_i denotes the Pearson correlation coefficient for each immune cell type i. Additional robust metrics used for the evaluation of deconvolution methods RMSE and mean absolute error (MAE). These are two well-known measures for evaluating the accuracy of a computational tool, yet their main difference from a mathematical perspective is sensitivity to outliers. Outliers in the estimated values can greatly impact RMSE, while MAE is less sensitive to such data. However, the RMSE metric seems to lack robustness when the concentrations of the cell types have a large variance in the bulk samples [28]. MAE is a robust measure in various settings; however, it only informs us about the absolute error of a method. Therefore, if used alone, it can be misleading for the performance of a deconvolution method applied to cell types with similar cell proportion [11]. It is evident that the evaluation of deconvolution methods relies on various metrics, each with distinct implications for accuracy and robustness, and the choice of metric can significantly influence the assessment of method performance.

4   Field Test of Deconvolution Methods

In this section, we aim at providing a practical example on how to perform a deconvolution analysis and examples of the impact of the software, processing and reference matrix on the final results. We first describe all steps leading to CIBERSORTx [29] analysis and then compare the results with those obtained using BayesPrism [30]. In a recent meta-analysis by Garmire et al., where they review on different benchmarking efforts, CIBERSORTx was one of the methods recommended by independent studies [12]. This method is widely used by the community thanks to its user-friendly web tool, which allows researchers to run it without having a computational background. Tran et al. evaluated the performance of nine different deconvolution methods and found that BayesPrism shows the best overall performance and prediction accuracy for nine major cell types in breast cancer samples, including normal epithelial, cancer epithelial, T cells, B cells, myeloid, endothelial, cancer-associated fibroblasts (CAFs), perivascular-like (PVL), and plasmablasts [13].

4.1   Example Analysis Using CIBERSORTx in TCGA

Here, we describe the main steps leading from pre-processed transcriptomic data to the deconvolution output. We will apply CIBERSORTx [29] in the context of TNBC, using publicly available data from The Cancer Genome Atlas (TCGA) [31] as bulk transcriptomics dataset to deconvolute and a single-cell RNA sequencing (scRNAseq) dataset [32] to derive the reference signature matrix.

Wu dataset [32] contains a total of 26 breast cancer patients belonging to all subtypes, for a total of over 100,000 cells, which have been assigned to 9 major cell types. The raw scRNA-seq of this dataset is available in the European Genome-Phenome Archive (EGA) under the accession code EGAS00001005173. The processed scRNA-seq data of this dataset is deposited in the Gene Expression Omnibus (GEO) with the accession number GSE176078. We manually downloaded the TAR format of processed transcription profiles from the supplementary file table (GSE176078_Wu_etal_2021_BRCA_scRNASeq.tar.gz).   The

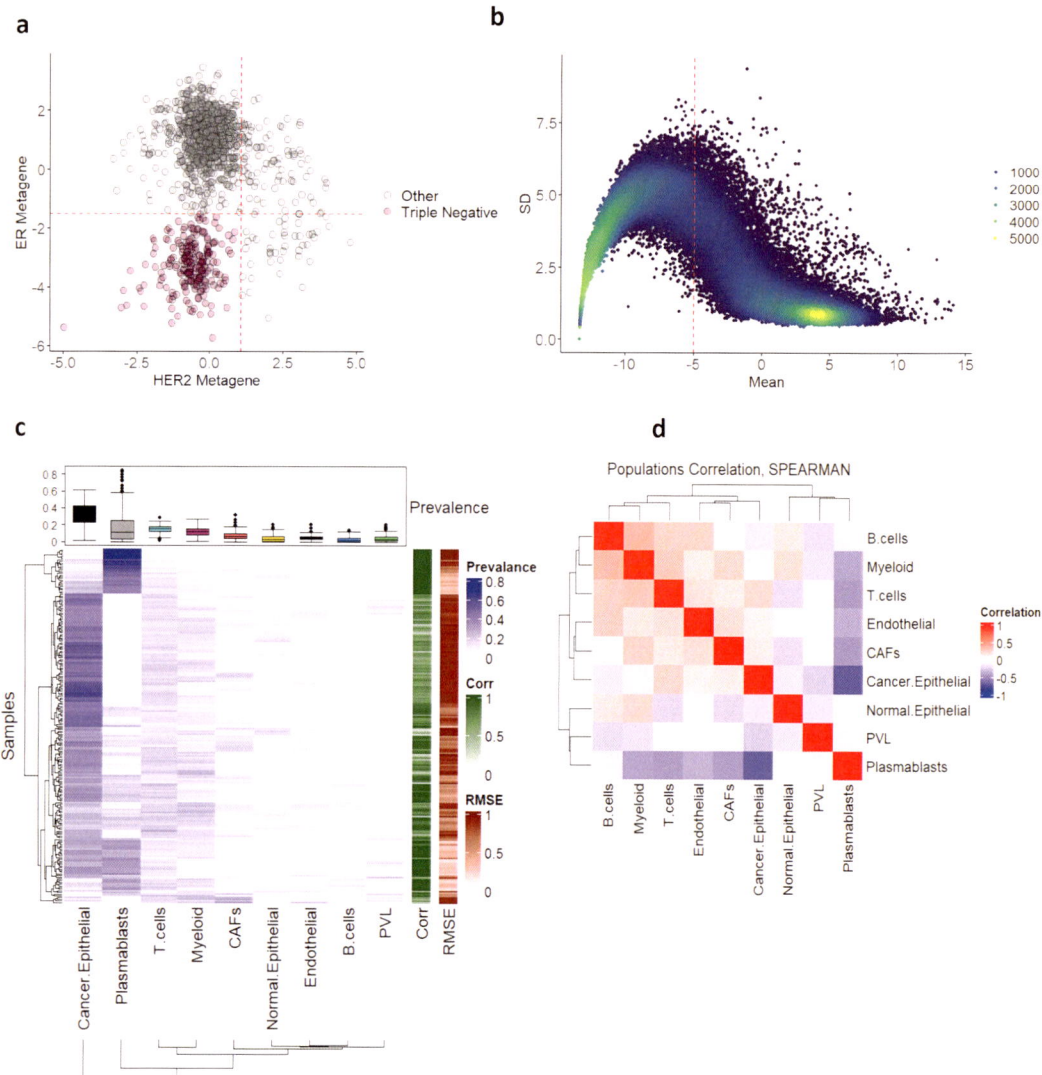

Fig. 3 TNBC TCGA data preparation and CIBERSORTx deconvolution. (**a**) Scatterplot of ER and HER2 metagenes used to identify the ER-HER2- or TNBC subtype in the breast cancer TCGA cohort. (**b**) Distribution of mean and standard deviation (SD) for each transcript in the TNBC TCGA cohort. Transcripts with a mean log2(TPM) value < -5 were discarded in downstream analyses. (**c**) Heatmap summarizing the output of CIBERSORTx deconvolution. Relative proportion for each cell type in each sample are shown. (**d**) Reciprocal correlation among all cell types detected in the TNBC TCGA dataset

patients' data was available in the supplementary file (1793222_Sup_Tab_1-11, Supplementary_table_1) of the article [32] or on the GEO page downloading it thought getGEO function (package GEOquery version 2.60.0).

The dataset was loaded and assembled in a Seurat object (version 5.0) in R/Bioconductor using the following code:

```
library(Seurat)

setwd(".../GSE176078_Wu_etal_2021_BRCA_scRNASeq")
Wu_em <- ReadMtx(
mtx = "matrix.mtx.gz", features = "features.tsv.gz",
cells = "barcodes.tsv.gz", feature.column = 1)

Wu_seurat <- CreateSeuratObject(counts = Wu_em)
```

Next, we added the patient and annotation data and selected TNBC tumors ($n = 9$) using the proper functions to manage Seurat object available on satijalab.org web site (https://satijalab.org/seurat/articles/essential_commands.html). We performed the standard workflow available on the same website to normalize, scale, and run the PCA and UMAP on the cell transcriptional profiles.

The TCGA dataset is accessible through the GDC Portal (https://portal.gdc.cancer.gov/) and/or by the R/Bioconductor TCGABiolinks package [33]. We downloaded TPM transcriptomic data related to breast cancer patients using the following commands:

```
library(TCGAbiolinks)

query <- GDCquery (
      project = "TCGA-BRCA",
      data.category = "Transcriptome Profiling",
      data.type = "Gene Expression Quantification",
      workflow.type = "STAR - Counts)

GDCdownload(query = query)

transcriptome <- GDCprepare(query = query)
TPM <- assays(transcriptome)$tpm_unstrand
```

After installing the TCGABiolinks package, we can access the data type and cancer type of interest by specifying them in the GDCquery() function. The data can later be downloaded from the GDC portal by using GDCdownload() function and stored and accessed locally by using GDCprepare(). Further details could be found at https://doi.org/10.18129/B9.bioc.TCGAbiolinks.

Sample filtering was required because the TCGA breast cancer transcriptomics dataset contains not only the expression profile from primary tumors but also from metastatic lesions and normal tissues. We used the sample ID to select solid tumor samples. Each sample in the TCGA repository has a unique barcode, which is the primary identifier of the biospecimen data within the TCGA project. For more information refer to https://docs.gdc.cancer.gov/Encyclopedia/pages/TCGA_Barcode/.

In TCGA-BRCA project, the solid tumor samples are identified by -01A- in the fourth block of the sample ID. The breast cancer project in TCGA contains 1231 samples and over 60,660 transcripts quantified. In this analysis, we specifically focused on the subset of TNBCc, identified by the lack of estrogen receptor (ER) expression and lack of human epidermal growth factor receptor 2 (HER2) amplification. Since immunohistochemistry (IHC)-based classification was not available for all cases, we used ER and HER2 metagene expression to identify the TNBC samples, as previously reported [34]. Metagene values were obtained by averaging the log10 TPM values of the genes belonging to the metagene. Based on the distribution of the metagenes, optimal thresholds were defined, and 213 samples were identified as TNBC (Fig. 3a).

To generate the input bulk transcriptomic matrix, a gene filtering was introduced. This had the double aim of removing genes with low/no expression and have unique gene symbols in the dataset. For all transcripts, we calculated the mean and standard deviation to characterize the overall data distribution (Fig. 3b). Transcripts with mean $\log10(\text{TPM})$ lower than -5 were filtered out. Some duplicated gene symbols were present after this filtering and the one with highest IQR was selected. This way, 25,700 unique genes remained in the TNBC TCGA bulk transcriptomics. Expression profiles were exported as unlogged TPM.

The CIBERSORTx analysis was run online, following the extensive documentation present for details on data format and structure. The primary output of CIBERSORTx deconvolution is a file containing the prevalence of each cell type defined in the reference matrix in each sample. Some additional information (i.e., RMSE and correlation) is provided and can help with quality control. Output can be represented as a heatmap, as shown in Fig. 3c for the TNBC TCGA dataset. Such representation provides a general overview of the results, relative abundance of the different cell types and a qualitative indication on the presence of groups of patients with similar patterns in terms of cell-type prevalence. Additionally, we performed a reciprocal correlation analysis among cell types, which could inform us on the tendency to specific TME populations to coexist or being mutually exclusive (Fig. 3d).

4.2 Comparison of the Outputs from Different Tools

To compare the results of the deconvolution outputs using two different software, we analyzed the TNBC TCGA dataset with BayesPrism [30]. This software has been optimized to work with raw read count data instead of TPM, although the authors suggest the possibility to use the normalized data if the only available. To extract the raw read counts in the object downloaded using TCGA-Biolinks, we can use the function assays() and choose the data type we need. For a fare comparison, the same samples and genes included in the CIBERSORTx analysis were included here. We

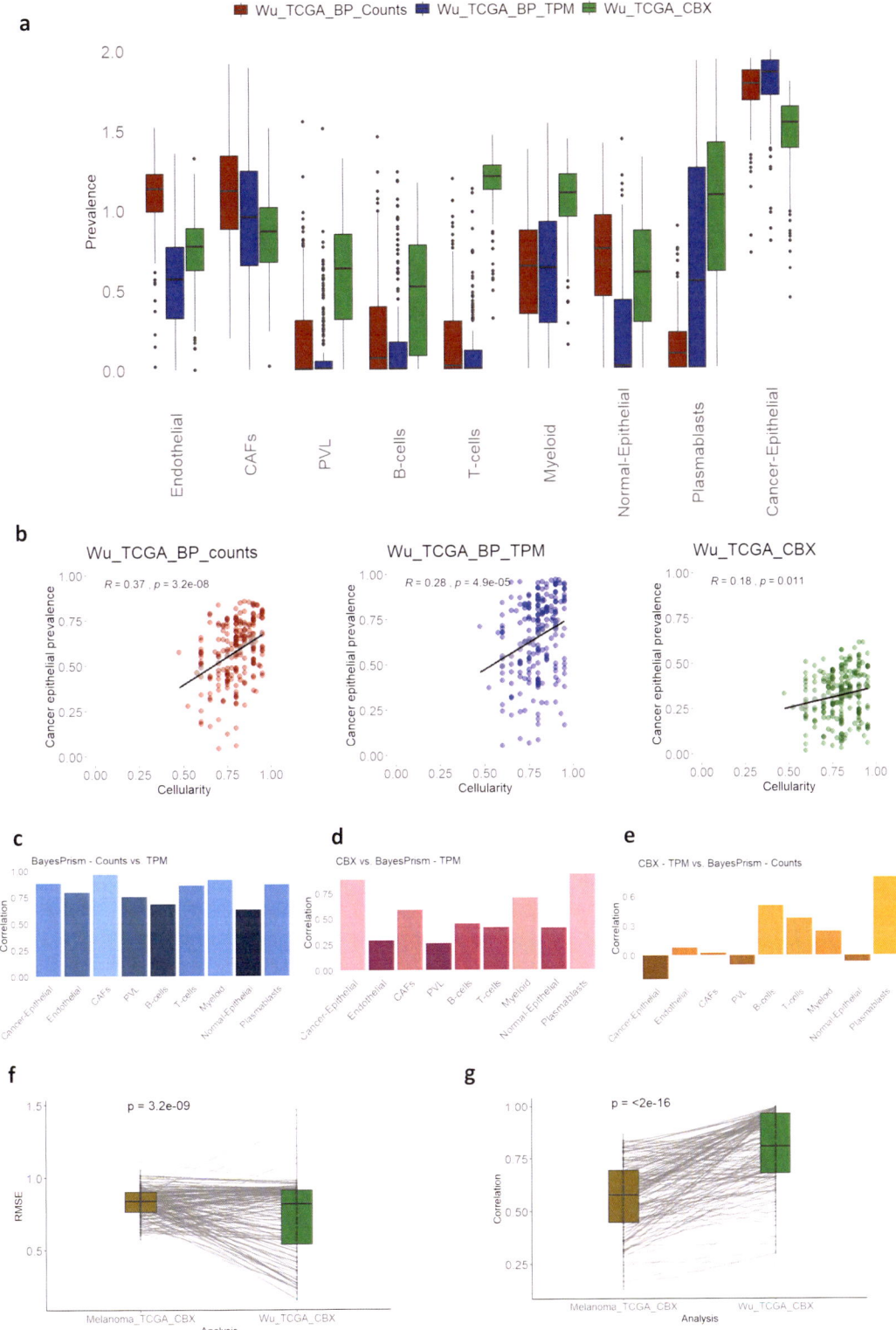

Fig. 4 Comparison of deconvolution results. (**a**) Boxplots showing cell-type prevalence distributions obtained with three deconvolution analyses applied to the tNBC TCGA dataset. (**b**) Correlation between pathologist estimated tumor cellularity and prevalence of cancer epithelial cells estimated by three deconvolution

remand to the online documentation for details on data format and structure and instructions on BayesPrism usage. For a thorough comparison with TPM-based deconvolution performed with CIBERSORTx, we additionally deconvoluted TNBC TCGA TPM data with BayesPrism.

As reported in Fig. 4a, prevalence of each cell type varied significantly depending on the software or data type used. For both methods cancer epithelial cells have the highest prevalence compared to other cell types; BayesPrism quantification of cancer cells were similar either starting from TPM or raw counts, but CIBERSORTx estimated lower prevalence. The same pattern can be seen for CAFs. A very noticeable difference can be seen in the T-cell prevalence estimation, where CIBERSORTx reported much higher prevalences than BayesPrism. For some cell types, namely endothelial, normal epithelial, and plasmablasts, prevalence estimated by BayesPrism starting from either raw counts or TPM was quite different. For the estimation of cancer epithelial cells, we could compare the deconvolution estimates with the tumor purity estimates obtained by the pathologists. Agreement between pathological and molecular estimation of tumor content has always shown low to moderate correlation [35]. Nevertheless, higher correlation values could be an indirect indication of higher performance of the deconvolution process. BayesPrism deconvolution starting from raw counts showed the highest agreement in our setting. This is in line with recent reports benchmarking multiple tools including BayesPrism [13] (Fig. 4b).

To further compare the results, we performed a correlation analysis between deconvolution results and for each cell type (Fig. 4c–e). Figure 4c, illustrates the correlation between BayesPrism results when using raw read counts or TPM as input. Overall, we found a good agreement with correlation reaching 0.9 for CAFs, but with the lowest correlation score being 0.7 for normal epithelial cells. Similarly, we compared CIBERSORTx results with BayesPrism results, for the latter starting either from TPM (Fig. 4d) or read counts (Fig. 4e). When comparing CIBERSORTx and BayesPrism outputs starting in both cases from TPM, cell-type correlations were remarkably lower for some cell types, reaching values around 0.25, except for plasmablasts, myeloids, and cancer epithelial (Fig. 4d). Correlation values went further down when CIBERSORT output was compared with BayesPrism output starting from read counts (Fig. 4e).

Fig. 4 (continued) analyses in the TNBC TCGA dataset. (c) Prevalence correlation for each cell type between BayesPrism results obtained starting from TPM or read counts. (d) Prevalence correlation for each cell type between CIBERSORTx and BayesPrism results using TPM as input. (e) Prevalence correlation for each cell type between CIBERSORTx results using TPM and BayesPrism results using read counts as input data

4.3 Effects of the Reference Data on the Output

Deconvolution tools usually provide reference matrices or signatures containing the expression profile of relevant genes driving the cell-type quantification in bulk samples. However, such reference data are often derived from quite different biological contexts. The context can affect cell phenotypes and, eventually, deconvolution performances when applied to bulk data from different biological contexts. To provide an example of how the choice of the reference matrix can affect the results, we repeated the CIBERSORTx analysis on TNBC TCGA data using the provided melanoma signature (https://doi.org/10.1126/science.aad0501). We compared the results in terms of RMSE and correlation values as provided by CIBERSORTx. Median RMSE was similar in the outputs obtained using the melanoma or the TNBC signature matrix, respectively. However, a strong reduction in RMSE was observed for 61.03% of the samples, while an increase was observed only in the 38.97% (Fig. 4f). Importantly, correlation between the original and the reconstructed bulk transcriptomic profile was significantly higher when using the TNBC matrix, matching the bulk transcriptome cancer type (median cor = 0.68 vs 0.84, $p < 2\text{e-}16$) (Fig. 4g).

5 Conclusions

Conducting a robust deconvolution analysis requires careful consideration of several factors. It is important to select the appropriate preprocessing method and normalization strategies, tailored to the specific dataset and software. Moreover, the choice of reference datasets and software tools significantly impacts deconvolution outcomes.

To ensure the quality of results, it is essential to validate findings using complementary experimental techniques and independent datasets whenever possible. Additionally, researchers should remain mindful of the limitations inherent in bulk transcriptomics-based deconvolution, including potential biases introduced by tissue heterogeneity, batch effects, and the reliance on predefined reference matrices. While deconvolution analysis offers valuable insights into tumor microenvironment dynamics, it is important to interpret results cautiously and consider the broader context of tumor biology.

Looking ahead, ongoing research efforts should focus on refining benchmarking methodologies, improving software tools, and addressing remaining limitations in deconvolution analysis. By advancing our understanding of the tumor microenvironment and enhancing the accuracy and reproducibility of deconvolution methods, we can pave the way for more effective precision oncology strategies and ultimately improve patient outcomes in cancer treatment.

Acknowledgments

This work has been supported by Fondazione Michelangelo (Milan, Italy) and Breast Cancer Research Foundation (grant BCRF 21-181), the Aragon Government (Group B29_23R), the Instituto de Salud Carlos III (ISCIII) grant PI22/01938, and by ASPANOA Foundation. This work is part of the CNS2022-136176 action, financed by MCIN/AEI/10.13039/501100011033 and for the European Union «Next Generation EU»/PRTR. This publication is based upon work from COST Action IMMUNO-model, CA21135, supported by COST (European Cooperation in Science and Technology). We would like to acknowledge, in memory of Sotiris, his early contributions to this work. His presence and spirit remain fondly remembered.

References

1. de Visser KE, Joyce JA (2023) The evolving tumor microenvironment: from cancer initiation to metastatic outgrowth. Cancer Cell 41: 374–403

2. Anderson NM, Simon MC (2020) The tumor microenvironment. Curr. Biol. 30:R921–R925

3. Lakshmi Narendra B, Eshvendar Reddy K, Shantikumar S, Ramakrishna S (2013) Immune system: a double-edged sword in cancer. Inflamm. Res. 62:823–834

4. Swanton C, Bernard E, Abbosh C, André F, Auwerx J, Balmain A et al (2024) Embracing cancer complexity: hallmarks of systemic disease. Cell 187:1589–1616

5. Dezem FS, Morosini NS, Arjumand W, DuBose H, Plummer J (2024) Spatially resolved single-cell omics: methods, challenges, and future perspectives. Annu Rev Biomed Data Sci 7(1)

6. Hackl H, Charoentong P, Finotello F, Trajanoski Z (2016) Computational genomics tools for dissecting tumour-immune cell interactions. Nat. Rev. Genet. 17:441–458

7. Kamal Y, Dwan D, Hoehn HJ, Sanz-Pamplona R, Alonso MH, Moreno V et al (2021) Tumor immune infiltration estimated from gene expression profiles predicts colorectal cancer relapse. Onco Targets Ther 10: 1862529

8. Brummel K, Eerkens AL, de Bruyn M, Nijman HW (2023) Tumour-infiltrating lymphocytes: from prognosis to treatment selection. Br. J. Cancer 128:451–458

9. Saleh R, Elkord E (2020) FoxP3+ T regulatory cells in cancer: Prognostic biomarkers and therapeutic targets. Cancer Lett. 490:174–185

10. García-Mulero S, Alonso MH, Pardo J, Santos C, Sanjuan X, Salazar R et al (2020) Lung metastases share common immune features regardless of primary tumor origin. J. Immunother. Cancer 8:e000491

11. Nguyen H, Nguyen H, Tran D, Draghici S, Nguyen T (2024) Fourteen years of cellular deconvolution: methodology, applications, technical evaluation and outstanding challenges. Nucleic Acids Res. 52:4761

12. Garmire LX, Li Y, Huang Q, Xu C, Teichmann SA, Kaminski N et al (2024) Challenges and perspectives in computational deconvolution of genomics data. Nat. Methods 21:391–400

13. Tran KA, Addala V, Johnston RL, Lovell D, Bradley A, Koufariotis LT et al (2023) Performance of tumour microenvironment deconvolution methods in breast cancer using single-cell simulated bulk mixtures. Nat. Commun. 14:5758

14. Im Y, Kim Y (2023) A comprehensive overview of RNA deconvolution methods and their application. Mol. Cells 46:99–105

15. Sturm G, Finotello F, List M (2020) Immunedeconv: an R package for unified access to computational methods for estimating immune cell fractions from bulk RNA-sequencing data. Methods Mol. Biol. 2120:223–232

16. Sturm G, Finotello F, Petitprez F, Zhang JD, Baumbach J, Fridman WH et al (2019) Comprehensive evaluation of transcriptome-based cell-type quantification methods for immuno-oncology. Bioinformatics 35:i436–i445

17. Zhong Y, Liu Z (2011) Gene expression deconvolution in linear space. Nat. Methods 9:8–9

18. Avila Cobos F, Alquicira-Hernandez J, Powell JE, Mestdagh P, De Preter K (2020) Benchmarking of cell type deconvolution pipelines for transcriptomics data. Nat. Commun. 11: 5650

19. Finotello F, Trajanoski Z (2018) Quantifying tumor-infiltrating immune cells from transcriptomics data. Cancer Immunol. Immunother. 67:1031–1040

20. Maden SK, Kwon SH, Huuki-Myers LA, Collado-Torres L, Hicks SC, Maynard KR (2023) Challenges and opportunities to computationally deconvolve heterogeneous tissue with varying cell sizes using single-cell RNA-sequencing datasets. Genome Biol. 24:288

21. Zappia L, Phipson B, Oshlack A (2017) Splatter: simulation of single-cell RNA sequencing data. Genome Biol. 18:174

22. Zhang X, Xu C, Yosef N (2019) Simulating multiple faceted variability in single cell RNA sequencing. Nat. Commun. 10:2611

23. Cao Y, Yang P, Yang JYH (2021) A benchmark study of simulation methods for single-cell RNA sequencing data. Nat. Commun. 12: 6911

24. Denisenko E, Guo BB, Jones M, Hou R, De Kock L, Lassmann T et al (2020) Systematic assessment of tissue dissociation and storage biases in single-cell and single-nucleus RNA-seq workflows. Genome Biol. 21:130

25. Subramanian A, Alperovich M, Yang Y, Li B (2022) Biology-inspired data-driven quality control for scientific discovery in single-cell transcriptomics. Genome Biol. 23:267

26. Sang-aram C, Browaeys R, Seurinck R, Saeys Y (2024) Spotless, a reproducible pipeline for benchmarking cell type deconvolution in spatial transcriptomics. Elife 12:RP88431

27. Miao YR, Zhang Q, Lei Q, Luo M, Xie GY, Wang H et al (2020) ImmuCellAI: a unique method for comprehensive T-cell subsets abundance prediction and its application in cancer immunotherapy. Adv Sci (Weinh) 7:1902880

28. Alonso-Moreda N, Berral-González A, De La Rosa E, González-Velasco O, Sánchez-Santos JM, De Las RJ (2023) Comparative analysis of cell mixtures deconvolution and gene signatures generated for blood, immune and cancer cells. Int. J. Mol. Sci. 24:10765

29. Newman AM, Steen CB, Liu CL, Gentles AJ, Chaudhuri AA, Scherer F et al (2019) Determining cell type abundance and expression from bulk tissues with digital cytometry. Nat. Biotechnol. 37:773–782

30. Chu T, Wang Z, Peer D, Danko CG (2022) Cell type and gene expression deconvolution with BayesPrism enables Bayesian integrative analysis across bulk and single-cell RNA sequencing in oncology. Nat Cancer 3:505–517

31. Hutter C, Zenklusen JC (2018) The cancer genome atlas: creating lasting value beyond its data. Cell 173:283–285

32. Wu SZ, Al-Eryani G, Roden DL, Junankar S, Harvey K, Andersson A et al (2021) A single-cell and spatially resolved atlas of human breast cancers. Nat. Genet. 53:1334–1347

33. Colaprico A, Silva TC, Olsen C, Garofano L, Cava C, Garolini D et al (2016) TCGAbiolinks: an R/Bioconductor package for integrative analysis of TCGA data. Nucleic Acids Res. 44: e71

34. Callari M, Cappelletti V, D'Aiuto F, Musella V, Lembo A, Petel F et al (2016) Subtype-specific metagene-based prediction of outcome after neoadjuvant and adjuvant treatment in breast cancer. Clin. Cancer Res. 22:337–345

35. Haider S, Tyekucheva S, Prandi D, Fox NS, Ahn J, Xu AW et al (2020) Systematic assessment of tumor purity and its clinical implications. JCO Precis. Oncol. 4:995–1005

36. Racle J, Gfeller D (2020) EPIC: a tool to estimate the proportions of different cell types from bulk gene expression data. Methods Mol. Biol. 2120:233–248

37. Becht E, Giraldo NA, Lacroix L, Buttard B, Elarouci N, Petitprez F et al (2016) Estimating the population abundance of tissue-infiltrating immune and stromal cell populations using gene expression. Genome Biol. 17:218

38. Li B, Li T, Liu JS, Liu XS (2020) Computational deconvolution of tumor-infiltrating immune components with bulk tumor gene expression data. Methods Mol. Biol. 2120: 249–262

39. Plattner C, Finotello F, Rieder D (2020) Deconvoluting tumor-infiltrating immune cells from RNA-seq data using quanTIseq. Methods Enzymol. 636:261–285

40. Jimenez-Sanchez A, Cast O, Miller ML (2019) Comprehensive benchmarking and integration of tumor microenvironment cell estimation methods. Cancer Res. 79:6238–6246

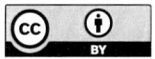

Chapter 17

Computational Methods for Cancer Neoantigen Prediction

Andrea Moreno-Manuel, Sotiris Ouzounis, Marius Eidsaa,
Roberto Fornelino-González, Pilar Ballesteros-Cuartero,
Daniel Gómez-Garrido, Esteban Veiga-Chacón, Theodora Katsila,
Maurizio Callari, Arrate Muñoz-Barrutia, and Rebeca Sanz-Pamplona

Abstract

Neoantigens are mutated peptides arising from tumor genomic alterations, which can be recognized and attacked by the immune system, leading to antitumor immune responses. In the last decades, many immunotherapeutic strategies have been developed, which has increased the interest in neoantigens. This led to the development of computational tools that facilitate neoantigen identification and prioritization, prior to their validation using experimental approaches. This chapter aims at explaining the key steps that need to be conducted to identify potential neoantigens in silico, including an example of the most frequently used tools. This is followed by a description and comparison of the cutting-edge tools and pipelines for neoantigen prediction both for human and mouse. The last aim of this chapter is to depict the technical challenges that limit neoantigen prediction using bioinformatics, as well as the expected improvements, given the current revolution of artificial intelligence, which is implemented in most of the neoantigen-related tools. As exposed in this book chapter, we believe that advances in immunomics and computational biology will be key to implement personalized cancer immunotherapy in the clinical practice, to improve outcomes of cancer patients.

Key words Neoantigen prediction, Bioinformatics, HLA-binding affinity, MHC, Mice, Immunomics, Immune microenvironment, Cancer

1 Introduction

Over the last decades, the emergence of immunotherapy has revolutionized cancer treatment and has offered new opportunities for precise and personalized interventions. Among others, one immunotherapy strategy is the identification and targeting of tumor-specific antigens (TSAs) including neoantigens, which are peptides resulting from genetic alterations. Aberrant proteins in tumors are

Andrea Moreno-Manuel, Sotiris Ouzounis and Marius Eidsaa have contributed equally to this work.

Maurizio Callari, Arrate Muñoz-Barrutia and Rebeca Sanz-Pamplona are senior co-authors of this work.

Sweta Rani and Lukasz Skalniak (eds.), *IMMUNO-model in Cancer: Methods and Protocols*, Methods in Molecular Biology, vol. 2959, https://doi.org/10.1007/978-1-0716-4734-9_17, © The Author(s) 2026

degraded by the proteasome and resulting peptides are transported to the endoplasmic reticulum (ER), where they are subsequently loaded onto major histocompatibility complex (MHC) molecules, known as human leukocyte antigens (HLAs) in humans [1]. There are a variety of sources of neoantigens. Although somatic mutations, especially missense (which change the amino acid codon), are the most studied; increasing evidence supports that neoantigens can also be derived from other events such as insertion/deletions of nucleotides (INDELs), frameshift mutations (insertion or deletion of a number of nucleotides not multiple of three, thus disrupting the reading frame), gene fusions (caused by joining parts of two different genes, leading to a new protein), endogenous retroviruses (ERVs) (ERV transcripts can be a source of tumor-specific neoantigens), RNA splicing anomalies (alternative splicing consists of different exon combinations, leading to proteins with different structure and function), post-transcriptional frameshift (e.g., ribosomal slippage) or post-translational frameshift (e.g., protein splicing) [2]. In fact, the more different the neoantigen versus the wild type, the more immunogenic [3].

Neoantigens are expressed in tumors but not in healthy tissues, thus they induce stronger effector responses than tumor-associated antigens (TAAs), which are overexpressed in tumor cells but also present at a lesser extent in nonmalignant cells [4]. To trigger antitumor immune responses, neoantigens need to be presented by MHC molecules. MHC Class I molecules primarily exhibits small protein fragments derived from degraded intracellular proteins, and its role in cancer neoantigen presentation is well established. On the contrary, MHC Class II molecules exhibit extracellular antigens typically captured by antigen-presenting cells (APCs). However, MHC class II pathway is also essential for effective immune responses against neoantigens since APCs can uptake neoantigens from dying cancer cells [5, 6]. Hence, the resulting neoantigen-MHC complexes are formed and transported to the surface of cancer cells to be recognized as nonself by T-cell receptor (TCR), leading to antitumor immune responses. This specific recognition allows the elimination of malignant cells without affecting healthy tissue [7] (Fig. 1a).

Traditionally, the discovery of neoantigens has relied on experimental approaches, which make the process tedious, thus offering limited results. However, the advances in computational biology and bioinformatics, such as the use of artificial intelligence and deep learning algorithms on next-generation sequencing (NGS) data, enable a possible strategy to predict potential neoantigens faster with high accuracy [4] (Fig. 1b). Optimal pipelines discussed below not only take into account the binding capacity of peptides to MHC but also the expression levels of the antigen of interest by tumor cells [8, 9].

A)

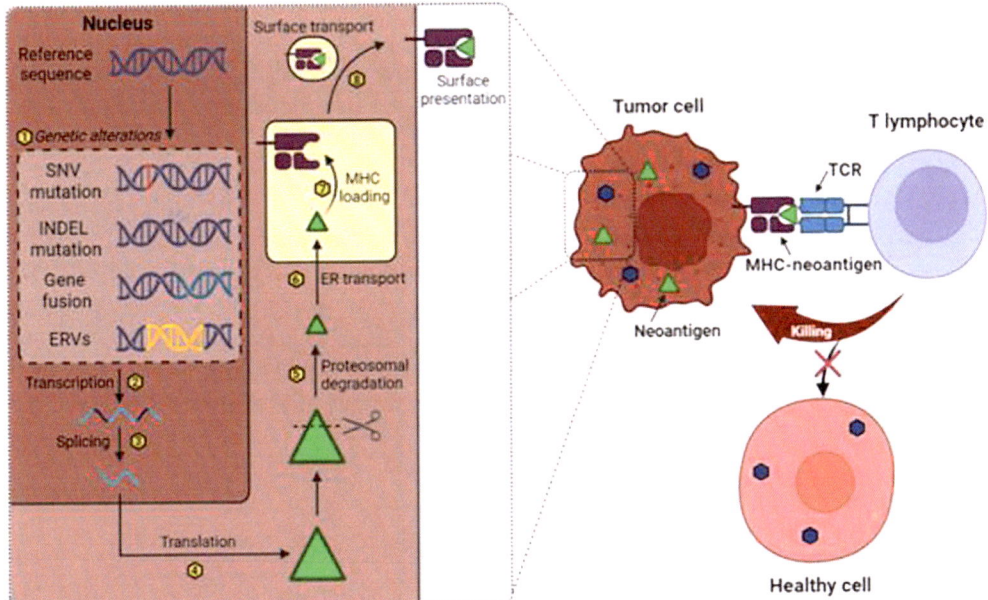

B)

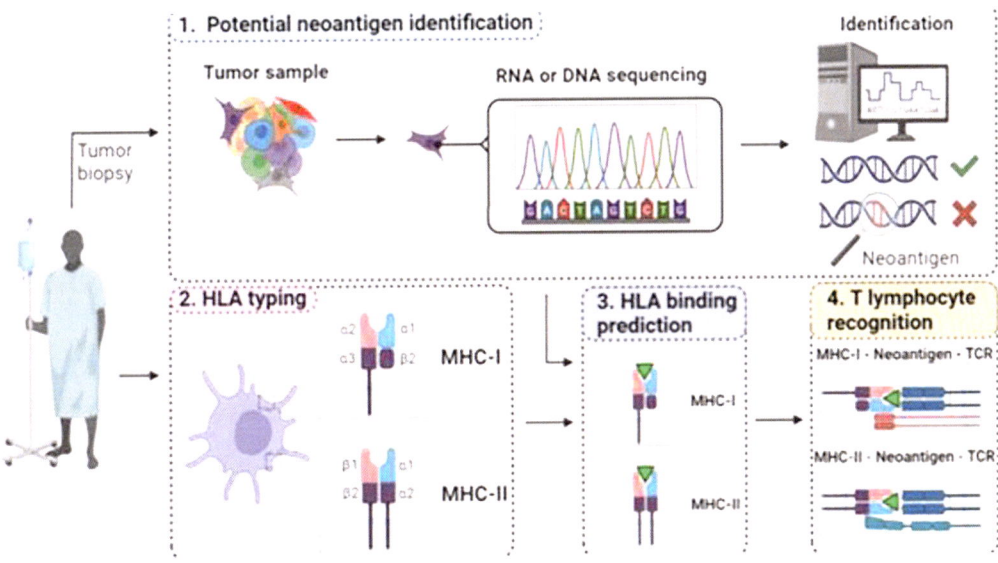

Fig. 1 (**a**) Key steps of neoantigens origin and processing until loaded in MHC molecules for their recognition by T cells: mutations can occur at a genomic level of the malignant cell (1), where they are transcribed (2) and spliced to form mRNA (3). During this process, alternative splicing can also produce splice variant mRNA. Translation of these variant mRNAs then leads to the synthesis of variant proteins (4). At this stage, post-transcriptional frameshifts, such as those caused by ribosomal slippage, can also produce variant proteins. These variant proteins can then undergo proteasomal degradation (5) and be transported to the endoplasmic reticulum (ER) (6), where they are subsequently loaded onto major histocompatibility complexes (MHCs) (7). After being loaded, the resulting neoantigen-MHC complexes can be transported to the cell surface (8), where they are exposed to recognition by the T-cell receptor (TCR) of lymphocytes. (**b**) Schematic representation of the overall process of identification of new neoantigens: Tumor samples are obtained and used to identify

Thus, the prediction of neoantigens is a critical process in the pursuit of truly personalized cancer immunotherapies, relying on advanced bioinformatics tools to integrate high-quality patient data with a rapidly expanding body of immunological knowledge. The overarching goal is to predict if patient-specific cancerous mutations can stimulate the immune system to target and eliminate the patient's own tumor.

In Subheading 2, an overview of the key steps in neoantigen prediction using NGS will be provided. Subheading 3 shows an example of neoantigenicity prediction comparing different methods over the same peptides. Afterwards, the available pipelines for neoantigen prediction and their characteristics will be listed in Subheading 4 for humans and in Subheading 5 for mouse models. Lastly, technical challenges and future improvements will be discussed in Subheading 6.

2 Key Steps of Neoantigen Prediction

The complex, multi-step process of neoantigen prediction involves several stages, each contributing to the final prediction. As explained before, the MHC Class I pathway is involved in presenting antigens originating from the inside of cells, for example, stemming from viruses and mutations, inducing CD8+ cytotoxic T cells. Traditionally, the MHC Class I antigen-presentation pathway has been recognized as the most restrictive, and consequently, the most predictive pathway for neoantigen prediction [10] and will thus be the main focus of this section. The key parts of neoantigen prediction process can be split into the following steps (Fig. 2):

2.1 Sample Collection

This is the initial, and arguably the most important, step in the process since all downstream results inadvertently depend on it. It involves obtaining high-quality patient samples from both tumor and representative normal tissues and comparing them to identify unique genetic alterations in the cancer cells that are not present in normal (germline) cells [11, 12]. These somatic mutations can potentially give rise to neoantigens, forming the basis for all downstream investigations. However, the mutations must be identified

Fig. 1 (continued) individualized neoantigens via RNA sequencing (RNAseq) or whole genome/exome sequencing (1). In parallel, HLA typing prediction is performed (2). Then a neoantigen-MHC complex binding prediction is evaluated (3). Once a suitable neoantigen-MHC complex is identified, the T-cell recognition via TCR is evaluated to check that a proper immune response can be triggered (4). In that case, the neoantigen discovered is classified as useful for therapeutic approaches. *SNV* single nucleotide variant, *INDEL* insertion/deletion, *ERV* endogenous retroviruses, *DNA* deoxyribonucleic acid, *MHC* major histocompatibility complex, *ER* endoplasmic reticulum, *TCR* T-cell receptor, *RNA* ribonucleic acid, *HLA* human leukocyte antigen. (Images created with BioRender)

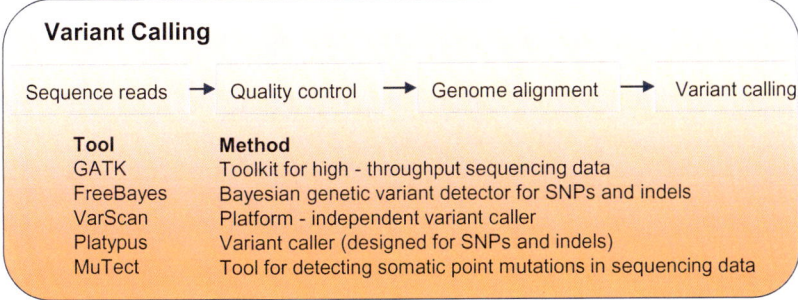

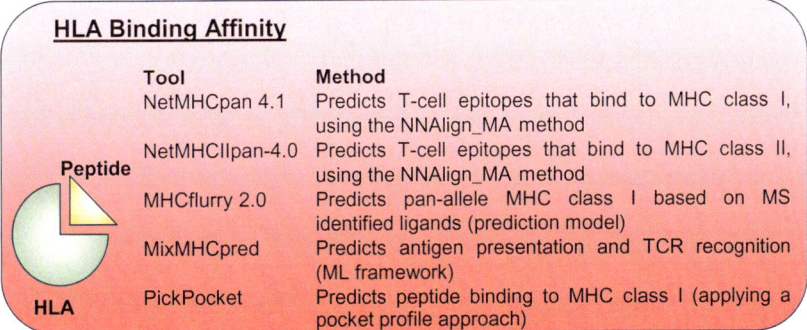

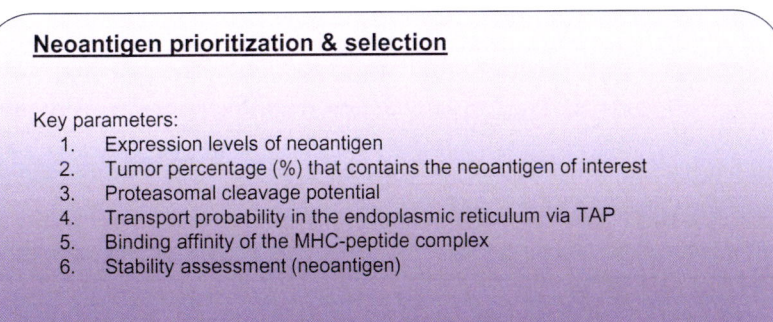

Fig. 2 Representation of a typical computational workflow integrating all the steps required for neoantigen prediction. Step 1 corresponds to variant calling where input data are processed to identify variants and annotate tumor-specific mutations. Step 2 refers to HLA typing where both Class I and Class II HLA alleles of

first, which requires the patient samples to be collected and stored in a manner that preserves the integrity of their genetic material.

2.2 Sequencing

These high-quality normal and tumor tissue samples are then typically sequenced using NGS techniques such as whole exome sequencing (WES) or whole genome sequencing (WGS). NGS can also be used for sequencing RNA, providing information on the expression level of specific somatic mutations [13].

2.3 Somatic Variant Calling

The sequenced reads from normal and tumor tissues are aligned to a reference genome, and the differences between them are identified. Specialized bioinformatics tools are used to perform this variant calling [14], and the identified somatic mutations are annotated and stored in variant call format (VCF) files, which contain essential details on each mutation. This includes information regarding nucleotide and amino acid changes, their genomic location, and additional annotations useful for downstream analyses and filtering, for example, variant allele frequency (VAF) scores, denoting the specific variant's prevalence.

2.4 In Silico Peptide Generation

Following the identification of patient-specific somatic variants, typically contained in VCF files, the next step is to construct all relevant peptides capable of containing these variants in silico. This involves using bioinformatics tools for transforming genomic nucleotide sequences into translated amino acid chains, constituting the proteins altered by the cancer. The subsequent splitting of proteins into mutation-containing peptides has no associated standard tool, but peptides of 8–12 amino-acid length, with a preference for 9-mers, are typically constructed for HLA Class I [15]. Longer peptides are constructed for HLA Class II, although the indicated range of relevant peptides can vary between studies, for example, 13–19 and 12–24 [16, 17].

2.5 Antigen Processing

The natural process emulated by in silico peptide generation occurs when proteins are damaged or decommissioned, and subsequently chopped up by proteasome enzymes into fragments. These peptide fragments are transported to the endoplasmic reticulum via transporter associated with antigen processing (TAP) proteins, where they can be further modified and finally loaded onto MHC molecules. This process is not random, however, and the uniformity

Fig. 2 (continued) patients are determined. Step 3 includes HLA binding affinity and stability prediction where in silico tools quantify the linkage among peptides-HLA alleles. Step 4 consists of neoantigen prioritization and selection aiming to facilitate the identification of immunogenic neoepitopes for personalized cancer immunotherapy. *SNP* single nucleotide polymorphism, *HLA* human leukocyte antigen, *NGS* next-generation sequencing, *MHC* major histocompatibility complex, *MS* mass spectrometry, *TCR* T-cell receptor, *ML* machine learning, *TAP* transporter associated with antigen processing

assumption of the in silico peptide generation needs modification. Computational immunology tools can help assess peptides, and their contextual flanking amino acids, by providing scores indicating the likelihood of, for example, cleavage sites and TAP compatibility [18, 19].

2.6 HLA Typing

The antigen-presentation pathway ultimately hinges on peptides binding to HLA molecules. Although in humans it is known as HLA, it is worth mentioning that the terms "MHC" and "HLA" are often used interchangeably. Thus, the patient's HLA alleles must be determined or typed [20]. There are three major HLA Class I genes: HLA-A, HLA-B, and HLA-C, with up to two alleles per gene, one from each biological parent. There are also several HLA Class II genes, which, unlike Class I, act as pairs forming heterodimer MHC molecules. HLA typing is performed by dedicated bioinformatics tools, providing allele identifiers denoting the amino acid composition of the resulting MHC molecules, and potentially also information affecting translation of the gene. The HLA genes are very polymorphic, and there are currently registered more than 27,000 Class I and 11,000 Class II allele variants ([21], v.3.56).

2.7 HLA Binding

The aim of HLA-binding prediction is estimating the binding affinity between all permutations of pairwise peptides and HLA alleles. This is a crucial step, since only peptides binding to HLA have a chance to be presented to the immune system. Machine learning, and neural networks in particular, have proven to be effective at this task, with well-known examples such as NetMHCpan [22] and MHCflurry [23]. These models are trained on large datasets of HLA-peptide pairs with associated experimentally determined binding affinities, typically given as half-maximal inhibitory concentration (IC50) values [24]. In the case of a competitive binding assay, an IC50 value represents the concentration of a candidate peptide required to outcompete a high-affinity reference peptide until only half of them remain bound to the HLA allele. There is a gradual transition from HLA-peptide pairs with strong binding affinities (small IC50 values) to weak binding affinities (large IC50 values), but a threshold of IC50 < 500 is often employed to denote Class I HLA-peptide pairs to be binders [25].

2.8 HLA-Peptide Stability

Similarly, measurements and predictions can be performed to assess the stability of HLA-peptide complexes. While closely related to HLA binding, stability revolves around measuring the HLA-peptide complex' ability to stay bound under perturbations, through, for example, thermal and kinetic stability assays [26]. Such stability assays work by subjecting the HLA-peptide complex to varying conditions and measuring how long it remains intact, providing valuable information about its durability. So, while HLA binding assesses the potential of a peptide to bind to an HLA allele, HLA-peptide stability assesses the half-life of an HLA-peptide complex. A more stable complex might have a higher chance of being recognized by T cells, potentially leading to a stronger immune response [27].

In the context of the HLA-peptide complexes, the affinity/stability for the HLA is defined in its majority as the anchor residues of the peptides. These residues are buried within the HLA pocket and create bonds with the residues within it to stabilize the docking. In 9-mer peptides, the anchoring residues can normally be found at positions 2 and 9, although peptides of different lengths can have anchor residues in different positions [28].

2.9 Antigen Presentation

Somatic mutations capable of navigating through the above steps, forming stable HLA-peptide complexes, are then transported to the surface of the cell for subsequent inspection by the immune system. In essence, this is the first main goal of neoantigen prediction: predict the somatic mutations with the right characteristics to be transported as peptides to the cell surface. Mass spectrometry techniques can be used to discover these presented peptides, or eluted ligands, but cannot ascertain which HLA allele it was bound to [29]. It provides verification that a peptide indeed was presented. There are several ways this information could be used to increase predictive power, such as reinforcing HLA binding scoring [22, 30].

2.10 T-Cell Recognition and Immunogenicity

Once the HLA-peptide complexes are presented on the cell surface, they can be recognized by T cells, each carrying a unique T-cell receptor (TCR) capable of recognizing a few specific HLA-peptide complexes [31]. If a TCR binds to an HLA-peptide complex containing a somatic mutation, it triggers a signaling cascade that can initiate an immune response against these cells. This is the second main goal of neoantigen prediction: to predict which of the presented peptides will likely trigger an immune response. Predicting T-cell recognition is a huge challenge; however, the TCR diversity is vast, and the rules governing TCR-peptide-HLA interaction are not fully understood [31]. Some bioinformatics tools attempt to predict T-cell recognition by modeling TCR-peptide-MHC interactions [32], and while predictive power is steadily increasing, these predictions are often uncertain and require experimental validation [10, 33]. Laboratory experiments can be performed to validate that the neoantigens can elicit an immune response, with assays such as ELISA and intracellular cytokine staining [34].

2.11 Neoantigen Prioritization

Following the above steps, there are several predictions, scores, and potential immune-response measurements associated with each neoantigen candidate. Ranking and prioritizing these candidates by their overall potential for inducing an immune response is challenging, and typically involves combining predictions of antigen processing, HLA binding and immunogenicity with gene expression and other relevant information into a single, combined score per neoantigen [10]. Recent advances within single-cell technologies and cutting-edge machine learning approaches are presumed to provide valuable insights for the future [35].

In conclusion, neoantigen prediction is a complex, multistep process that integrates numerous bioinformatics tools and data types in elaborated pipelines. There are several factors omitted in this section that could further increase the complexity, such as HLA Class II, posttranslational modifications, immune escape, mutated HLA genes, and alternative sequencing methods [7, 34, 36]. Despite the challenges, neoantigen prediction holds great promise for the transition toward truly personalized cancer immunotherapies.

3 Examples of Neoantigen Prediction Applying Different Tools to Cancer Driver Mutations

In order to illustrate the key steps described in the previous section and show how different tools perform on neoantigen prediction, an example using driver mutations will be developed in this section.

A variety of tools including those predicting binding affinity, stability, peptide cleavage, and TAP transportation will be tested. Although many tools focus on predicting HLA-binding affinity of mutated peptides, the two considered as gold standard will be used (NetMHCpan and MHCflurry, as discussed below) [22, 23]. The other tested tools focus on prediction of binding stability of the peptide-MHC complex (netMHCstabpan) [37], prediction of cleavage sites (netChop 3.1) [38], and TAP transport of the chopped peptides (TAP) [39]. Three well-known mutations have been selected: *KRAS* p.G12C, *TP53* p.H179R, and *GNAQ* p. Q209L. For the sake of clarity, only one allele (HLA-A*03–01) will be tested.

First, the mutated peptides (17-mers) need to be generated and written in FASTA format:

```
> sp|P01116|RASK_HUMAN - G12C
YKLVVVGACGVGKSALT


> sp|P04637|P53_HUMAN TP53 - H179R
EVVRRCPHRERCSDSDG


> sp|P50148|GNAQ_HUMAN Q209L
FRMVDVGGLRSERRKWI
```

3.1 Predicting Affinity and Stability

Many deep learning-based tools have been developed over the last years, but they all share the main functionality of predicting the HLA-binding affinity.

A work by Zhao et al. tested 18 antigen prediction tools and compared their capacity to accurately find binders by testing peptides of different lengths in a variety of HLAs [40]. In summary, MHCflurry and NetMHCpan outperformed other tools in peptide-MHC-binding prediction. Both tools are based on artificial neural networks (ANN) and exhibited superior performance in binary classification compared to logistic regression-based methods. This is because ANN-based approaches are favored for their ability to capture complex interactions between MHC-binding residues and for better regularization, reducing overfitting. MHCflurry consistently demonstrated robust performance in binder prediction. Moreover, MHCflurry was superior in three-class classification, suggesting its efficacy not only in identifying MHC binders but also in distinguishing strong binders. Nevertheless, one of the downsides of using this type of tools is the available data used for their training. The performance of AI-based tools largely depends on the quality and comprehensiveness of their training data. These tools use both quantitative (binding affinity) and qualitative (eluted ligand) assays. The latter yield binary outcomes, indicating only whether a peptide binds or not, without quantifying the strength of that binding in traditional affinity units such as nM. This poses a challenge for prediction tools like MHCflurry and NetMHCpan, which predict affinity values. The researchers who developed the tools came up with different strategies to assign affinity values to data lacking precise measurements, but these estimates may not always align with reality. Despite these shortcomings, NetMHCpan 4.1 and MHCflurry are still considered the gold standard in the field. Both tools can predict the affinity between the peptides and HLA allele input, among other neoantigen presentation related scores. They also have a very useful feature which is the splitting of protein sequences in all the possible peptides of a specified length. For these reasons, the examples below will focus on these tools.

3.1.1 NetMHCpan 4.1

NetMHCpan is one of the most well-known tools for MHC affinity predictions. It allows the user to predict the affinity of peptides for the different existing HLAs in different scores. In netMHCpan, the important information to define a binder or not, and to distinguish between strong and weak binders, comes from the predicted binding affinity and eluted ligand score. Apart from the raw score NetMHCpan provides %Rank scores, which indicate whether a predicted binding score stands relative to a set of random natural peptides. Unlike some scoring methods that can be skewed by the tendency of certain molecules to generally have higher or lower predicted affinities, the rank values are designed to be bias-free,

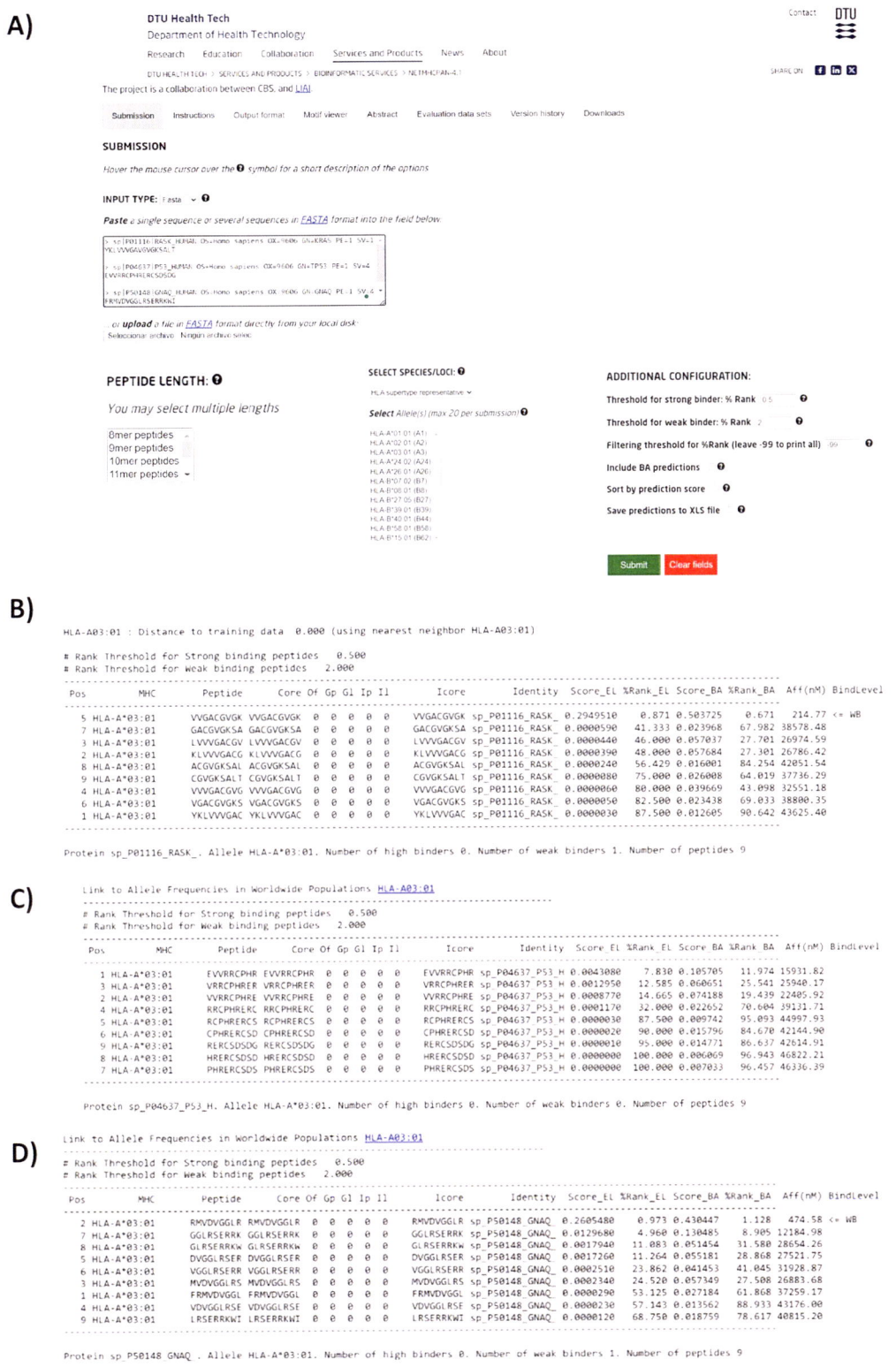

Fig. 3 (**a**) User interface for the NetMHCpan tool for MHC affinity prediction. Input box to enter the full protein sequence containing the neoantigen of interest as FASTA, or directly input the peptide, to select peptide length and HLA alleles, as well as other filters and optional settings for the output. (**b**–**d**) Predictions from mutated

ensuring an accurate comparison across different peptides. If the % Rank score for either binding affinity or eluted ligand is above 2.0, the peptide is considered a non-binder. If the score falls between 2.0 and 0.5 (exclusive), the peptide is classified as a weak binder. If the score is equal to or under 0.5, the peptide is labeled as a strong binder. NetMHCpan also offers a column called "Binding level," which points to the binding strength based on the later values, classifying peptides as weak binder (WB), and strong binder (SB). The evaluation of peptide binding to MHC molecules is often assessed through various scoring systems such as the IC50. The IC50 value represents the peptide's binding affinity to MHC, with lower values indicating stronger binding. For instance, an IC50 of 500 nM or 50 nM typically denotes peptide binders or strong binders to MHC, respectively [22].

NetMHCpan can be used through the interface available or the command line version. The interface version is shown in Fig. 3a. NetMHCpan outputs the result in tables containing information of all the evaluated 9-mer peptides, their affinity, and their ranks both for binding affinity and for eluted ligand, as well as a final column indicating whether the peptide is a strong or weak binder. Figure 3b–d shows the resulting predictions of the mutated peptides used for this example. Evaluation of the selected 17-mers resulted in two potential neoantigens. The 9-mer peptides were RMVDVGGLR, VVGACGVGK, from *GNAQ* p.Q209L and *KRAS* p.G12C, respectively. These peptides passed both %Rank (BA and EL) scores as Weak Binders (under 2.0, but above 0.5). Since the different tools might have discrepancies, the same peptides were evaluated using MHCflurry to confirm their neoantigenicity.

3.1.2 MHCflurry 2.0   MHCflurry implements Class I peptide/MHC-binding affinity prediction. MHCflurry also includes two experimental predictors: an "antigen processing" predictor that attempts to model MHC allele-independent effects such as proteasomal cleavage and a "presentation" predictor that integrates processing predictions with binding affinity predictions to give a composite "presentation score." Both models are trained using binding affinity and mass spectrometry eluted ligand assays [23].

MHCflurry has the same functionality as netMHCpan, but runs in Python. The input can be a full protein sequence, which is

Fig. 3 (continued) peptides by NetMHCpan for (**b**) *KRAS* p.G12C, (**c**) *TP53* p.H179R, and (**d**) *GNAQ* p.Q209L mutations. Pos, indicates the residue number of the peptide in the protein sequence, starting from 0; MHC, specifies the HLA allele or supertipe; Score_EL, is the raw prediction score for eluted ligand; %Rank_EL, is the rank of the predicted binding score compared to a set of random natural peptides; Aff, affinity; BindLevel, indicates the binding level, where SB stands for strong binder and WB for weak binder; *HLA* human leukocyte antigen, *MHC* major histocompatibility complex, *nM* nanoMolar

A)

pos	peptide	n_flank	c_flank	sample_name	affinity	best_allele	affinity_percentile	processing_score	presentation_score	presentation_percentile
4	VVGACGVCK	YKLV	SALT	sample1	88.1087177956	A0301	0.356625	0.2948311158	0.7180030017	0.407826087
2	LVVVGACGV	YK	GKSAL	sample1	24764.5673555715	A0301	11.878	0.0460864494	0.0040635644	62.744673913
6	GACGVGKSA	KLVVV	LT	sample1	27047.3267352356	A0301	15.252375	0.0641564511	0.0039947597	99.2866032609
3	VVVGACGVG	YKL	KSALI	sample1	27446.6044791236	A0301	15.813875	0.0424762408	0.0036278675	99.2866032609
1	KLVVVGACG	Y	VGKSA	sample1	27516.1414633246	A0301	15.813875	0.0911028546	0.0043507799	62.744673913
7	ACGVGKSAL	LVVVG	T	sample1	27768.0887766753	A0301	16.440875	0.0409491413	0.0035664157	99.2866032609
5	VGACGVGKS	YKLVV	AIT	sample1	30137.2671019385	A0301	24.726625	0.0064701785	0.0028904508	100
8	CGVGKSALT	VVVGA		sample1	30978.0759969185	A0301	28.558125	0.0559852204	0.0033952934	99.2866032609
0	YKLVVVGAC		GVGKS	sample1	33569.7738385478	A0301	71.81975	0.1942298999	0.0053010713	46.2246713913

B)

pos	peptide	n_flank	c_flank	sample_name	affinity	best_allele	affinity_percentile	processing_score	presentation_score	presentation_percentile
0	EVVRRCPHR		FRCSD	sample1	5744.16002...	A0301	2.862	0.4129955769	0.0639445992	4.1571195652
2	VRRCPHRER	EV	CSDSD	sample1	17211.5580...	A0301	6.47125	0.0830098669	0.0066467655	37.359048913
1	VVRRCPHRE	E	RCSDS	sample1	23378.3835...	A0301	10.26625	0.019987814	0.0038926161	99.2866032609
3	RRCPHRERC	EVV	SDSDG	sample1	30418.5527...	A0301	26.48575	0.0106666694	0.0029104374	100
4	RCPHRERCS	EVVR	DSDG	sample1	31189.8780...	A0301	31.022125	0.0004339218	0.0027324261	100
8	RERCSDSDG	RRCPH		sample1	32154.5158...	A0301	41.914375	0.0048288169	0.0026973716	100
5	CPHRERCSD	EVVRR	SDG	sample1	32232.4733...	A0301	41.914375	0.0005860818	0.0026480847	100
7	HRERCSDSD	VRRCP	G	sample1	32570.1713...	A0301	47.31825	0.0001834681	0.0026174171	100
6	PHRERCSDS	VVRRC	DG	sample1	33219.3063...	A0301	62.27625	0.0009916644	0.0025756128	100

C)

pos	peptide	n_flank	c_flank	sample_name	affinity	best_allele	affinity_percentile	processing_score	presentation_score	presentation_percentile
1	RMVDVGGLR	F	SERRK	sample1	54.6607075396	A0301	0.1915	0.5723558851	0.920906192	0.0904347826
6	GGLRSERRK	RMVDV	WI	sample1	6936.977180565	A0301	3.153625	0.002089716	0.0117762514	20.2322554348
4	DVGGLRSER	FRMV	RKWI	sample1	7467.0617919316	A0301	3.301	0.9150099531	0.2630452771	1.5116032609
5	VGGLRSERR	FRMVD	KWI	sample1	18239.7721678958	A0301	6.912875	0.0085001605	0.0047409168	62.744673913
7	GLRSERRKW	MVDVG	I	sample1	23208.061240231	A0301	10.26625	0.0522665373	0.00443	62.744673913
3	VDVGGLRSE	FRM	RRKWI	sample1	27228.3615168625	A0301	15.252375	0.4686669018	0.0182147959	12.8054619565
2	MVDVGGLRS	FR	FRRKW	sample1	27577.4211648356	A0301	16.440875	0.2779251873	0.0087942378	27.6173913043
0	FRMVDVGGL		RSERR	sample1	29585.2449192134	A0301	21.8915	0.4013217771	0.0130729844	17.3055978261
8	LRSERRKWI	VDVGG		sample1	31189.2817495858	A0301	31.022125	0.0810565602	0.003709077	99.2866032609

Fig. 4 Predictions from mutated peptides by MHCflurry for peptides containing (**a**) *KRAS* p.G12C mutation, (**b**) *TP53* p.H179R, and (**c**) *GNAQ* p.Q209L mutations. Pos, indicates the residue number of the peptide in the protein sequence, starting from 0

splitted into all the possible peptides of the specified length (9-mers in this example) to predict the binding affinities and calculate the scores of each resulting peptide. The sequences have to be input as a Python dictionary using the argument "sequences." Then, the argument "alleles" takes a list with the HLA alleles that are going to be used for the predictions. The length of the peptides is called "peptide_lengths," which takes a list with the desired input lengths. An example of how to run MHCflurry is shown below:

```
from mhcflurry import Class1PresentationPredictor
predictor = Class1PresentationPredictor.load()

predictor.predict_sequences(
```

```
sequences={'RASK_HUMAN - G12C': "YKLVVVGACGVGKSALT",
'P53_HUMAN TP53 - H179R': "EVVRRCPHRERCSDSDG",
'GNAQ_HUMAN Q209L': "FRMVDVGGLRSERRKWI"},

alleles={"sample1": ["A0301"] },
result="all",
peptide_lengths= [9],
throw = False,
verbose=0)
```

In this case, it does not calculate %Rank like NetMHCpan but outputs a percentile, which can be used to define a binder or not. Any peptide with an affinity and/or presentation percentiles that falls between 0 and 5 can be considered a binder or a presented peptide. However, this is not a validated range. The well-validated threshold is affinity of 500 nM. Figure 4 shows the resulting predictions of the mutated peptides used for this example. The two peptides classified as HLA-A*03–01 binders with NetMHCpan were also classified as binders by MHCflurry, showing concordance between these two tools.

In summary, only one out of the 9-mers generated from *KRAS* p.G12C mutation has been identified as a potential neoantigen, although classified as weak. Also, one 9-mer from the *GNAQ* p. Q209L mutation has been identified as a potential neoantigen. In the case of *TP53* p.H179R, none of the generated 9-mers had affinity for the tested HLA. Therefore, it will be excluded from downstream analyses. Next, the stability of the peptide-MHC complex in *KRAS* p.G12C and *GNAQ* p.Q209L putative neoantigens will be evaluated.

3.1.3 NetMHCstabpan 1.0

NetMHCstabpan is a computational tool designed to predict the stability of peptide-MHC Class I (pMHC-I) complexes. It uses a machine learning approach to forecast the half-life of peptides bound to MHC molecules, an essential step in antigen presentation by the immune system. It is possible to run this tool using the interface or the command line version [37] (Fig. 5a).

As in netMHCpan, the %rank values are not affected by the inherent bias of certain molecules toward higher or lower mean predicted affinities. Strong binders are defined as having %rank <0.5, and weak binders with %rank <2. Of note, this tool also includes a combined score using the affinity and stability values. In fact, the output information is similar to netMHCpan, except for the two new parameters related to stability and combined scores of affinity and stability (Fig. 5b, c).

As a result, the two peptides from *KRAS* p.G12C and *GNAQ* p.Q209L mutations, RMVDVGGLR and VVGACGVGK, were predicted as stable binders. Thus, netMHCstabpan confirmed

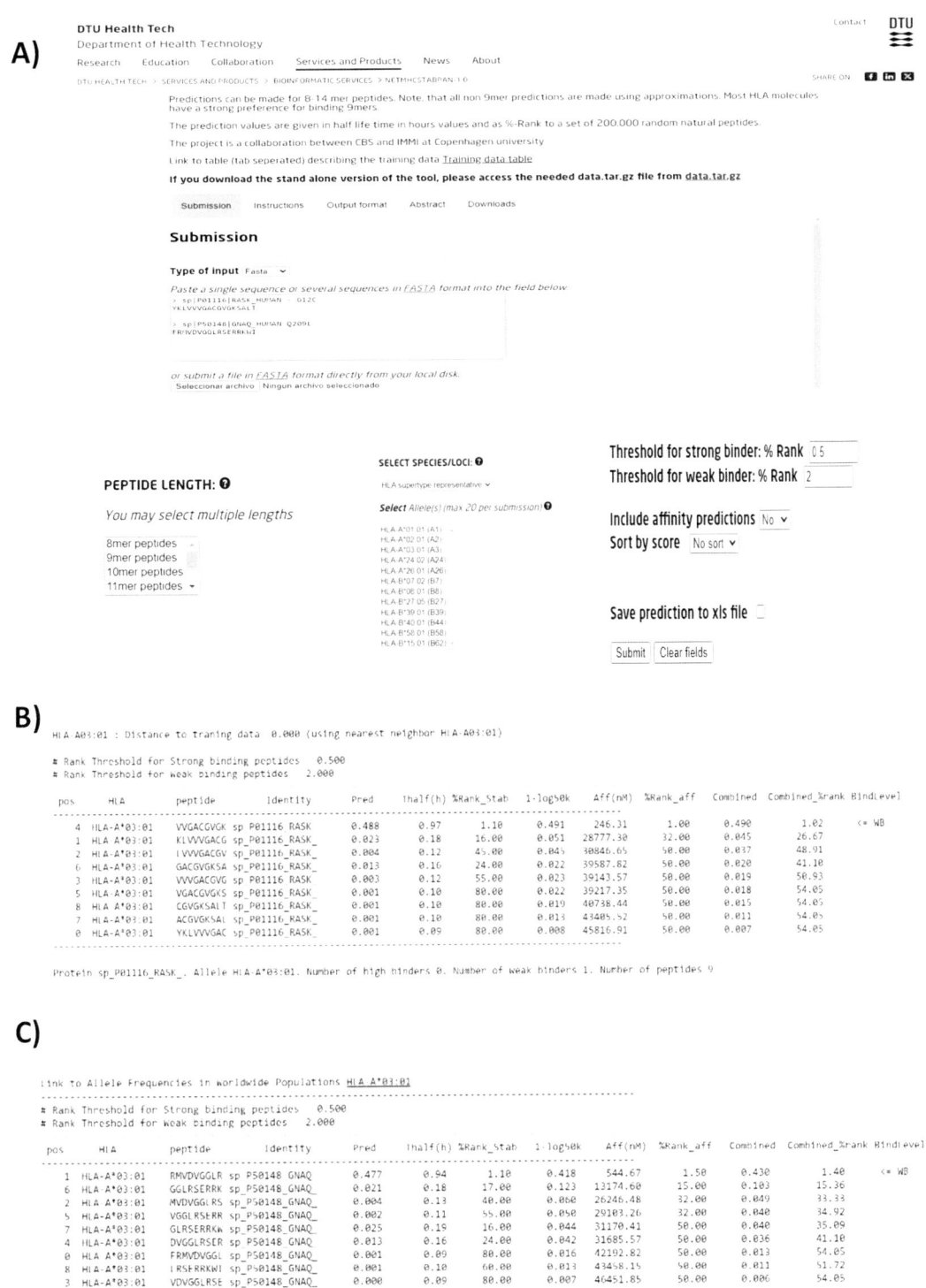

Fig. 5 (**a**) User interface for the NetMHCstabpan tool for prediction of the stability of peptide-MHC Class I complexes: Input box to enter the full protein sequence containing the neoantigen of interest as FASTA, or directly input the peptide, to select peptide length and HLA allele, as well as other filters and optional settings for the output. (**b–c**) Predictions from mutated peptides by netMHCstabpan for peptides containing

that those mutations could produce potential neoantigens, with affinity and stability for HLA-A*03:01. Nevertheless, additional steps are required to evaluate whether these peptides will be presented on the cell surface, such as prediction of cleavage sites.

3.2 Predicting Cleavage and Transport

3.2.1 NetChop 3.1

NetChop is a computational tool designed to predict cleavage sites for processing protein precursors into mature peptides by proteases within the MHC Class I antigen presentation pathway. It operates by using a neural network trained on a dataset of experimentally verified cleavage sites, learning patterns indicative of protease specificity. When provided with an amino acid sequence, NetChop assesses the likelihood of each residue being part of a cleavage site based on its surrounding sequence context and outputs a probability score for cleavage at each position [38].

NetChop also offers an interface closely similar to netMHCpan and netMHCstabpan (Fig. 6a). In this example, the prediction method was "C term 3.0," with the default threshold of "0.5" and output set to "Short output." NetChop gives as a result the input sequence marked with the predicted cleavage sites. The residue where the cleavage is most likely happening is marked with an "S," whereas, if the cleavage is not occurring, the residue is marked with a ".". If a residue is assigned with an "S" the peptide bond on the C-terminal side is cleaved.

The cleavage sites are selected based on the value output by the tool. This value can go from 0 to 1 and everything above 0.5 is selected as a cleavage site. To access the predicted values per amino acid "Short output" option needs to be unselected.

Figure 6b shows the resulting cleavage predictions of the mutated peptides. In the case of *KRAS*, the 9-mer VVGACGVGK was not found within the array of peptides produced after chopping the mutated protein. On the contrary, the predicted cleavage pattern of the 17-mer *GNAQ* p.Q209L can produce the peptide RMVDVGGLR, which had binding affinity for HLA-A*03:01 allele (as shown above). It is important to note that the 9-mer RMVDVGGLR also contains internal cleavage sites, which could lead to the generation of shorter peptides.

Therefore, only the peptide RMVDVGGLR from *GNAQ* p. Q209L remains as a potential neoantigen and will be tested in the

---

Fig. 5 (continued) KRAS p.G12C and *GNAQ* p.Q209L mutations. Pos, indicates the residue number of the peptide in the protein sequence, starting from 0; HLA, specifies the MHC molecule or allele name; Pred, Stability prediction score; Thalf(h), The predicted half-life of the pMHC complex (in hours); %Rank_Stab, %Random - % Rank of predicted stability score to a set of 200,000 random natural 9-mer peptides; 1-log50K, Affinity Prediction score (called 1-log50K(aff)); Aff(nM), Affinity as IC50 value in nM (only for white-listed alleles); % Rank_aff, %Random - %Rank of predicted affinity score to a set of 200,000 random natural 9-mer peptides; Combined, Prediction score combining Affinity and Stability predictions; Combined_%rank, %Rank approximation using both stability and affinity %Rank; BindLevel, Binding level (*SB* strong binder, *WB* weak binder)

A)

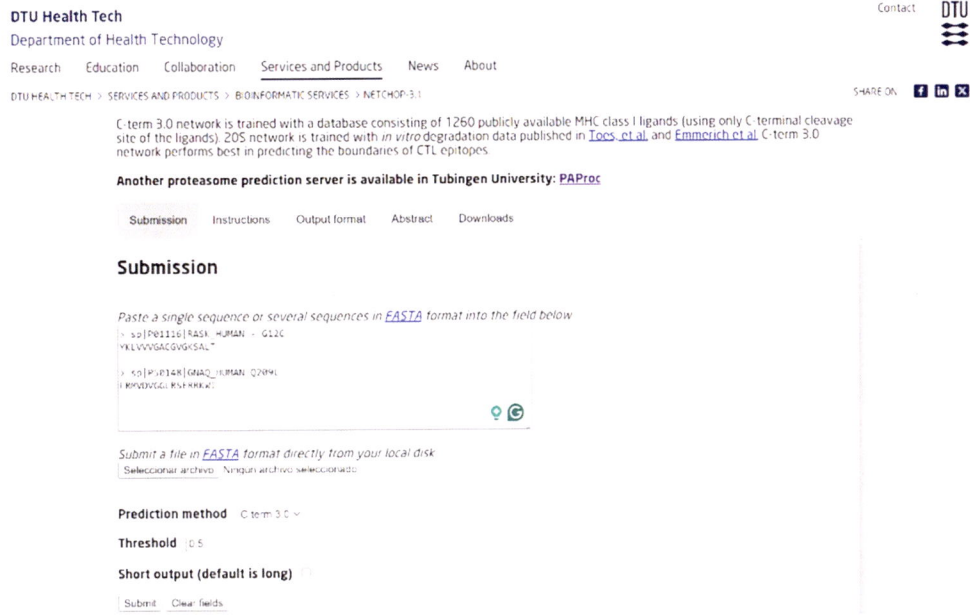

B)

```
NetChop 3.0 predictions using version C-term. Threshold 0.500000

17   sp_P01116
YKLVVVGACGVGKSALT
S.S.SS.S..S......
----------------------------------------

Number of cleavage sites 6. Number of amino acids 17. Protein name  sp_P01116

----------------------------------------
17   sp_P50148
FRMVDVGGLRSERRKWI
S..S....SS.....SS
----------------------------------------

Number of cleavage sites 6. Number of amino acids 17. Protein name  sp_P50148
```

Fig. 6 (**a**) User interface for the netChop 3.1 tool for prediction of the peptide cleavage sites: Input box to enter the full protein sequence containing the neoantigen of interest as FASTA, or input the peptide directly, together with optional settings. (**b**) Predictions of cleavage sites by netChop 3.1 for the 17-mer containing the *GNAQ* p. Q209L mutation

last step, intending to predict if this peptide could be presented on the cell surface of cancer cells by being transported to the ER by TAP protein.

3.2.2 TAP Transport Predictions

For the TAP transport prediction, many AI-based tools have recently been developed. A validated method described by Peters et al. will be used in this example. The scoring matrix and how the values are assigned for every amino acid at each position of a 9-mer (calculated from experimental data) and formula used to score each 9-mer can be found in the original work [39].

The TAP score using this method on RMVDVGGLR was −1.97. Since the authors specified that any TAP score below 1 would be considered a potential neoantigen, this peptide would pass all thresholds to be considered as a potential neoantigen.

In summary, according to our findings; from the three evaluated mutations, only *GNAQ* p.Q209L mutation would have a potential neoantigen, in agreement with previous reports. Interestingly, *GNAQ* p.Q209L mutation is harboured by approximately 70% patients with uveal melanoma so it could represent a therapeutic opportunity [41, 42]. In contrast, none of the peptides resulting from *TP53* p.H179R mutation had sufficient affinity to bind HLA so would not be immunogenic, in agreement with previous studies [42]. Whilst other mutations arising from *TP53* could lead to potential neoantigens [43], it has been reported that *TP53* mutations with greater oncogenic potential would be less immunogenic [44]. Finally, although one peptide derived from *KRAS* p.G12C mutation scored as a potential HLA-binding peptide, this 9-mer would not be generated according to the cleavage prediction tool. Of note, more potential neoantigens would have been found if more HLA genotypes had been interrogated. In that sense, the fact that neoantigens are restricted to certain HLA alleles limits the applicability for immunotherapeutic approaches [45, 46].

4 Overview of Available Computational End-to-End Workflows for Neoantigen Identification

Computational workflows for neoantigen prediction consist of four main steps, which can be categorized as (1) variant calling and annotation for tumor-specific mutations, (2) HLA genotyping of patients' alleles, (3) prediction of HLA-binding affinity and stability of peptide epitopes, and (4) neoantigen prioritization and identification of immunogenic neoepitopes for personalized cancer immunotherapy (Fig. 2). Those steps, explained in Subheading 2, are typically integrated into a sophisticated bioinformatics pipeline provided as a ready-to-use software. With the advent of AI, some of the steps are being replaced or facilitated by machine learning algorithms, whereas recent state-of-the-art approaches utilize end-to-end deep learning models. Over the past years, several methods have been proposed to conduct each step of the neoantigen prediction process. As an example, in Subheading 3 an extensive description of the available methods for HLA-binding affinity and stability prediction has been provided. Herein, an overview of the methods providing unified pipelines and workflows for neoantigen prediction will be presented. Since several end-to-end pipelines are available, this section will focus on those that provide unique features to users aimed at improving neoantigen identification, facilitating clinical implementation, reducing computation time, and inclusiveness in the user group.

CloudNeo [47]: It was the initial effort to introduce a cloud-based neoantigen prediction workflow with the scope of identifying patient-specific tumor neoantigens. The CloudNeo workflow requires non-synonymous mutations in VCF format and RNA or DNA sequencing data in BAM format for HLA typing. Then, the VEP tool [48] and a custom R script named Protein_Translator are utilized to convert genomic variants into amino acid changes. The Protein_Translator generates a list of N-amino-acid-long peptide sequences in FASTA format, with the single peptide change positioned in the middle of the N-mer. Additionally, it generates another FASTA file for homologous N-mers without peptide mutations. Users can select either HLAminer [49] or Polysolver [50] to calculate six predicted HLA types (top two predictions each for HLA-A, HLA-B, and HLA-C). Then, the NetMHCpan tool [22, 51] computes binding affinities between the six HLA types and each ($[N/2] + 1$)-mer peptide subsequence within the N-mers. The platform's output includes peptide subsequences and MHC-binding affinity scores for all six HLA types. The CloudNeo pipeline, implemented in Common Workflow Language (CWL), is publicly available on GitHub. It can be executed using Rabix, enabling deployment on various platforms such as AWS, Google Compute Engine, and Azure.

Antigen.garnish [52] is a workflow featuring unique characteristics. The first is ensemble neoantigen prediction, while the second is utilizing the dissimilarity to the non-mutated (reference) proteome to identify high-quality predicted neoantigens. More specifically, the antigen.garnish workflow input options include VCFs, peptide sequences, or ensemble transcript IDs with HGVS-style cDNA annotations. Mutated sequences undergo prediction and filtering against the non-mutated proteome. The main function of the tool, "garnish_affinity," is to conduct ensemble MHC affinity prediction. The ensemble method generates a unified affinity score by averaging the affinities from all models predicting the peptide-MHC binding. The pipeline provides both the ensemble value and the individual algorithm prediction affinities from each model. Dissimilarity analysis integrates Smith-Waterman alignments against the reference proteome, with a cutoff of dissimilarity metric >0.75 applied to identify high dissimilarity neoantigens, enhancing identification of immunogenic peptides. The workflow is provided as an open-source tool, implemented in R, designed for Linux, and utilizes the "mclapply" function for parallelization.

NeoFuse [53] was proposed as the first fully unified workflow for the prediction of fusion neoantigens from tumor RNA-seq data. The unique characteristic of this tool lies in the integration of the preprocessing steps required for fusion transcript prediction in an end-to-end pipeline, which yields IC50 annotation for each neoantigen, percentile rank, confidence score, binding HLA type, expression of both HLA genes and fusion. Additionally, it identifies premature stop codons that could lead to nonsense-mediated decay of the fusion transcript. NeoFuse is a command line tool with five modules. Initially, data is imported in FASTQ format, and the first module performs HLA Class I typing using OptiType [54]. The second module utilizes Arriba [55] to predict fusion peptides, while the binding affinity of fusion peptides to HLA types is predicted by MHCflurry [23, 56] in the third module. Afterward, the fourth module quantifies gene expression levels as transcripts per million by utilizing both STAR [57] and feature-Counts [58]. The fifth and final module filters and prioritizes based on the binding affinity and confidence score resulting from the fourth step. In this way, it produces a set of peptides that indicate potential fusion neoantigens. The tool is provided through two major container technologies, Docker and Singularity.

DeepHLApan [59] in contrast with the other methods is not a unified neoantigen prediction pipeline since it requires some preprocessing steps, yet it provides the distinctive feature of an end-to-end deep learning scheme for neoantigen prediction based on peptide-HLA binding and the immunogenicity of the complex. Specifically, DeepHLApan utilizes recurrent neural networks (RNN) and consists of two models, the first for predicting the probability of the peptide binding to the HLA in the tumor cell membrane and the second immunogenicity model for predicting the capacity of the peptide-HLA complex to induce T-cell activation. The immunogenicity score is used as a filter to rank the binding prediction score to yield a high confidence neoantigen identification. The model works only for HLA Class I neoantigens (A, B, and C alleles). Moreover, preprocessing steps are required since the model's input data should be in CSV format with the columns' heads being "Annotation, HLA, Peptide." DeepHLApan is provided as a ready-to-use model through a web platform or as a docker image.

pVACtools [60–62] is not a pipeline itself but a toolkit with several modules that can be integrated into one workflow to create an end-to-end neoantigen prediction tool. It is a modularized toolkit that provides the independent use of its module while facilitating multiple input types. It can also be integrated with external tools. The main feature of this toolkit is pVACseq, a pipeline for identifying and prioritizing neoantigens from a VCF file, which can be coupled with the pVACviz GUI for the visualization and selection of data resulting from pVACseq. The pVACbind is used for FASTA files, while the pVACfuse is utilized for neoantigen prediction in gene fusions. Another tool is the pVACvector, which is employed to optimize the design of DNA-based cancer vaccines that prevent high-affinity junction neoantigens. Finally, the pVACapi offers a Rest-API for the pVACtools suite.

NextNEOpi [63] is a fully automated pipeline for neoantigen prediction with some special characteristics, such as quantification of neoepitope and patient-specific features associated with tumor immunogenicity and response to immunotherapy. NextNEOpi is a command line tool that utilizes raw DNA and RNA sequencing data, and a list of known patients' HLA types can also be imported. The first step of the pipeline after sequencing data pre-processing is HLA typing for both Class I using the OptiType and HLA-HD [64] for Class II. Then, variant calling is performed with several different independent algorithms, and variants called by more than one tool are marked as having high confidence. All variants are then annotated by the VEP tool, and the pVACseq tool is used to predict neoantigens from SNVs and INDELs, whereas NeoFuse is used to predict neoantigens from gene fusions. For peptide-HLA Class I binding prediction, NextNEOpi uses by default netMHCpan [65], MHCFlurry [23], and NetMHCIIpan [22]. For peptide-HLA II binding prediction mixMHC2pred [66] is employed. MiXCR [67] is used to predict T- and B-cell receptor repertoires, while clonality, tumor mutational burden, and CSiN scores are computed for the individual neoantigens and samples. NextNEOpi is implemented in NextFlow, providing reproducibility and scalability as a user-friendly tool.

NeoSplice [68] is another neoantigen prediction method, yet its unique characteristic is the use of splice variants. This method utilizes RNA-seq data as input and generates tumor-specific k-mers by comparing tumor cells with normal cells. Hence it identifies k-mer sequences abundant in the tumor transcriptome but rare in normal cells. Then, splice variant transcripts are predicted by constructing a splice graph using tumor cell RNA-seq data. Tumor-specific k-mers identified in the first step are then mapped to these splice variant transcripts. Annotations from Gencode are utilized to ascertain if the novel splice occurs within a protein-coding region and to determine the reading frame of the transcript. Finally, it translates novel splice junctions found within each splice variant transcript into peptide sequences based on the inferred open reading frame. Following translation, HLA Class I-binding affinity prediction is carried out on these peptide sequences employing NetMHCpan-4.0 [65] to identify regions that may produce neoepitopes. This tool is provided as a command line tool implemented in Python 2 while also shipping in a docker image.

Seq2Neo [69] provides a one-stop solution pipeline for neoantigen immunogenicity prediction and specifically for neoepitope feature prediction through raw sequencing data. The major distinctive characteristic of this pipeline is the use of a convolutional neural network (CNN) that predicts the immunogenicity of neoepitopes. Seq2Neo is a command line tool that automates workflows for predicting immunogenic peptides. It integrates mutation labeling, HLA typing, and HLA affinity-binding prediction tools, along with a (CNN)-based model for immunogenicity prediction. The workflow begins with importing raw sequencing data in FASTQ, SAM, or BAM format and then selecting the workflow of interest. For point mutation and INDEL detection, Mutect2 [70] was utilized, while for gene fusion detection STAR-Fusion [71] was employed. VCF format was used for the somatic variant data generated. HLA-HD is used for MHC genotyping, and ANNOVAR [72] or Agfusion [73] were utilized to annotate somatic variants to identify mutated peptides. Seq2Neo uses NetMHCpan for peptide-HLA-binding affinity prediction, while TPMCalculator [74] was used to detect gene expression and NetCTLpan [19] to obtain TAP transport efficiency. The tool outputs various peptide features, aiding in neoantigen prediction and immunogenicity assessment. Seq2Neo is provided as a Conda package or a docker image.

PGNneo [75] is another unique pipeline that performs neoantigen prediction in noncoding regions based on proteogenomics. The overall computational framework of PGNneo comprises the following components. First, there is noncoding somatic variant calling and HLA typing, this involves using paired tumor and normal samples for somatic variant calling, filtering out low-quality mutations, and extracting noncoding mutations. HLA typing is determined based on RNA-seq data from tumor samples. Second, nucleotide sequences are obtained and translated into proteins via six-frame translation. Tumor mutated peptides are extracted, and a customized protein database is constructed by combining these mutated protein sequences with reference proteins. Third, variant peptide identification involves filtering resulting peptides using MS datasets, providing evidence for their presence at protein levels and their binding to MHC molecules. Finally, neoantigen prediction and selection are conducted. Candidate neoantigens are predicted based on peptides and HLA types using NetMHCpan 4.1 [22]. These candidates undergo filtering using the dbPepNeo 2.0 database, which contains 746 experimental immunogenic peptides as a reference. The tool is provided both in a command line version and GUI versions, while for its implementation, Python, R, Java, and Perl were used.

NeoMUST [76] employs multitask learning, representing a novel approach to neoantigen prediction. The primary task of the model is neoantigen presentation classification, while the secondary task is binding affinity prediction between HLA Class I molecules and eluted peptides. It effectively captures and utilizes task-specific information from both tasks, identifying similarities and distinctions to enhance performance. Additionally, it optimizes individual loss functions to balance the two tasks effectively while significantly reducing training time and enhancing scalability for large datasets. Although it is not an end-to-end pipeline, it features some novel capabilities. The model is available either as a Conda package or a docker image.

ImmuneMirror [77] is another recent method that provides an integrative pipeline for neoantigen prediction enhanced by machine learning. The machine learning model was constructed utilizing the balanced random forest algorithm to predict neoantigens. It integrates multiple biological features pertinent to neoantigen processes, including biogenesis, transportation, presentation, and T-cell recognition (such as agretopicity, foreignness, hydrophobicity, binding stability, peptide processing, and transportation scores). This machine learning model was then integrated into the ImmuneMirror bioinformatics pipeline, which also operates as a web server for predicting and prioritizing neoantigens from multiomics sequencing data. The pipeline accepts raw FASTQ reads as input, while the web server requires VCF files containing somatic mutations. The web server produces a visual report that incorporates the following: tumor mutational burden (TMB), HLA types, neoantigen load for HLA Class I and II, mismatch repair (MMR) status, germline and somatic mutations, ImmuneMirror prediction score, and IPRES gene expression signature.

GraphMHC [78] is one of the most recent approaches for neoantigen prediction, utilizing a graph neural network applied to molecular structure to simulate the binding between peptide and MHC proteins. The pipeline begins by converting HLA into MHC amino acid sequences. Next, both MHC and peptide sequences are transformed into SMILES structures using the RDKit 2022.03.2 library. Then, these two SMILES strings are combined using non-bond notation. Afterward, the combined structure is converted into a molecular structure using RDKit, ensuring that any omitted hydrogen atoms are included. Following this, the molecular structure is transformed into a graph structure using the RDKit library, allowing for the encoding of vectors and matrices. Each feature is encoded using one-hot encoding and assembled into a sparse matrix. Finally, the graph dataset is converted using the PyTorch Geometric (PyG) 2.1.0 library.

Table 1 summarizes all the methods discussed. The table provides the name of each tool, the intended function of the software and specifies the input data utilized in neoantigen prediction. Additionally, it provides neoantigen classification, the method employed to evaluate the binding affinity between the neoantigen and HLA molecules and the outcomes obtained from the analysis. A link to

Table 1
Computational tools, pipelines, and workflows for neoantigen prediction

Name	Purpose	Input type	HLA Class	HLA binding affinity method	Output	Source	Year of publication	Last Update
CloudNeo	Cloud-based pipeline to streamline neoantigen prediction	VCF, BAM	HLA Class I	NetMHCpan 3.0	Peptide subsequences and MHC-binding affinity scores for all six HLA types	https://github.com/TheJacksonLaboratory/CloudNeo/tree/master	June 2017	2019
Antigen. garnish	An R package to predict neoantigen immunogenicity based on dissimilarity to self-proteome	VCFs or ensemble transcript IDs or HGVS-style cDNA annotations	HLA Class I & II	Ensemble affinity score utilizing: NetMHCI/II, netMHCI/IIpan, MHCflurry, and MHCnuggets	Ensemble binding affinity and peptide immunogenicity	https://github.com/andrewrech/antigen.garnish	October 2019	2022
NeoFuse	An automated workflow for the identification of fusion neoantigens	FASTQ files	HLA Class I	MHCflurry	Neoantigen prioritization based on IC50 binding affinity, confidence score, and annotation of each neoantigen	https://github.com/icbi-lab/NeoFuse	November 2019	2022
DeepHLApan	A deep learning method for predicting neoantigens based on peptide-HLA binding and the immunogenicity of the complex	CSV file with annotations, HLA alleles and peptides	HLA Class I & II	Recurrent Neural Network-based approach integrating HLA-peptide binding and pHLA immunogenicity	Neoantigen prediction and immunogenicity	https://github.com/jiujiezz/deephlapan	November 2019	2022
pVACtools	A modularized toolkit for neoantigen predictions with an interactive display for review by the end user. Highly compatible with external tools	BAM, VCF, FASTA	HLA Class I & II	Utilizes the algorithms supported in pVACseq	Neoantigen prediction and ranking	https://github.com/griffithlab/pVACtools	March 2020	2024

Name	Description	Input	HLA	Binding predictor	Output	URL	Date	Year
NextNEOpi	Automated bioinformatics pipeline for predicting tumor neoantigens from raw DNA and RNA sequencing	Raw FASTQ or BAM files	HLA Class I & II	NetMHCpan 4.0 and MHCflurry 2.0	Tumor mutational burden, canonical neontigens, fusion neoantigens	https://github.com/icbi-lab/nextNEOpi	November 2021	2023
NeoSplice	An end-to-end workflow for splice variant neoantigen prediction	BAM files	HLA Class I & II	NetMHCpan 4.0	HLA binding prediction, with predicted binders representing putative splice variant neoantigens	https://github.com/pirl-unc/NeoSplice	May 2022	2024
Seq2Neo	A comprehensive pipeline to predict the immunogenicity of neoepitopes derived from somatic DNA alterations, aiding in cancer immunotherapy	Files in FASTQ, SAM and BAM format	HLA Class I	NetMHCpan 4.1 & NetMHCIIpan-4.0	Binding affinity, TAP transport efficiency, gene expression, and immunogenicity score	https://github.com/XSLiuLab/Seq2Neo	October 2022	2023
PGNneo	An integrated pipeline for neoantigen prediction in noncoding region based on proteogenomics	FASTQ and raw MS data	HLA Class I	NetMHCpan 4.1	Neoantigen prediction and selection	https://github.com/tanxiaoxiu/PGNneo	March 2023	2023
NeoMUST	A deep learning model utilizing multitask learning	CSV file with columns "hla,peptide," BLOSUM62 file and a CSV file for HC_pseudo-sequences with columns "allele, sequence"	HLA Class I	Multitask learning (MTL) approach to predict the neoantigen presentation as its main task and the neoantigen–MHC binding as an auxiliary task	Binding affinity, eluted peptide, and the rank of the peptide	https://github.com/Freshwind-Bioinformatics/NeoMUST	January 2024	2024
ImmuneMirror	A web server for an integrative pipeline for neoantigen prediction leveraging machine learning	FASTQ for the CLI and VCF for the web app	HLA Class I & II	pVACtools	TMB, HLA types, neoantigen load for HLA Class I and II, MMR status, germline and somatic mutations,	https://github.com/weidai2/ImmuneMirror/	February 2024	2024

(continued)

Table 1
(continued)

Name	Purpose	Input type	HLA Class	HLA binding affinity method	Output	Source	Year of publication	Last Update
					ImmuneMirror prediction score, and IPRES gene expression signature			
GraphMHC	A Graph Neural Network utilizing molecular structure to model the binding affinity for neoantigen prediction-based	CSV HLA type, peptide sequence	HLA Class I and II	Graph neural network for MHC-peptide-binding prediction	Neoantigen binding	https://github.com/ recognizability/ GraphMHC	March 2024	2024

VCF Variant call format, *BAM* binary alignment map, *HGVS* human genome variation society, *CSV* comma-separated values, *SAM* sequence alignment/map format, *HLA* human leukocyte antigens, *MHC* major histocompatibility complex, *MS* mass spectrometry, *CLI* command-line interface, *TBM* tumor mutation burden, *MMR* DNA mismatch repair, *IPRES* A transcriptional signature related to innate anti-PD-1 resistance, *TAP* transporter associated with antigen processing, *IC50* half-maximal inhibitory concentration

the source code or user interface of the software is also provided along with its publication date and the date of its last update.

The above methods provide only an overview of the distinctive utilities offered by available tools and pipelines. However, there are several other methods available for neoantigen prediction. The choice of method depends on factors such as the specific use, the user's level of bioinformatics expertise, and the ease of pipeline implementation. Therefore, users should consider both the input and output data of each pipeline based on their needs. Additionally, users can choose among command-line interface (CLI) tools or web applications with user-friendly interfaces, depending on their proficiency in utilizing informatics tools. It is important to note that a direct comparison of the prediction accuracy of tools can only be made when the prediction endpoint of the pipeline is the same.

In the last decade, deep learning models have flourished due to their high prediction accuracy across several fields. Thus, they have been widely adopted in biomedical research. This trend is particularly evident in the field of neoantigen prediction, where deep learning methods have been introduced for binding affinity prediction. While machine learning models were predominantly utilized for neoantigen-peptide binding, there has been a noticeable transition in many pipelines toward deep learning methods. This shift is strongly correlated with the continuous expansion of available training data and the emergence of additional features. As a result, the complexity of the data is increasing, favouring deep learning models due to their enhanced capacity to capture and process this wealth of information compared to traditional machine learning models.

5   Neoantigen Prediction in Mouse Models

In silico prediction of neoantigens represents a pivotal phase in unlocking the therapeutic potential of cancer immunotherapy. As described in the previous section, a plethora of software for neoantigen discovery is available. However, these pipelines are mainly tailored to human data with a focus on predicting the binding affinity between epitope and HLA. Nevertheless, models specific to murine systems are crucial for facilitating in vivo experimentation and further translation of immunotherapies into clinical practice. The availability of these pan-specific software solutions remains limited, posing a significant challenge in preclinical immunotherapy research. Consequently, some human-centric software platforms have undergone adaptation to include binding affinity predictions for mouse MHC. Moreover, efforts have also been made to develop murine-specific models aimed at bridging this gap in experimental settings.

When evaluating the collection of available software tools, it is important to recognize that neoantigen presentation and recognition by T cells entail a complex process comprising various steps. Many existing neoantigen prediction tools primarily focus on predicting the binding affinity between the epitope and the MHC molecule while overlooking other critical steps, leading to a high false positive rate of predicted epitopes [64]. Emerging software solutions are now considering these additional steps to yield more robust predictions. First, the different software platforms specializing in binding affinity prediction within murine models will be examined. These tools exhibit variations in training data modalities, training methodologies, and input data types. While some tools exclusively predict binding affinity for user-identified neoepitopes, others offer end-to-end platforms capable of processing RNA-seq data to predict neoantigens directly. These latter tools enable users to input raw data directly without having to create and apply variant calling pipelines. In terms of training data, it is common to utilize either binding affinity data or mass spectrometry-eluted ligands. However, studies have demonstrated that combining both input data types enhances predictive performance [22]. Additionally, predictive models have transitioned from earlier methodologies, such as support vector machine regression [79] or profiles [80], to more advanced approaches like ANNs and RNNs, which have shown superior performance.

Among the reviewed software solutions, only two are explicitly designed for murine models. The first, NetH2Pan [81], employs an ANN architecture to predict binding affinity. It performs the prediction based on user-provided peptides, leveraging both binding affinity and eluted ligand data during training. Conversely, NAP-CNB [9] operates as an end-to-end platform, using RNA-seq for neoantigen prediction. The tool integrates a variant calling pipeline that returns SNVs and INDELs unique to the tumor. This method implements a more advanced neural network with long-short-term memory (LSTM) units, albeit trained solely on binding affinity data. Additionally, several software platforms initially developed for human data have been adapted to incorporate murine H2 alleles. Examples of such software include NetMHC [25], NetMHCpan [65], and MHCflurry [23]. Both NetMHC and NetMHCpan utilize an ANN architecture and were trained on binding affinity and eluted ligand data. Moreover, they accept user-generated tumor-specific peptides as input. However, NetMHC employs an allele-specific training approach, while NetMHCpan adopts a "pan-specific" strategy, combining information from both data modalities and diverse MHC molecules into a unified network. The authors reported that the novel training strategy employed by NetMHCpan enhances predictive accuracy. In contrast, MHCflurry uses binding affinity and eluted ligand data in a more sequential manner. The method initially conducts binding predictions using an ensemble of ANNs trained on binding affinity data and subsequently integrates mass spectrometry data into another ensemble of ANNs to account for the antigen processing steps, particularly focusing on proteasomal cleavage. The outputs of these two models are then aggregated to generate a comprehensive presentation score. Furthermore, certain tools seek to bridge the gap between RNA-seq data and tumor-specific peptides by integrating some of the prediction methods mentioned above with variant calling pipelines, offering end-to-end solutions for neoantigen prediction. Examples include Epi-Seq [82], a bioinformatics pipeline utilizing NetMHC, and pVAC-Seq [62], which incorporates various prediction methods like NetMHC or MHCflurry. A general summary of these methods can be found in Table 2.

Newly developed methods are taking into consideration additional steps of the neoantigen processing pipeline, aiming to reduce the occurrence of false positives. One such tool, DeepNeo [83], a neural network-based tool, integrates predictions on MHC binding affinity and T-cell reactivity, a crucial factor for the success of neoantigen vaccines. The tool accepts peptide sequences from both mouse and human data and generates a binary prediction for MHC binding alongside a quantification of T-cell reactivity. While the prediction of T-cell reactivity holds promise for designing more effective neoantigen-based treatments, it is worth noting that the authors do not provide validation of the tool's performance on murine data in the paper. Another recently introduced tool, Neo-Intiline [84], similarly accounts for various stages of peptide presentation and recognition. The tool is designed to be used with WGS data. The tool's optimal performance is observed when analyzing melanoma data, although its applicability extends to any relevant dataset of interest.

Although these methods have demonstrated efficacy in silico, in vivo validations are imperative to assess their real-world performance. Both NetH2pan and NAP-CNB, validated in clinical settings, have proven effective in neoantigen discovery [85].

6 Technical Challenges and Future Improvements

The field of neoantigen prediction has evolved significantly, propelled by advancements in computational biology, high-throughput sequencing technologies, and the integration of machine learning approaches. Despite these advancements, several technical challenges persist, and addressing these challenges is crucial for enhancing the predictive accuracy and clinical utility of neoantigen prediction methods.

Table 2
Methods for MHC Class I-binding affinity prediction

Name	Input type	Encoding	Type of data for training	Prediction method	Mouse-specific?	Source	Year of publication
NetH2Pan	Peptides or protein sequence	BLOSUM encoding	BA + EL	ANN	Yes	Web server: https://services.healthtech.dtu.dk/services/NetH2pan-1.0/	March, 2018
NAP-CNB	RNA-seq or peptides	One-hot encoding	BA	LSTM units and dense units	Yes	Web server: https://biocomp-cnb.csic.es/NeoantigensApp/	May, 2021
NetMHC 4.0	Peptides or protein sequence	BLOSUM encoding	BA + EL	ANN	No	Web server: https://services.healthtech.dtu.dk/services/NetMHC-4.0/	February, 2016
NetMHCpan 4.1	Peptides or protein sequence	BLOSUM encoding	BA + EL	ANN	No	Web server: https://services.healthtech.dtu.dk/services/NetMHCpan-4.1/	July, 2020
MHCflurry 2.0	Peptides or proteins	45-mer representation and BLOSUM	BA + EL	ANN	No	Command line tool: https://github.com/openvax/mhcflurry	July, 2020
Epi-seq	RNA-seq	–	–	NetMHC	No	Software available at https://dna.engr.uconn.edu/?page_id=470	October, 2014
pVAC-Seq	VCF file	–	–	Different softwares available	No	Software available at https://github.com/griffithlab/pVACtools	January, 2016

VCF variant call format, *BLOSUM* BLOcks SUbstitution Matrix, *BA* binding affinity, *EL* eluted ligand, *ANN* artificial neural network, *LSTM* long short-term memory

6.1 Technical Challenges

The main challenges we have identified are:

1. High false positive rates: One of the enduring challenges in neoantigen prediction is the high rate of false positives. Many predicted neoantigens are not genuinely immunogenic, which can lead to inefficient or ineffective therapeutic strategies. This challenge stems primarily from the limitations in accurately modeling the complex interplay of factors that contribute to the immunogenicity of neoantigens, such as peptide-MHC-binding affinity, TCR recognition, and the expression and presentation dynamics in tumor microenvironment.

2. HLA allelic diversity: The genetic diversity of HLA alleles poses a significant challenge due to its impact on binding affinity predictions. Current prediction tools often have reduced accuracy for less common HLA alleles, which are underrepresented in training datasets. This limitation affects the generalizability of prediction models across different populations. In addition, most tools are specific to MHC Class I molecules, although it has been demonstrated that MHC Class II is also essential for effective antitumor immune responses.

3. Integration of epitope processing: Neoantigen prediction tools primarily focus on the binding affinity of peptides to MHC molecules. However, the entire process of antigen presentation, including proteasomal processing, transport by TAP proteins, and trimming by ER aminopeptidases, significantly influences the presence of peptides on the cell surface. The lack of comprehensive integration of these steps can lead to inaccuracies in predicting true neoantigens.

4. Scalability and computational efficiency: As genomic datasets grow in size and complexity, the computational demands of neoantigen prediction also increase. Scalability and efficiency become critical, especially for real-time or near-real-time analysis in clinical settings. Many existing tools require substantial computational resources, which can be a barrier to routine clinical use.

6.2 Future Improvements

As future improvements to be accomplished, we propose the following:

1. Enhanced machine learning models: Future advancements should include the development of more sophisticated machine learning models integrating multiple aspects of antigen presentation and immune recognition. Deep learning approaches that can learn complex patterns from large datasets may offer improvements in predicting the immunogenicity of neoantigens beyond mere peptide-MHC binding and development of neoantigen-based therapies.

2. Incorporation of tumor microenvironment factors: Incorporating data from the tumor microenvironment, such as cytokine profiles, immune infiltration, and checkpoint expression, could enhance the prediction of neoantigen immunogenicity. Understanding the interaction between neoantigens and the tumor microenvironment will aid in prioritizing neoantigens that are more likely to elicit a robust immune response.

3. Expanding training datasets: To address the issue of HLA diversity, it is essential to expand training datasets to include a broader array of HLA types, particularly those that are less common globally. This expansion would improve the accuracy of the model and its applicability to diverse populations.

4. Integrative multiomics approaches: Future tools should aim to integrate multi-omics data, including genomics, transcriptomics, and proteomics, to provide a more holistic view of neoantigen presentation and potential immunogenicity. This integration will help in understanding the complex dynamics of cancer biology and immune responses.

5. Cloud-based platforms and real-time analysis: Developing cloud-based platforms that can perform real-time analysis of neoantigen predictions would significantly benefit clinical applications. Such platforms should be designed to handle large-scale data efficiently, providing accessible and rapid insights for personalized cancer immunotherapy.

7   Discussion and Conclusions

The prediction of neoantigens represents a cornerstone in the development of personalized cancer immunotherapies. It leverages the power of computational biology, genomics, and immunology to identify tumor-specific antigens that can be targeted by the immune system, offering a highly personalized approach to cancer treatment. The insights gained from this research area are critical in guiding the design of vaccines and cell-based therapies that have the potential to significantly improve patient outcomes.

Throughout this chapter, various computational methods and tools developed for neoantigen prediction have been explored. These tools have evolved from basic sequence alignment techniques to sophisticated machine learning models that predict peptide-MHC-binding affinities and assess immunogenic potential. The integration of deep learning has particularly enhanced the accuracy and predictive power of these tools, reflecting broader trends in biomedical research where advanced computational methods are increasingly pivotal.

However, despite these technological advancements, several challenges remain. The prediction of neoantigens still contends with issues such as high false positive rates, limited understanding of the immunogenicity landscape, and the need for better integration of comprehensive antigen processing pathways. Moreover, the diversity of HLA alleles presents a significant hurdle in achieving universally applicable prediction tools, necessitating ongoing efforts to expand and diversify the training datasets used in model development.

Looking forward, the field of neoantigen prediction is poised for transformative growth. Key areas for future improvement include the development of integrative multi-omics platforms that can provide a more complete picture of tumor immunogenicity and the microenvironmental factors influencing immune recognition. Additionally, the expansion of machine learning models to include more diverse data types and training sets will enhance the accuracy and applicability of predictions across different populations and cancer types.

Ultimately, the integration of neoantigen prediction into clinical practice promises to revolutionize cancer immunotherapy. By tailoring treatments to the specific immunogenic landscape of the tumor of each patient, neoantigen prediction paves the way for more effective and less toxic therapies. It holds the promise of turning the immune system into a precise tool for targeting cancer, fundamentally changing the way we approach cancer treatment and heralding a new era of precision oncology. As we continue to refine and improve computational methods for neoantigen prediction, we move closer to realizing the full potential of immunotherapy in providing durable and potent cancer treatments.

Acknowledgments

We would like to acknowledge, in memory of Sotiris, his early contributions to this work. His presence and spirit remain fondly remembered. This work has been supported by the Aragon Government (Group B29_23R), the Instituto de Salud Carlos III (ISCIII) grant PI22/01938, and by ASPANOA Foundation. This work is part of the CNS2022-136176 action, financed by MCIN/AEI/10.13039/501100011033 and for the European Union «Next Generation EU»/PRTR. This publication is based upon work from COST Action IMMUNO-model, CA21135, supported by COST (European Cooperation in Science and Technology).

References

1. Jhunjhunwala S, Hammer C, Delamarre L (2021) Antigen presentation in cancer: insights into tumour immunogenicity and immune evasion. Nat Rev Cancer 21:298–312. https://doi.org/10.1038/s41568-021-00339-z

2. Smith CC, Selitsky SR, Chai S et al (2019) Alternative tumour-specific antigens. Nat Rev Cancer 19:465–478. https://doi.org/10.1038/s41568-019-0162-4

3. Turajlic S, Litchfield K, Xu H et al (2017) Insertion-and-deletion-derived tumour-specific neoantigens and the immunogenic phenotype: a pan-cancer analysis. Lancet Oncol 18:1009–1021. https://doi.org/10.1016/S1470-2045(17)30516-8

4. Li J, Xiao Z, Wang D et al (2023) The screening, identification, design and clinical application of tumor-specific neoantigens for TCR-T cells. Mol Cancer 22:141. https://doi.org/10.1186/s12943-023-01844-5

5. Neefjes J, Jongsma MLM, Paul P, Bakke O (2011) Towards a systems understanding of MHC class I and MHC class II antigen presentation. Nat Rev Immunol 11:823–836. https://doi.org/10.1038/nri3084

6. Marty Pyke R, Thompson WK, Salem RM et al (2018) Evolutionary pressure against MHC class II binding cancer mutations. Cell 175:416–428.e13. https://doi.org/10.1016/j.cell.2018.08.048

7. Xie N, Shen G, Gao W et al (2023) Neoantigens: promising targets for cancer therapy. Signal Transduct Target Ther 8:9. https://doi.org/10.1038/s41392-022-01270-x

8. Méndez-Pérez A, Acosta-Moreno AM, Wert-Carvajal C et al (2023) Unraveling the power of NAP-CNB'S machine learning-enhanced tumor neoantigen prediction. Life 13:RP95010. https://doi.org/10.7554/eLife.95010.1

9. Wert-Carvajal C, Sánchez-García R, Macías JR et al (2021) Predicting MHC I restricted T cell epitopes in mice with NAP-CNB, a novel online tool. Sci Rep 11:10780. https://doi.org/10.1038/s41598-021-89927-5

10. Borden ES, Buetow KH, Wilson MA, Hastings KT (2022) Cancer neoantigens: challenges and future directions for prediction, prioritization, and validation. Front Oncol 12:836821. https://doi.org/10.3389/fonc.2022.836821

11. Griffith M, Miller CA, Griffith OL et al (2015) Optimizing cancer genome sequencing and analysis. Cell Syst 1:210–223. https://doi.org/10.1016/j.cels.2015.08.015

12. Bhagwate AV, Liu Y, Winham SJ et al (2019) Bioinformatics and DNA-extraction strategies to reliably detect genetic variants from FFPE breast tissue samples. BMC Genomics 20:689. https://doi.org/10.1186/s12864-019-6056-8

13. Holtsträter C, Schrörs B, Bukur T, Löwer M (2020) Bioinformatics for cancer immunotherapy. Methods Mol Biol 2120:1–9. https://doi.org/10.1007/978-1-0716-0327-7_1

14. Koboldt DC (2020) Best practices for variant calling in clinical sequencing. Genome Med 12:91. https://doi.org/10.1186/s13073-020-00791-w

15. Gfeller D, Guillaume P, Michaux J et al (2018) The length distribution and multiple specificity of naturally presented HLA-I ligands. J Immunol 201:3705–3716. https://doi.org/10.4049/jimmunol.1800914

16. Osterbye T, Nielsen M, Dudek NL et al (2020) HLA class II specificity assessed by high-density peptide microarray interactions. J Immunol 205:290–299. https://doi.org/10.4049/jimmunol.2000224

17. Saha I, Mazzocco G, Plewczynski D (2013) Consensus classification of human leukocyte antigen class II proteins. Immunogenetics 65:97–105. https://doi.org/10.1007/s00251-012-0665-6

18. Saxová P, Buus S, Brunak S, Keşmir C (2003) Predicting proteasomal cleavage sites: a comparison of available methods. Int Immunol 15:781–787. https://doi.org/10.1093/intimm/dxg084

19. Stranzl T, Larsen MV, Lundegaard C, Nielsen M (2010) NetCTLpan: pan-specific MHC class I pathway epitope predictions. Immunogenetics 62:357–368. https://doi.org/10.1007/s00251-010-0441-4

20. Baxter-Lowe LA (2021) The changing landscape of HLA typing: understanding how and when HLA typing data can be used with confidence from bench to bedside. Hum Immunol 82:466–477. https://doi.org/10.1016/j.humimm.2021.04.011

21. Barker DJ, Maccari G, Georgiou X et al (2023) The IPD-IMGT/HLA database. Nucleic Acids Res 51:D1053–D1060. https://doi.org/10.1093/nar/gkac1011

22. Reynisson B, Alvarez B, Paul S et al (2020) NetMHCpan-4.1 and NetMHCIIpan-4.0: improved predictions of MHC antigen presentation by concurrent motif deconvolution and integration of MS MHC eluted ligand data. Nucleic Acids Res 48:W449–W454. https://doi.org/10.1093/nar/gkaa379

23. O'Donnell TJ, Rubinsteyn A, Laserson U (2020) MHCflurry 2.0: improved pan-allele prediction of MHC class I-presented peptides by incorporating antigen processing. Cell Syst 11:42–48.e7. https://doi.org/10.1016/j.cels.2020.06.010

24. Vita R, Mahajan S, Overton JA et al (2019) The immune epitope database (IEDB): 2018 update. Nucleic Acids Res 47:D339–D343. https://doi.org/10.1093/nar/gky1006

25. Lundegaard C, Lamberth K, Harndahl M et al (2008) NetMHC-3.0: accurate web accessible predictions of human, mouse and monkey

MHC class I affinities for peptides of length 8-11. Nucleic Acids Res 36:W509–W512. https://doi.org/10.1093/nar/gkn202

26. Hellman LM, Yin L, Wang Y et al (2016) Differential scanning fluorimetry based assessments of the thermal and kinetic stability of peptide-MHC complexes. J Immunol Methods 432:95–101. https://doi.org/10.1016/j.jim.2016.02.016

27. Blaha DT, Anderson SD, Yoakum DM et al (2019) High-throughput stability screening of neoantigen/HLA complexes improves immunogenicity predictions. Cancer Immunol Res 7:50–61. https://doi.org/10.1158/2326-6066.CIR-18-0395

28. Zhang H, Lund O, Nielsen M (2009) The PickPocket method for predicting binding specificities for receptors based on receptor pocket similarities: application to MHC-peptide binding. Bioinforma 25:1293–1299. https://doi.org/10.1093/bioinformatics/btp137

29. Paul S, Grifoni A, Peters B, Sette A (2019) Major histocompatibility complex binding, eluted ligands, and immunogenicity: benchmark testing and predictions. Front Immunol 10:3151. https://doi.org/10.3389/fimmu.2019.03151

30. Gfeller D, Bassani-Sternberg M (2018) Predicting antigen presentation-what could we learn from a million peptides? Front Immunol 9:1716. https://doi.org/10.3389/fimmu.2018.01716

31. Marrer-Berger E, Nicastri A, Augustin A et al (2024) The physiological interactome of TCR-like antibody therapeutics in human tissues. Nat Commun 15:3271. https://doi.org/10.1038/s41467-024-47062-5

32. Zvyagin IV, Tsvetkov VO, Chudakov DM, Shugay M (2020) An overview of immunoinformatics approaches and databases linking T cell receptor repertoires to their antigen specificity. Immunogenetics 72:77–84. https://doi.org/10.1007/s00251-019-01139-4

33. Ji H, Wang X-X, Zhang Q et al (2024) Predicting TCR sequences for unseen antigen epitopes using structural and sequence features. Brief Bioinform 25:bbae210. https://doi.org/10.1093/bib/bbae210

34. Roudko V, Greenbaum B, Bhardwaj N (2020) Computational prediction and validation of tumor-associated neoantigens. Front Immunol 11:27. https://doi.org/10.3389/fimmu.2020.00027

35. Shah RK, Cygan E, Kozlik T et al (2023) Utilizing immunogenomic approaches to prioritize targetable neoantigens for personalized cancer immunotherapy. Front Immunol 14:1301100. https://doi.org/10.3389/fimmu.2023.1301100

36. Martin MV, Aguilar-Rosas S, Franke K et al (2024) The neo-open reading frame peptides that comprise the tumor framome are a rich source of neoantigens for cancer immunotherapy. Cancer Immunol Res 12:759. https://doi.org/10.1158/2326-6066.CIR-23-0158

37. Rasmussen M, Fenoy E, Harndahl M et al (2016) Pan-specific prediction of peptide-MHC class I complex stability, a correlate of T cell immunogenicity. J Immunol 197:1517–1524. https://doi.org/10.4049/jimmunol.1600582

38. Nielsen M, Lundegaard C, Lund O, Keşmir C (2005) The role of the proteasome in generating cytotoxic T-cell epitopes: insights obtained from improved predictions of proteasomal cleavage. Immunogenetics 57:33–41. https://doi.org/10.1007/s00251-005-0781-7

39. Peters B, Bulik S, Tampe R et al (2003) Identifying MHC class I epitopes by predicting the TAP transport efficiency of epitope precursors. J Immunol 171:1741–1749. https://doi.org/10.4049/jimmunol.171.4.1741

40. Zhao W, Sher X (2018) Systematically benchmarking peptide-MHC binding predictors: from synthetic to naturally processed epitopes. PLoS Comput Biol 14:e1006457. https://doi.org/10.1371/journal.pcbi.1006457

41. García-Mulero S, Fornelino R, Punta M et al (2023) Driver mutations in GNAQ and GNA11 genes as potential targets for precision immunotherapy in uveal melanoma patients. Onco Targets Ther 12:2261278. https://doi.org/10.1080/2162402X.2023.2261278

42. Ragone C, Cavalluzzo B, Mauriello A et al (2024) Lack of shared neoantigens in prevalent mutations in cancer. J Transl Med 22:344. https://doi.org/10.1186/s12967-024-05110-0

43. Hsiue EH-C, Wright KM, Douglass J et al (2021) Targeting a neoantigen derived from a common *TP53* mutation. Science 371:eabc8697. https://doi.org/10.1126/science.abc8697

44. Hoyos D, Zappasodi R, Schulze I et al (2022) Fundamental immune–oncogenicity trade-offs define driver mutation fitness. Nature 606:172–179. https://doi.org/10.1038/s41586-022-04696-z

45. Choi J, Goulding SP, Conn BP et al (2021) Systematic discovery and validation of T cell targets directed against oncogenic KRAS mutations. Cell Rep Methods 1:100084. https://doi.org/10.1016/j.crmeth.2021.100084

46. Hartmaier RJ, Charo J, Fabrizio D et al (2017) Genomic analysis of 63,220 tumors reveals insights into tumor uniqueness and targeted cancer immunotherapy strategies. Genome

Med 9:16. https://doi.org/10.1186/s13073-017-0408-2

47. Bais P, Namburi S, Gatti DM et al (2017) CloudNeo: a cloud pipeline for identifying patient-specific tumor neoantigens. Bioinforma 33:3110–3112. https://doi.org/10.1093/bioinformatics/btx375

48. McLaren W, Gil L, Hunt SE et al (2016) The Ensembl variant effect predictor. Genome Biol 17:122. https://doi.org/10.1186/s13059-016-0974-4

49. Warren RL, Choe G, Freeman DJ et al (2012) Derivation of HLA types from shotgun sequence datasets. Genome Med 4:95. https://doi.org/10.1186/gm396

50. Shukla SA, Rooney MS, Rajasagi M et al (2015) Comprehensive analysis of cancer-associated somatic mutations in class I HLA genes. Nat Biotechnol 33:1152–1158. https://doi.org/10.1038/nbt.3344

51. Nielsen M, Andreatta M (2016) NetMHCpan-3.0; improved prediction of binding to MHC class I molecules integrating information from multiple receptor and peptide length datasets. Genome Med 8:33. https://doi.org/10.1186/s13073-016-0288-x

52. Richman LP, Vonderheide RH, Rech AJ (2019) Neoantigen dissimilarity to the self-proteome predicts immunogenicity and response to immune checkpoint blockade. Cell Syst 9:375–382.e4. https://doi.org/10.1016/j.cels.2019.08.009

53. Fotakis G, Rieder D, Haider M et al (2020) NeoFuse: predicting fusion neoantigens from RNA sequencing data. Bioinforma 36:2260–2261. https://doi.org/10.1093/bioinformatics/btz879

54. Szolek A, Schubert B, Mohr C et al (2014) OptiType: precision HLA typing from next-generation sequencing data. Bioinforma 30:3310–3316. https://doi.org/10.1093/bioinformatics/btu548

55. Uhrig S, Ellermann J, Walther T et al (2021) Accurate and efficient detection of gene fusions from RNA sequencing data. Genome Res 31:448–460. https://doi.org/10.1101/gr.257246.119

56. O'Donnell TJ, Rubinsteyn A, Bonsack M et al (2018) MHCflurry: open-source class I MHC binding affinity prediction. Cell Syst 7:129–132.e4. https://doi.org/10.1016/j.cels.2018.05.014

57. Dobin A, Davis CA, Schlesinger F et al (2013) STAR: ultrafast universal RNA-seq aligner. Bioinforma 29:15–21. https://doi.org/10.1093/bioinformatics/bts635

58. Liao Y, Smyth GK, Shi W (2014) featureCounts: an efficient general purpose program for assigning sequence reads to genomic features. Bioinforma 30:923–930. https://doi.org/10.1093/bioinformatics/btt656

59. Wu J, Wang W, Zhang J et al (2019) DeepHLApan: a deep learning approach for neoantigen prediction considering both HLA-peptide binding and immunogenicity. Front Immunol 10:2559. https://doi.org/10.3389/fimmu.2019.02559

60. Hundal J, Kiwala S, Feng Y-Y et al (2019) Accounting for proximal variants improves neoantigen prediction. Nat Genet 51:175–179. https://doi.org/10.1038/s41588-018-0283-9

61. Hundal J, Kiwala S, McMichael J et al (2020) pVACtools: a computational toolkit to identify and visualize cancer Neoantigens. Cancer Immunol Res 8:409–420. https://doi.org/10.1158/2326-6066.CIR-19-0401

62. Hundal J, Carreno BM, Petti AA et al (2016) pVAC-Seq: a genome-guided in silico approach to identifying tumor neoantigens. Genome Med 8:11. https://doi.org/10.1186/s13073-016-0264-5

63. Rieder D, Fotakis G, Ausserhofer M et al (2022) nextNEOpi: a comprehensive pipeline for computational neoantigen prediction. Bioinforma 38:1131–1132. https://doi.org/10.1093/bioinformatics/btab759

64. Kawaguchi S, Higasa K, Shimizu M et al (2017) HLA-HD: an accurate HLA typing algorithm for next-generation sequencing data. Hum Mutat 38:788–797. https://doi.org/10.1002/humu.23230

65. Jurtz V, Paul S, Andreatta M et al (2017) NetMHCpan-4.0: improved peptide-MHC class I interaction predictions integrating eluted ligand and peptide binding affinity data. J Immunol 199:3360–3368. https://doi.org/10.4049/jimmunol.1700893

66. Racle J, Michaux J, Rockinger GA et al (2019) Robust prediction of HLA class II epitopes by deep motif deconvolution of immunopeptidomes. Nat Biotechnol 37:1283–1286. https://doi.org/10.1038/s41587-019-0289-6

67. Bolotin DA, Poslavsky S, Mitrophanov I et al (2015) MiXCR: software for comprehensive adaptive immunity profiling. Nat Methods 12:380–381. https://doi.org/10.1038/nmeth.3364

68. Chai S, Smith CC, Kochar TK et al (2022) NeoSplice: a bioinformatics method for prediction of splice variant neoantigens. Bioinforma Adv 2:vbac032. https://doi.org/10.1093/bioadv/vbac032

69. Diao K, Chen J, Wu T et al (2022) Seq2Neo: a comprehensive pipeline for cancer Neoantigen immunogenicity prediction. Int J Mol Sci 23: 11624. https://doi.org/10.3390/ijms231911624

70. Chen Z, Yuan Y, Chen X et al (2020) Systematic comparison of somatic variant calling performance among different sequencing depth and mutation frequency. Sci Rep 10:3501. https://doi.org/10.1038/s41598-020-60559-5

71. Haas BJ, Dobin A, Li B et al (2019) Accuracy assessment of fusion transcript detection via read-mapping and de novo fusion transcript assembly-based methods. Genome Biol 20: 213. https://doi.org/10.1186/s13059-019-1842-9

72. Wang K, Li M, Hakonarson H (2010) ANNOVAR: functional annotation of genetic variants from high-throughput sequencing data. Nucleic Acids Res 38:e164. https://doi.org/10.1093/nar/gkq603

73. Murphy C, Elemento O (2016) AGFusion: annotate and visualize gene fusions. bioRxiv. https://doi.org/10.1101/080903

74. Vera Alvarez R, Pongor LS, Mariño-Ramírez L, Landsman D (2019) TPMCalculator: one-step software to quantify mRNA abundance of genomic features. Bioinforma 35:1960–1962. https://doi.org/10.1093/bioinformatics/bty896

75. Tan X, Xu L, Jian X et al (2023) PGNneo: a proteogenomics-based neoantigen prediction pipeline in noncoding regions. Cells 12:782. https://doi.org/10.3390/cells12050782

76. Ma W, Zhang J, Yao H (2024) NeoMUST: an accurate and efficient multi-task learning model for neoantigen presentation. Life Sci Alliance 7:e202302255. https://doi.org/10.26508/lsa.202302255

77. Chuwdhury GS, Guo Y, Chiang C-L et al (2024) ImmuneMirror: a machine learning-based integrative pipeline and web server for neoantigen prediction. Brief Bioinform 25:

bbae024. https://doi.org/10.1093/bib/bbae024

78. Jeong H, Cho Y-R, Gim J et al (2024) GraphMHC: Neoantigen prediction model applying the graph neural network to molecular structure. PLoS One 19:e0291223. https://doi.org/10.1371/journal.pone.0291223

79. Wan J, Liu W, Xu Q et al (2006) SVRMHC prediction server for MHC-binding peptides. BMC Bioinform 7:463. https://doi.org/10.1186/1471-2105-7-463

80. Reche PA, Reinherz EL (2007) Prediction of peptide-MHC binding using profiles. Methods Mol Biol 409:185–200. https://doi.org/10.1007/978-1-60327-118-9_13

81. DeVette CI, Andreatta M, Bardet W et al (2018) NetH2pan: a computational tool to guide MHC peptide prediction on murine tumors. Cancer Immunol Res 6:636–644. https://doi.org/10.1158/2326-6066.CIR-17-0298

82. Duan F, Duitama J, Al Seesi S et al (2014) Genomic and bioinformatic profiling of mutational neoepitopes reveals new rules to predict anticancer immunogenicity. J Exp Med 211: 2231–2248. https://doi.org/10.1084/jem.20141308

83. Kim JY, Bang H, Noh S-J, Choi JK (2023) DeepNeo: a webserver for predicting immunogenic neoantigens. Nucleic Acids Res 51: W134–W140. https://doi.org/10.1093/nar/gkad275

84. Li B, Jing P, Zheng G et al (2023) Neo-intline: integrated pipeline enables neoantigen design through the in-silico presentation of T-cell epitope. Signal Transduct Target Ther 8:397. https://doi.org/10.1038/s41392-023-01644-9

85. DeVette CI, Gundlapalli H, Lai S-CA et al (2020) A pipeline for identification and validation of tumor-specific antigens in a mouse model of metastatic breast cancer. Onco Targets Ther 9:1685300. https://doi.org/10.1080/2162402X.2019.1685300

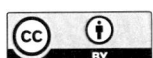

Chapter 18

Bioinformatics Analysis of Transcriptomic Data (Bulk and scRNA-Seq) for Immuno-Oncology

Mai Hanh Nguyen and Nguyen Quoc Khanh Le

Abstract

Bioinformatics plays a pivotal role in immunology by enabling the analysis of large-scale datasets generated from high-throughput technologies, such as next-generation sequencing (NGS), single-cell RNA sequencing (scRNA-seq), and mass cytometry. These methods provide deep insights into immune system dynamics, helping to decode immune cell heterogeneity, gene expression patterns, and immune receptor repertoires. Key bioinformatics approaches include transcriptomic analysis to identify immune-related gene signatures, single-cell sequencing tools for profiling immune cell states, immune repertoire analysis to understand T-cell and B-cell diversity, and multiomics integration to uncover regulatory networks. By leveraging these methods, researchers can better understand immune responses in health and disease, identify therapeutic targets, and develop precision immunotherapies. This chapter will offer a comprehensive guide to the essential bioinformatics tools and techniques used in immunological research, facilitating effective data analysis and interpretation.

Key words Bioinformatics, Immunology, Transcriptomic, Oncology, Immunotherapy

1 Introduction

Bioinformatics has emerged as a cornerstone in the field of immuno-oncology, providing the computational frameworks necessary to analyze and interpret vast amounts of biological data [1]. As cancer therapies increasingly focus on leveraging the immune system to target tumors, understanding the complex interactions between immune cells and cancer cells has become critical. Bioinformatics bridges this gap by enabling the integration and analysis of multidimensional datasets, shedding light on the molecular mechanisms of immune responses within the tumor microenvironment. It is used to identify immune-related biomarkers [2, 3], map the immune landscape within tumors [4], and predict patient responses to immunotherapies such as immune checkpoint inhibitors [5, 6]. By integrating multiomics data, including genomic, transcriptomic, and proteomic datasets, bioinformatics helps to

Sweta Rani and Lukasz Skalniak (eds.), *IMMUNO-model in Cancer: Methods and Protocols*, Methods in Molecular Biology, vol. 2959, https://doi.org/10.1007/978-1-0716-4734-9_18, © The Author(s) 2026

reveal the mechanisms of immune evasion and tumor-immune interactions. Furthermore, it enables the identification of novel therapeutic targets, supports the design of personalized immunotherapies, and enhances our understanding of tumor heterogeneity and immune infiltration.

This chapter will provide an overview of key bioinformatics methods that are applied in immunological studies, with a focus on their role in high-throughput data analysis, immune cell profiling, functional genomics, and the integration of multi-omics datasets (Fig. 1). By understanding these methods, researchers can gain a deeper insight into immune system dynamics and their implications for disease development and therapy.

2   Materials

1. Fresh, frozen, or formalin-fixed paraffin-embedded (FFPE) tumor tissue from patients or experimental models.

2. RNAlater (for fresh tissues) or access to a −80 °C freezer (for frozen tissue storage).

3. RNA isolation kit.

4. RNase-free pipette tips, tubes, and other consumables to prevent RNA degradation.

5. Spectrophotometer to measure RNA concentration.

6. Agilent Bioanalyzer or TapeStation for assessing RNA Integrity Number (RIN) and RNA quality.

7. Poly(A) enrichment or rRNA depletion kits for bulk RNA-seq library preparation.

8. Reverse transcription kit and reverse transcriptase enzymes for cDNA synthesis.

9. PCR reagents and thermal cycler for library amplification.

10. Agilent Bioanalyzer or equivalent tool to check library size distribution and adapter ligation.

11. Access to a high-throughput sequencing platform.

12. Software for alignment, quantification and normalization.

13. A robust computing environment with adequate CPU, GPU, RAM, and storage capacity to handle large transcriptomic datasets.

3   Methods

Step 1: Tissue Collection and RNA Extraction

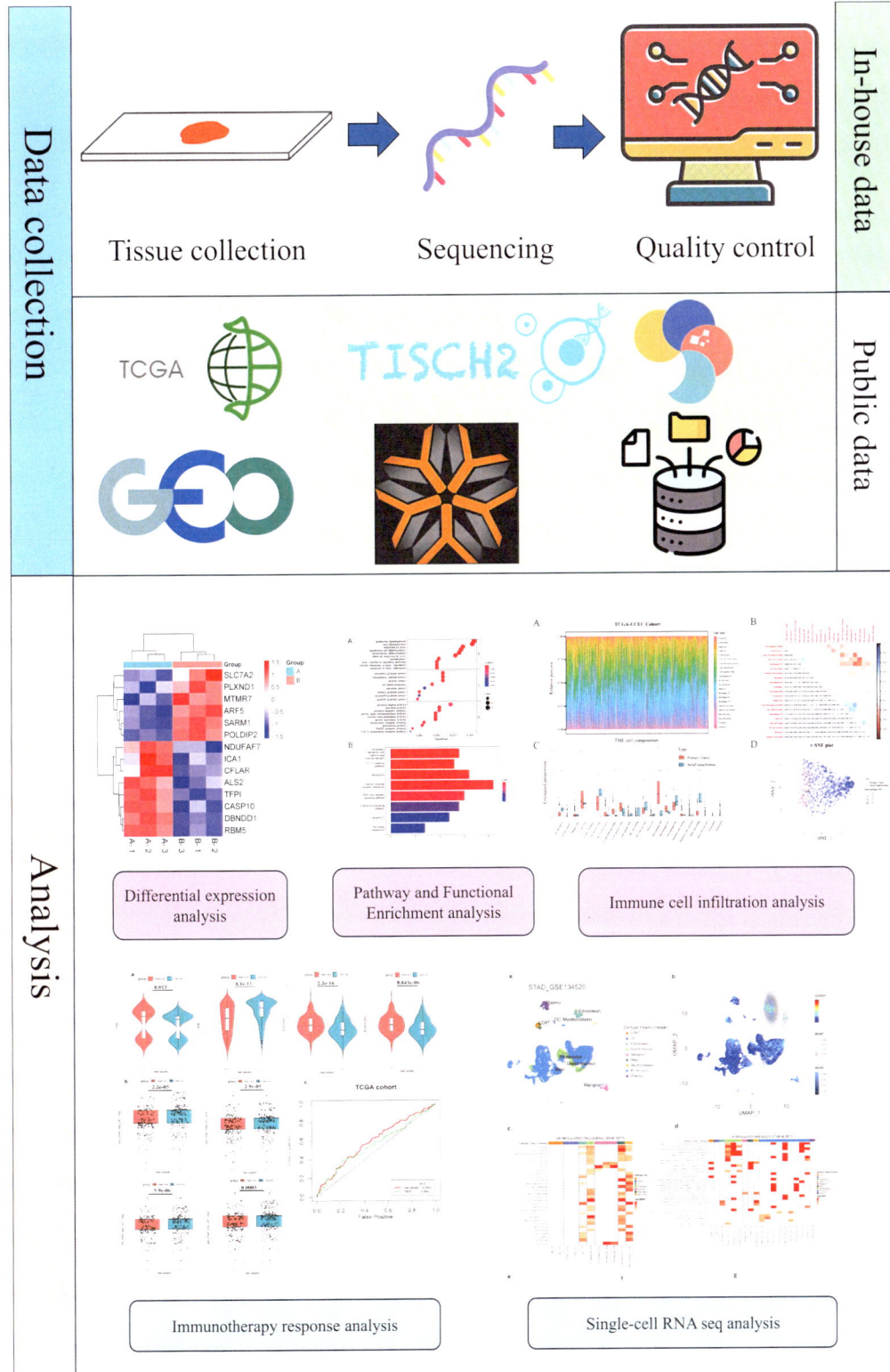

Fig. 1 Workflow of bioinformatics analysis of transcriptomic data for immuno-oncology

3.1 Data Collection

3.1.1 In-House Data Collection

1. Collect tumor tissue samples:
   - Collect fresh, frozen, or formalin-fixed paraffin-embedded (FFPE) tumor tissues from patients or experimental models (*see* **Note 1**).

2. Isolate RNA:
   - Extract total RNA from the tumor tissue using an appropriate RNA isolation kit (e.g., TRIzol or column-based methods).
   - Measure RNA concentration and quality using a spectrophotometer (e.g., Nanodrop) and check RNA integrity using an Agilent Bioanalyzer or Tape Station. High-quality RNA should have an RNA Integrity Number (RIN) above 7.

Step 2: Library Preparation

3. Prepare cDNA library:
   - For bulk RNA-seq, the extracted RNA is typically poly(A)-enriched (to select for mRNA) or rRNA-depleted (to remove ribosomal RNA) using commercial kits (*see* **Note 2**).
   - Reverse-transcribe the mRNA into complementary DNA (cDNA) using reverse transcriptase enzymes.

4. Fragmentation and adapter ligation:
   - Fragment the cDNA into smaller pieces (around 200–300 bp) for sequencing.
   - Add sequencing adaptors to both ends of the cDNA fragments to allow their binding to the sequencing platform. Indexes or barcodes are also added to allow multiplexing of multiple samples in a single sequencing run.

5. Amplification:
   - Amplify the cDNA library using PCR to ensure sufficient material for sequencing.
   - Perform quality control checks on the library using an Agilent Bioanalyzer or similar tool to confirm proper size distribution and adapter ligation.

Step 3: Sequencing

6. Select sequencing platform:
   - Use a high-throughput sequencing platform such as Illumina NovaSeq or HiSeq for paired-end sequencing, depending on the required depth and coverage.

7. Set the sequencing parameters:

- For typical bulk RNA-seq experiments, aim for a sequencing depth of 30–50 million reads per sample to obtain sufficient coverage of the transcriptome.

8. Perform sequencing:

- Run the sequencing experiment. Once completed, confirm that the quality control metrics (e.g., Q30 score, duplication rate) meet the required thresholds before moving to the bioinformatics analysis (*see* **Note 3**).

Step 4: Data preprocessing

9. Quality control of raw sequencing data:

- Check the quality of the raw sequencing reads using tools like FastQC. This step includes assessing parameters such as:
  - Per base quality scores.
  - GC content.
  - Adapter contamination.
  - Read length distribution.

10. Trimming of low-quality reads and adapters:

- Use a tool like Trimmomatic or Cutadapt to remove low-quality bases and any residual adapter sequences from the reads. This ensures that only high-quality data is used for downstream analysis (*see* **Note 4**).

Step 5: Alignment to reference genome

11. Align reads to the reference genome:

- Map the cleaned reads to a reference genome (e.g., GRCh38 for humans) using alignment tools such as STAR or HISAT2. This step aligns each read to its corresponding location on the genome.

12. Generate BAM files:

- The aligned reads are saved in BAM (binary alignment map) format, which contains both the sequence information and the genomic coordinates.

13. Assess alignment quality:

- Use tools like Samtools or Picard to assess alignment quality metrics, such as the percentage of mapped reads, number of uniquely mapped reads, and presence of duplicates (*see* **Note 5**).

Step 6: Transcript quantification

14. Quantify gene expression:
   - Count the number of reads mapped to each gene using tools such as Feature Counts or HTSeq. This generates a gene expression matrix, where each entry corresponds to the number of reads aligned to a particular gene in a sample (*see* **Note 6**).

15. Normalize gene expression:
   - Normalize the raw read counts to account for sequencing depth and library size differences between samples. Common normalization methods include FPKM (fragments per kilobase of transcript per million mapped reads), TPM (transcripts per million), or DESeq2's size factor normalization (*see* **Note 7**).

3.1.2 Public Data Collection

There are many public databases for transcriptomic, the following database are commonly used:

1. TCGA database: comprehensive public database that provides multiomics data across over 30 cancer types, encompassing genomic, transcriptomic, epigenomic, and proteomic profiles that enables researchers to investigate the molecular basis of cancer, facilitating insights into tumor heterogeneity, identifying biomarkers, and supporting precision oncology [7].
   - Access the data portal https://portal.gdc.cancer.gov/, choose the organ and the project of interest (*see* **Note 8**).
   - Download the manifest file with the GDC data transfer tool.
   - Or use the "TCGA biolinks" R package [8] to download the data.

2. GEO: a public repository for high-throughput gene expression data that contains a vast array of datasets, including transcriptomic, epigenomic, and proteomic data from diverse organisms, supporting studies in gene expression and molecular biology [9].
   - Access the portal https://www.ncbi.nlm.nih.gov/geo.
   - Use the search bar at the top to search for the transcriptomic data such as datasets, experiments, or specific terms.
   - Clicking on an accession number (e.g., GSE or GDS) to access the dataset's page, where providing details about the study, including the types of data available, number of samples, and platform used.
   - Scroll down to the "Series Matrix File(s)" section.
   - Under the "Series Matrix File(s)" section, click the download link for the matrix file. This file usually contains expression data for all samples in a matrix format (e.g., .txt or .csv).

- Or using "GEOquery" R package [10] to download the data.

3. ImmPort database: a publicly available resource for sharing immunological data funded by the NIH. It provides access to datasets on immune responses, diseases, and treatments, helping researchers analyze and accelerate discoveries in immunology [11].

   - Visit the ImmPort website: https://www.immport.org/shared/home.

   - Browse through the search results and click on a study or gene list of interest.

   - Click on the "Download" button next to the specific data file or type of data that interested.

4. TISCH (tumor immune single-cell hub): a database specifically for single-cell RNA-seq data, focusing on tumor microenvironments, including immune and nonimmune cells [12].

   - Visit the TISCH website http://tisch.comp-genomics.org/ .

   - Click on "Datasets" to browse the available single-cell RNA-seq datasets.

5. CancerSEA: CancerSEA is a database that focuses on single-cell functional states in cancer, providing data related to different functional states such as proliferation, metastasis, differentiation for various cancer types [13].

   - Visit the CancerSEA website http://biocc.hrbmu.edu.cn/CancerSEA/.

   - In the search bar, you can input keywords related to a specific cancer type, functional state, or gene of interest.

   - Scroll down to the "Data Download" section, click on the corresponding Download links to download the data files.

3.2 Differential Expression Analysis

- Filter out lowly expressed genes.
- Use tools such as DESeq2, edgeR, or limma-voom to perform differential expression analysis (*see* **Note 9**):

   - DESeq2: Uses a negative binomial distribution to model count data and find differentially expressed genes (DEGs) [13].

   - edgeR: Another popular tool for RNA-seq differential expression based on count data [14].

   - limma-voom: Uses linear models and precision weights for RNA-seq data [15].

- Apply false discovery rate (FDR) correction to control for multiple testing and report significant genes using the corrected p-values (e.g., FDR < 0.05).

• Visualize DEGs: Create a volcano plot to visualize DEGs. Using "ggplot2" or "EnhancedVolcano" R package to highlight significant genes by fold change and adjusted p value.

• Create heatmaps of expression data: Use "pheatmap" or "ComplexHeatmap" R packages to generate heatmaps of normalized gene expression data. Include the most highly variable genes or DEGs for visualization.

3.3   Pathway and Functional Enrichment Analysis

The first step in pathway and functional enrichment analysis is to identify DEGs from the dataset. These DEGs represent genes that show statistically significant changes in expression between conditions, such as treated vs. control groups. Once identified, these gene sets form the basis for downstream functional and pathway analysis to uncover the biological relevance of the observed changes in gene expression (see Subheading 3.2).

3.3.1   Identify Gene Sets for Enrichment

3.3.2   Perform Pathway Enrichment

Use tools such as GSEA (gene set enrichment analysis), DAVID, or enrich to perform pathway enrichment analysis:

- Input the DEGs into enrichment analysis tools to find overrepresented biological pathways or molecular functions:

• GSEA (gene set enrichment analysis):

- GSEA does not require a predefined set of DEGs, but instead ranks all genes based on their differential expression and looks for coordinated expression changes in predefined gene sets.

- It calculates an enrichment score that reflects whether genes from a particular pathway or function are mostly over- or underrepresented at the top or bottom of the ranked gene list [16].

• DAVID (database for annotation, visualization, and integrated discovery):

- DAVID takes a list of DEGs and maps them to pathways or functions using various annotation sources, such as GO and KEGG. It performs overrepresentation analysis to identify pathways that contain more DEGs than expected by chance [17].

- The tool also provides visualization options, including functional clustering and heatmaps, to aid in interpreting the results.

• EnrichR:

- EnrichR is a web-based tool that simplifies the process of functional enrichment by allowing users to input gene sets and retrieve results from multiple databases like KEGG, Reactome, and GO. It provides ranked enrichment terms based on a variety of statistical metrics, helping users identify the most relevant pathways and processes [18].

- Use pathway databases such as:
  - KEGG: (Kyoto Encyclopedia of Genes and Genomes): A resource for understanding high-level biological functions, pathways, and utilities of cells, organisms, and ecosystems [19].

  - GO (Gene Ontology): Provides structured vocabularies for annotating gene products across three categories- biological processes, molecular functions, and cellular components [20].

  - Reactome: A curated database of pathways and reactions in human biology, providing insights into molecular interactions and biological processes [21].

- Plot pathway enrichment results: Use bar plots or bubble plots to visualize enriched pathways from your gene set enrichment analysis. Tools like "ggplot2" R package can be used to create informative visualizations.

3.4 Analyzing Tumor-Immune Interactions

- Use tools like CIBERSORT, EPIC, or xCell to estimate the proportions of different immune cell types in the tumor microenvironment based on the gene expression matrix.

  - CIBERSORT: Uses known immune cell gene signatures to infer immune cell types and quantities [22].

  - EPIC: Estimates the proportions of tumor, immune, and stromal cell types in solid tumors [23].

  - xCell: Provides enrichment scores for a variety of immune and stromal cell types in tissue samples [24].

- Visualize immune cell composition: Create bar plots or heatmaps using "ggplot2" or "pheatmap" R packages to display the estimated immune cell fractions across samples.

- Analyze how immune infiltration differs between different groups, such as responders vs. nonresponders to immunotherapy.

3.5 Predicting Immunotherapy Response

3.5.1 Calculate Immune Scores

- Calculate immune scores such as immunophenoscore (IPS) or tumor immune dysfunction and exclusion (TIDE) to predict the likelihood of a patient's response to immune checkpoint inhibitors.

  – TIDE: Predicts immunotherapy response by modeling two mechanisms of immune evasion (T-cell dysfunction and T-cell exclusion) [25]. Access http://tide.dfci.atherard.edu/ to get the TIDE score.

  – IPS: A scoring system that integrates multiple immune-related parameters to predict sensitivity to immunotherapy [26]. The IPS score were sourced from The Cancer Immunome Atlas (TCIA) https://tcia.at/home/.

3.5.2 Evaluate Tumor Mutational Burden

- TMB is a measure of the total number of mutations per mega base in a tumor's DNA, often used as a biomarker to predict response to immunotherapies [27].

- Higher TMB is often associated with better responses to immune checkpoint blockade therapies.

  – Download the MAF (Mutation annotation format).

  – Calculate TMB using the "Maftools" R package.

3.6 Single-Cell RNA-Seq Analysis

3.6.1 Dimensionality Reduction

- Perform principal component analysis (PCA):

  – Use PCA to reduce the dimensionality of the gene expression data. Select the top principal components (PCs) that explain the most variation in the dataset. This step helps prepare the data for clustering and visualization (*see* **Note 10**).

- Apply nonlinear dimensionality reduction:

  – Use t-SNE (t-distributed stochastic neighbor embedding) or UMAP (uniform manifold approximation and projection) to visualize the high-dimensional data in 2D or 3D space (*see* **Note 11**).

  – Each point in the plot represents a single cell, with cells grouped based on gene expression similarities.

3.6.2 Clustering of Cells

- Cluster cells based on gene expression:

  – Use clustering algorithms such as Louvain, Leiden, or K-means to group cells into distinct clusters based on their gene expression profiles.

  – Each cluster is expected to represent a specific cell population or cell state.

- Visualize cell clusters:
  - Use UMAP or t-SNE plots to visualize how the clusters of cells are grouped. Colors can be used to differentiate between clusters in the plot.

3.6.3 Identification of Cell Types

- Identify marker genes for each cluster:
  - Perform differential gene expression analysis to find marker genes that are uniquely expressed in each cell cluster.
  - Use tools like Seurat or Scanpy to find genes that are significantly upregulated in each cluster compared to others.
- Annotate cell types:
  - Based on the marker genes identified for each cluster, annotate the clusters with known cell types (e.g., T-cells, B-cells, macrophages) by comparing them to known marker gene lists from the literature or public databases (*see* **Note 12**).

4   Notes

1. Ensure samples are handled under appropriate conditions to maintain RNA integrity (use RNAlater for fresh tissues or store at −80 °C if using frozen tissues).
2. Ensure efficient poly(A) enrichment or rRNA depletion for accurate mRNA representation.
3. Monitor sequencing run progress to quickly identify and troubleshoot any potential quality issues.
4. Adjust trimming parameters if excessive adapter content or low-quality bases are detected.
5. Choose alignment parameters carefully to maximize mapping accuracy, particularly for unique reads and review alignment quality metrics before proceeding to ensure sufficient data coverage.
6. Optionally, use a pseudo-alignment tool like Salmon or Kallisto for faster transcript quantification without the need for full alignment.
7. Check normalization outcomes to ensure they align with the intended comparative analyses.
8. If the TCGA dataset is small enough, download directly from the portal by clicking the download button.
9. Normalize the data again if necessary, using methods specific to your chosen differential expression tool.

10. Select the most informative principal components from PCA to capture primary data variation, preparing it for more precise clustering. Adjust the number of PCs based on explained variance and dataset complexity.

11. Choose between t-SNE and UMAP for visualizing cell relationships in a simplified 2D/3D space. UMAP is often favored for preserving global structure, while t-SNE emphasizes local similarities.

12. Use marker gene profiles to classify clusters into known cell types, referencing reliable marker databases or literature to ensure accurate annotations.

Acknowledgments

This publication is based upon work from COST Action IMMUNO-model, CA21135, supported by COST (European Cooperation in Science and Technology). It was also supported by the National Science and Technology Council, Taiwan [grant number MOST111–2628-E-038-002-MY3].

References

1. Holträter C, Schrörs B, Bukur T, Löwer M (2020) Bioinformatics for cancer immunotherapy: methods and protocols, pp 1–9

2. Xiao Y, Yu X, Wang Y, Song G, Liu M, Wang D, Wang H (2024) A novel immune-related gene signature for diagnosis and potential immunotherapy of microsatellite stable endometrial carcinoma. Sci Rep 14(1):3738

3. Mei J, Xing Y, Lv J, Gu D, Pan J, Zhang Y, Liu J (2020) Construction of an immune-related gene signature for prediction of prognosis in patients with cervical cancer. Int Immunopharmacol 88:106882

4. Zhou J, Shi S, Qiu Y, Jin Z, Yu W, Xie R, Zhang H (2023) Integrative bioinformatics approaches to establish potential prognostic immune-related genes signature and drugs in the non-small cell lung cancer microenvironment. Front Pharmacol 14:1153565

5. Jiang Y, Hammad B, Huang H, Zhang C, Xiao B, Liu L, Liu Q, Liang H, Zhao Z, Gao Y (2024) Bioinformatics analysis of an immunotherapy responsiveness-related gene signature in predicting lung adenocarcinoma prognosis. Transl Lung Cancer Res 13(6): 1277

6. Xu Q, Cao D, Fang B, Yan S, Hu Y, Guo T (2022) Immune-related gene signature predicts clinical outcomes and immunotherapy

response in acute myeloid leukemia. Cancer Med 11(17):3364–3380

7. Tomczak K, Czerwińska P, Wiznerowicz M (2015) Review the cancer genome atlas (TCGA): an immeasurable source of knowledge. Contemp Oncol/Współczesna Onkologia 1:68–77

8. Colaprico A, Silva TC, Olsen C, Garofano L, Cava C, Garolini D, Sabedot TS, Malta TM, Pagnotta SM, Castiglioni I (2016) TCGAbiolinks: an R/Bioconductor package for integrative analysis of TCGA data. Nucleic Acids Res 44(8):e71–e71

9. Clough E, Barrett T (2016) The gene expression omnibus database. In: Statistical genomics: methods and protocols, pp 93–110

10. Davis S, Meltzer PS (2007) GEOquery: a bridge between the gene expression omnibus (GEO) and BioConductor. Bioinformatics 23(14):1846–1847

11. Bhattacharya S, Dunn P, Thomas CG, Smith B, Schaefer H, Chen J, Hu Z, Zalocusky KA, Shankar RD, Shen-Orr SS (2018) ImmPort, toward repurposing of open access immunological assay data for translational and clinical research. Sci Data 5(1):1–9

12. Sun D, Wang J, Han Y, Dong X, Ge J, Zheng R, Shi X, Wang B, Li Z, Ren P (2021) TISCH: a comprehensive web resource

enabling interactive single-cell transcriptome visualization of tumor microenvironment. Nucleic Acids Res 49(D1):D1420–D1430

13. Yuan H, Yan M, Zhang G, Liu W, Deng C, Liao G, Xu L, Luo T, Yan H, Long Z (2019) CancerSEA: a cancer single-cell state atlas. Nucleic Acids Res 47(D1):D900–D908

14. Robinson MD, McCarthy DJ, Smyth GK (2010) edgeR: a Bioconductor package for differential expression analysis of digital gene expression data. Bioinformatics 26:139–140

15. Law CW, Chen Y, Shi W, Smyth GK (2014) Voom: precision weights unlock linear model analysis tools for RNA-seq read counts. Genome Biol 15:1–17

16. Subramanian A, Tamayo P, Mootha VK, Mukherjee S, Ebert BL, Gillette MA, Paulovich A, Pomeroy SL, Golub TR, Lander ES (2005) Gene set enrichment analysis: a knowledge-based approach for interpreting genome-wide expression profiles. Proc Natl Acad Sci 102(43):15545–15550

17. Dennis G, Sherman BT, Hosack DA, Yang J, Gao W, Lane HC, Lempicki RA (2003) DAVID: database for annotation, visualization, and integrated discovery. Genome Biol 4:1–11

18. Kuleshov MV, Jones MR, Rouillard AD, Fernandez NF, Duan Q, Wang Z, Koplev S, Jenkins SL, Jagodnik KM, Lachmann A (2016) Enrichr: a comprehensive gene set enrichment analysis web server 2016 update. Nucleic Acids Res 44(W1):W90–W97

19. Kanehisa M, Goto S (2000) KEGG: Kyoto encyclopedia of genes and genomes. Nucleic Acids Res 28(1):27–30

20. Ashburner M, Ball CA, Blake JA, Botstein D, Butler H, Cherry JM, Davis AP, Dolinski K, Dwight SS, Eppig JT (2000) Gene ontology: tool for the unification of biology. Nat Genet 25(1):25–29

21. Fabregat A, Jupe S, Matthews L, Sidiropoulos K, Gillespie M, Garapati P, Haw R, Jassal B, Korninger F, May B (2018) The reactome pathway knowledgebase. Nucleic Acids Res 46(D1):D649–D655

22. Newman AM, Liu CL, Green MR, Gentles AJ, Feng W, Xu Y, Hoang CD, Diehn M, Alizadeh AA (2015) Robust enumeration of cell subsets from tissue expression profiles. Nat Methods 12(5):453–457

23. Racle J, Gfeller D (2020) EPIC: a tool to estimate the proportions of different cell types from bulk gene expression data. In: Bioinformatics for cancer immunotherapy: methods and protocols, pp 233–248

24. Aran D, Hu Z, Butte AJ (2017) xCell: digitally portraying the tissue cellular heterogeneity landscape. Genome Biol 18:1–14

25. Jiang P, Gu S, Pan D, Fu J, Sahu A, Hu X, Li Z, Traugh N, Bu X, Li B (2018) Signatures of T cell dysfunction and exclusion predict cancer immunotherapy response. Nat Med 24(10):1550–1558

26. Charoentong P, Finotello F, Angelova M, Mayer C, Efremova M, Rieder D, Hackl H, Trajanoski Z (2017) Pan-cancer immunogenomic analyses reveal genotype-immunophenotype relationships and predictors of response to checkpoint blockade. Cell Rep 18(1):248–262

27. Sha D, Jin Z, Budczies J, Kluck K, Stenzinger A, Sinicrope FA (2020) Tumor mutational burden as a predictive biomarker in solid tumors. Cancer Discov 10(12):1808–1825

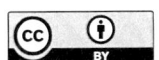

Correction to: IMMUNO-model in Cancer

Sweta Rani and Lukasz Skalniak

Correction to:
Sweta Rani and Lukasz Skalniak (eds.), *IMMUNO-model in Cancer: Methods and Protocols*, Methods in Molecular Biology, vol. 2959, https://doi.org/10.1007/978-1-0716-4734-9

The original version of the book, *IMMUNO-model in Cancer*, was previously published without the EU emblem placed in the Acknowledgments section. The book has now been updated with this change.

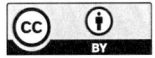
The updated version of this book can be found at
https://doi.org/10.1007/978-1-0716-4734-9

Sweta Rani and Lukasz Skalniak (eds.), *IMMUNO-model in Cancer: Methods and Protocols*, Methods in Molecular Biology, vol. 2959, https://doi.org/10.1007/978-1-0716-4734-9_19, © The Author(s) 2026

INDEX

Sweta Rani and Lukasz Skalniak (eds.), *IMMUNO-model in Cancer: Methods and Protocols*, Methods in Molecular Biology,
vol. 2959, https://doi.org/10.1007/978-1-0716-4734-9, © The Editor(s) (if applicable) and The Author(s) 2026

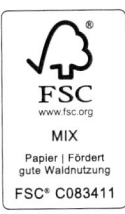

Zeitfracht Medien GmbH
Ferdinand-Jühlke-Straße 7
99095 Erfurt, Deutschland
produktsicherheit@kolibri360.de